Culturally and Linguistically Responsive Intervention and Assessment Practices with Emergent Bilingual Students

Desiree Vega • Jaclyn N. Wolf
Editors

Culturally and Linguistically Responsive Intervention and Assessment Practices with Emergent Bilingual Students

Springer

Editors
Desiree Vega
Department of Disability &
Psychoeducational Studies
University of Arizona
Tucson, AZ, USA

Jaclyn N. Wolf
Psychology Department
San Francisco State University
San Francisco, CA, USA

ISBN 978-3-032-02083-3 ISBN 978-3-032-02084-0 (eBook)
https://doi.org/10.1007/978-3-032-02084-0

This Springer imprint is published by the registered company Springer Nature Switzerland AG
The registered company address is: Gewerbestrasse 11, 6330 Cham, Switzerland

This book is dedicated to all of the emergent bilingual learners who are navigating an educational system that views their culture and language as limiting. We see you and celebrate your many strengths!

Preface

Culturally and Linguistically Responsive Intervention and Assessment Practices with Emergent Bilingual Students was written in response to the limited research and practical support available to school-based practitioners, such as school psychologists, who work with bilingual youth. While much guidance is available on evidence-based interventions, there is a dearth of resources available on culturally adapted and culturally responsive intervention practices, specific to emergent bilingual (EB) students. Additionally, much of the assessment literature for EB youth tends to focus on specific learning disabilities, with little to no support for identifying other disabilities. Therefore, we sought to collaborate with experts in the profession to disseminate much-needed content, helping school-based practitioners effectively and equitably serve EB students.

This book addresses the general and special education needs of EB students from a holistic and strengths-based lens. It focuses on interventions to support their academic and social-emotional needs, as well as conducting culturally responsive assessments to determine eligibility for special education services. The book is divided into three main parts, which center on (1) the educational experiences and needs of EB students, (2) implementing a multi-tiered system of supports with culturally adapted and responsive interventions, and (3) utilizing culturally responsive assessment practices to differentiate between language differences and disability.

Part I of the book begins with contextual information defining EB students and their educational experiences, followed by an overview of the instructional opportunities available to them, as well as a discussion of acculturation and its impact on educational experiences and outcomes. This part of the book provides foundational background information that influences how practitioners should approach intervention and assessment practices.

Part II of the book describes the application of a culturally and linguistically responsive multi-tiered system of supports, including specialized considerations related to literacy and language needs, as well as the importance of culturally adapted behavioral, social-emotional, and academic interventions. Additionally, this section emphasizes the importance of collaborating with families to address the needs of EB students during the intervention process. It also provides an overview of best practices to work with interpreters throughout the intervention process.

Part III of this book provides guidance on the evaluation process for special education and related services, including considerations for differentiating language, culture, and disability across various eligibility categories, such as Speech and Language Impairment, Specific Learning Disability, Intellectual Disability, and Autism. It also discusses opportunities for collaborating with speech-language pathologists throughout the assessment process.

While geared primarily toward school psychologists, this book offers practical recommendations for K-12 education professionals, including general education teachers, special educators, and speech-language pathologists, to support EB students in the intervention and assessment processes. Additionally, this book will aid graduate students, instructors, and researchers in their practice. It fills a critical need and will be a must-have resource for educators seeking to advance the educational success of EB students.

Tucson, AZ Desiree Vega
San Francisco, CA Jaclyn N. Wolf

Acknowledgments

We must begin by thanking Judy Jones and the publication team at Springer for their support in the development and production of this project. This book would not have been possible without the expertise of our authors, to whom we are so incredibly grateful. Thank you for sharing your knowledge and for your dedication to enhancing the educational experiences of emergent bilingual youth! Last but certainly not least, we extend our gratitude to our family, friends, and mentors whose support carried us through this process.

Contents

Notes on Contributors

Wualú Altamira, M.A., is a doctoral candidate in the School Psychology program at Texas A&M University. She is a Licensed Professional Counselor (LPC) in the state of Texas and Doctoral Candidate. She earned a B.A. in Psychology and M.A. in Counseling Psychology from Texas A&M International University. Her research focuses on promoting social-emotional competencies and sense of belonging of Latine newcomer youth through culturally sensitive interventions and mentoring relationships.

Genesis D. Arizmendi, PhD, CCC-SLP, is an Assistant Professor in the College of Science at the University of Arizona, with appointments in Speech, Language, and Hearing Sciences and Cognitive Science, and is the director of the Multicultural Bilingual Certificate Program. As an interdisciplinary clinician-scientist, she is dedicated to community-centered, representative science that drives systemic change across disciplines and into practice. She is a certified and licensed bilingual speech-language pathologist with over 10 years of clinical experience in the Southwest, committed to improving clinical research practices and educational outcomes for Spanish-English speaking communities. Dr. Arizmendi earned her PhD in Speech, Language, and Hearing Sciences from the University of Arizona and expanded her expertise through postdoctoral training in Educational Psychology at the University of New Mexico and in Special Education at the University of Texas at Austin and the Texas Center for Equity Promotion. Within the framework of her research program, Dr. Arizmendi aims to mitigate disparities and advance equity within the educational and healthcare systems. Dr. Arizmendi interrogates how policy and social context influence bilingual development, educational outcomes, and healthcare access. Drawing from her research and clinical training, she integrates implementation science frameworks to examine the intersection of cognition, language, and academic achievement in bilingual children with diverse learning profiles, spanning typical development, developmental language disorder, and difficulties with mathematics and reading.

Fedra A. Calderón, Ed.S., NCSP, is a nationally and Arizona-certified school psychologist with experience in public education since 2017. Her professional work is grounded in serving diverse student populations, with a particular focus on supporting children and families from ethnically, racially, culturally, and linguistically minoritized backgrounds. She has provided services across preschool, elementary, and middle school settings. Fedra is an Indigenous member of the Tohono O'odham Nation and a queer Mexican woman who has lived in the United States since 2008. Her intersecting identities profoundly shape her approach to school psychology and social justice, and as a bilingual and biliterate practitioner in Spanish and English, she is committed to delivering culturally responsive services to the communities she serves. Currently, Fedra is pursuing a Ph.D. in School Psychology with a minor in American Indian Studies at the University of Arizona. Her research and practice are deeply intertwined, as she actively works to advocate for marginalized voices and challenge systemic oppression within public education. Fedra believes in the power of community, collaboration, and agency in transforming oppressive systems. Her work reflects a commitment to equity, community, and inclusive practices across all aspects of education and mental health services.

Sara Castro-Olivo, Ph.D., is an Associate Professor in the Educational Psychology Department at Texas A&M University. She is a Nationally Certified School Psychologist and a Licensed Specialist in School Psychology in the state of Texas. She has worked with Latinx communities in Texas, California, and Oregon since 2001 as a bilingual community health educator, bilingual parent trainer, and school psychologist. She earned a Master's in Special Education and Ph.D. in School Psychology from the University of Oregon. Her research focuses on the development and validation of community and school-based culturally responsive social-emotional and behavioral interventions for culturally and linguistically diverse populations.

Linda O. Cavazos, Ph.D., is the Executive Director and founder of ELLAS Consulting (English Learner Leadership Advocacy Support). She is a technical assistance provider and researcher with 32 years of experience in education, focusing on the needs of English Learners. She began her professional journey as a bilingual English and Spanish teacher before transitioning to a bilingual reading interventionist and coach. For a decade, she developed curricula for English Learners in both English and Spanish, covering reading, writing, math, and science for grades K-8. Dr. Cavazos founded and led the English Learners Research Alliance, as well as the New Mexico Achievement Gap Research Alliance, at the Regional Education Laboratory Southwest. She has served as an English Learner content expert for various US Department of Education Regional Education Laboratories and Comprehensive Centers. She was the principal investigator and a co-investigator on two federally funded projects on Multi-Tiered Systems of Support (MTSS) for English Learners in grades 3–5 and for English Learners in grades K-3. She provides biliteracy expertise to state and local education agencies on the Science of Reading for English Learners, MTSS, and biliteracy. Dr. Cavazos has extensive experience in enhancing academic outcomes for English Learners, including those with learning difficulties or disabilities. She conducts research on English Learner programs, MTSS, and biliteracy development. Her research examines the intersections of these topics and aims to improve the academic outcomes of English Learners. Dr. Cavazos earned her doctorate in Multicultural Special Education from the University of Texas at Austin.

Meagan Dorman, is an educator and researcher with expertise in culturally and linguistically responsive pedagogy, special education, and teacher preparation. At the time of writing this chapter, she was a doctoral candidate in the Department of Special Education and Clinical Sciences at the University of Oregon, where she recently completed her Ph.D. Her research explores how educators support multilingual learners and students with disabilities, with particular focus on language development, instructional practice, and teacher learning. She has contributed to projects examining the visibility of Indigenous languages in data systems, the relationship between executive functioning and writing development among emergent bilinguals, and the design of culturally responsive multi-tiered systems of support (MTSS). Dr. Dorman draws on her experience as a special education teacher and consultant to bridge research and practice. Her work emphasizes equity, inclusive instructional design, and systems-level approaches to professional learning.

Anisa N. Goforth, Ph.D., ABPP, is a Professor in the Department of Psychology at the University of Montana and directs the Culturally Responsive Evidence-based Practices in School Psychology (CRESP) Lab. An Australian and American citizen, she was born in Yemen and raised in Asia and Latin America. Dr. Goforth earned her M.A. and Ph.D. in School Psychology from Michigan State University. Her research focuses on culturally responsive evidence-based practices for children and their families, grounded in cultural humility. She has published over 100 articles and book chapters and co-authored a book (with Dr. Andy Pham) titled *Culturally Responsive School-based Practices: Supporting Mental Health and Learning of Diverse Youth*. Dr. Goforth is Board Certified in School Psychology, a licensed psychologist (MT), and a Nationally Certified School Psychologist.

Bryn Harris, PhD, is a Professor in the School Psychology doctoral program in the School of Education and Human Development at the University of Colorado Denver. She has a secondary appointment in the Department of Pediatrics (Developmental Pediatrics) at the University of Colorado Denver Anschutz Medical Campus. Her primary research interests include the psychological assessment of multilingual learners, culturally and linguistically responsive assessment of autism spectrum disorder, health disparities among children with autism spectrum disorder, and improving mental health access and opportunity within traditionally underserved populations. Dr. Harris is the director and founder of the bilingual school psychology program at the University of Colorado Denver. She is also a bilingual (Spanish) licensed psychologist and nationally certified school psychologist. Dr. Harris practices as a bilingual school psychologist part-time in Denver Public Schools.

Jennifer E. Kong, PhD, is an Assistant Professor of Special Education in the Attallah College of Educational Studies at Chapman University. Her research focuses on mathematical and cognitive development of elementary-aged children who are English learners, with the goal of developing effective math interventions for these children. Her research interests were inspired by her experience as a Special Education teacher in the Chicago area. Dr. Kong primarily teaches in teacher education programs and is also appointed to the faculty of the Ph.D. in Education programs.

Izabela Konopko, is a certified bilingual school psychologist in New York. Her training has focused extensively on culturally and linguistically informed practices, particularly in the assessment of specific learning disabilities (SLD). She completed the bilingual track in her school psychology program at St. John's University, served as a teaching assistant for a graduate course in psychoeducational assessment, and conducted dissertation research on school psychologists' understanding of SLD identification methods. Dr. Konopko's professional interests include bilingual and equitable assessment, SLD identification, and the development of inclusive practices that honor students' linguistic and cultural identities. As an emerging professional in the field, she is committed to advancing best practices in school psychology through collaboration, advocacy, and ongoing professional development. With experience in assessment, consultation, and therapeutic intervention, she supports students from diverse backgrounds by integrating culturally responsive frameworks into her work. Dr. Konopko remains deeply dedicated to fostering educational equity and ensuring that all students receive fair, comprehensive, and supportive psychological services.

Kelsey Kuperman, is a bilingual (Spanish/English) Consultation-Liaison Psychologist on an interdisciplinary treatment team in the Department of Psychiatry at Denver Health Medical Center. She holds a Ph.D. in Counseling Psychology with a specialization in Spanish Language Psychological Services and Research from the University of Oregon. Dr. Kuperman is dedicated to providing culturally responsive, trauma-informed, and evidence-based behavioral health services to historically underserved communities in a safety-net hospital. Her clinical work primarily focuses on supporting patients with severe chronic pain, acute injuries, trauma histories, and co-occurring psychiatric and complex medical conditions. She also works closely with subspecialty medicine teams to provide wrap-around services to patients, including diagnostic and risk assessment, psychotherapy at bedside, and end-of-life care. With a passion for supervision and teaching, Dr. Kuperman co-facilitates a Spanish Supervision and Consultation Group for bilingual Psychology Interns at Denver Health and is an Affiliate Instructor at the University of Colorado School of Medicine. Her research focuses on a range of topics, including complex trauma, psychosocial development, and psychological treatment for patients with serious and terminal illness. She has been published in the peer-reviewed Journal of Aggression, Maltreatment, and Trauma, and is currently in the process of being published in the Journal of Palliative Medicine. This will be Dr. Kuperman's first publication of a book chapter. Beyond the professional world, Dr. Kuperman feels most alive while traveling, learning new languages, and getting lost in creative projects.

Tamika P. La Salle-Finley, is a Professor in the Georgia State University College of Education and Human Development. Dr. La Salle-Finley serves as Editor-in-Chief of the International Journal of School & Educational Psychology (IJSEP), and the Director of the Center for Research on School Climate. She joined the Society for the Study of School Psychology in 2023. In the same year, she received the "40 under 40" award from the Georgia State Alumni Association. In 2022, she was awarded the Perry A. Zirkel Distinguished Teacher Award at the University of Connecticut. Dr. La Salle-Finley's scholarship, service and teaching focuses on creating equitable environments for youth with minoritized and marginalized identities engages in research, consultation, and service focused on creating equitable environments for youth with minoritized and marginalized identities.

Sylvia Linan-Thompson, Ph.D., is Associate Dean for Academic Affairs, an associate professor at the University of Oregon in the Department of Special Education and Clinical Sciences, and is affiliated with the Center on Teaching and Learning. Her teaching and research focus on teaching and assessing the reading development of struggling readers who are monolingual English speakers, bilingual students acquiring Spanish and English literacy, and literacy in a second or additional language. Her research includes longitudinal intervention projects that developed and examined reading interventions and examined the implementation of RtI/MTSS in dual language schools. She has authored articles, chapters, and books on these topics. Dr. Thompson also works as a literacy specialist on international development projects in education in collaboration with the World Bank, UNESCO, and the US Agency for International Development to develop reading curriculum and assessments worldwide, including extensive academic and field expertise in mother-tongue and second language literacy in Africa, the Middle East, Asia, Latin America, and the Caribbean and she chairs the Advisory Committee on Exceptional Children and Youth of the Office of Overseas Schools, US State Department.

Emilia C. Lopez, PhD, graduated from Fordham University with a specialization in bilingual school psychology. She is a Professor in the Graduate Program in School Psychology within the Department of Educational and Community Programs at Queens College, City University of New York. She created the bilingual specialization within the program. Her scholarly work focuses on culturally responsive practices, multicultural competencies for school psychologists, working with interpreters in school settings, and multicultural consultation. She served as editor of the *Journal of Educational and Psychological Consultation*. She is one of the co-editors of the *Handbook of Multicultural School Psychology: An Interdisciplinary Perspective*.

Jesslynn Rocha Neves-McCain, is an Assistant Professor in the Department of Counseling, School Psychology, and Sport at the University of Massachusetts, Boston. Dr. Neves' scholarship and practice focus on school climate, measuring school quality, and culturally responsive school psychology. She is currently a member of the lead team for the International School Climate Collaborative (ISCC), a research collective that advocates for a positive school climate worldwide. Dr. Neves currently serves as an Editorial Fellow for the *International Journal of Educational and School Psychology*. Dr. Neves engages in applied consultation and practice related to psychoeducational assessment, bilingual assessment, and culturally responsive education.

Trianna K. Oglivie, PhD, CCC-SLP, is a research speech-language pathologist at the University of Arizona. She earned her master's degree in speech-language pathology and her doctoral degree in Speech, Language, and Hearing Sciences both from the University of Arizona. Dr. Oglivie is licensed speech-language pathologist and holds the Certificate of Clinical Competence from the American Speech-Language-Hearing Association (ASHA). Dr. Oglivie's research centers on multilingual speech and language assessment, with particular emphasis on addressing health and educational disparities affecting multilingual children. Her clinical experience spans diverse settings, including public schools, home health, hospitals, and research environments, where she has focused primarily on evaluating and treating pediatric speech and language disorders. Overall, Dr. Oglivie's work aims to improve the quality and accessibility of speech and language services for individuals from culturally and linguistically minoritized backgrounds, ensuring that assessment and intervention strategies are not only evidence-based but also contextually and culturally relevant.

Alexandro Ornelas, M.Ed., M.S., Ed.S., is a bilingual School Psychologist currently serving students in San Diego, California. He grew up in the border communities of Tijuana and San Diego, which shaped his deep understanding of multilingual and multicultural populations. Prior to his current role, he worked as an English Language Learner (ELL) teacher for fifth and sixth grades and as a third-grade classroom teacher in Kansas City, Missouri. His professional experiences continue to inform his commitment to supporting diverse student needs through culturally responsive psychoeducational services.

Monica E. Romero, Ph.D., NCSP, LSSP, is an Assistant Professor in the School and Clinical Child Psychology program at the University of Texas at Austin. A nationally certified and bilingual school psychologist, Dr. Romero's work is grounded in a commitment to advancing equity and social justice for Latine and multilingual children and families. Her research focuses on culturally and linguistically responsive practices in school psychology, including interventions, assessments, and family-school-home collaboration within Multi-Tiered Systems of Support (MTSS). Dr. Romero leads multiple community-based research projects in collaboration with schools, nonprofits, and organizations serving Latine multilingual communities. Her work includes co-designing and evaluating interventions that promote academic, social-emotional learning, and mental health well-being for Latine and multilingual learners. She employs mixed-methods, participatory action research, and critical frameworks to center the lived experiences of Latine youth and families. Drawing from her practice-based experience as a bilingual school psychologist, Dr. Romero informs her research, teaching, and mentorship of future school psychologists. She collaborates with local districts to strengthen culturally and linguistically sustaining MTSS frameworks and to implement inclusive universal screening systems for multilingual students. Dr. Romero earned her Ph.D. in School Psychology from the University of Missouri. Through her scholarship, she seeks to reimagine school psychology as a field that uplifts the voices, strengths, and aspirations of Latine and multilingual communities.

Patricia Sánchez Lizardi, PhD, NCSP, is an Associate Professor in the School Psychology program at San Diego State University. She has been a bilingual school psychologist in Arizona, California, and New Jersey, and has conducted research internationally in Brazil and Mexico. Currently, her scholarly work focuses on preparing bilingual school psychologists to provide psychoeducational services to the increasing population of Multilingual Learners in K-12 schools in the United States.

Rachel T. Santiago, Ph.D., NCSP, is an Assistant Professor in the Department of Educational, School & Counseling Psychology at the University of Missouri and a Faculty Affiliate at the Missouri Prevention Science Institute. Dr. Santiago earned her Ph.D. in School Psychology from the University of Oregon and completed her postdoctoral training at the University of Wisconsin–Madison. Her research focuses on social-emotional and mental health outcomes for youth, with an emphasis on culturally responsive practices, implementation science, family–school–community partnerships, and community-engaged scholarship. Dr. Santiago is a licensed school psychologist (MO), provisionally licensed psychologist (MO), and a Nationally Certified School Psychologist.

Marlene Sotelo-Dynega, is a licensed psychologist and certified bilingual school psychologist in New York State with extensive experience in assessment and training. She currently serves as the Director of the Master of Science Program in School Psychology and Associate Professor in the Department of Psychology at St. John's University. Dr. Sotelo-Dynega's expertise lies in school neuropsychology, learning disability assessment, and culturally responsive practices like non-discriminatory assessment. A diplomate in School Neuropsychology, Dr. Sotelo-Dynega maintains a private practice and consults with school districts, providing neuropsychological assessments and professional development. Her research interests include orthographic processing and the neuropsychological underpinnings of learning disabilities. She has published in peer-reviewed journals and contributed chapters to leading textbooks in the field. A sought-after speaker, Dr. Sotelo-Dynega presents at national and regional conferences on topics such as dyslexia, neuropsychological assessment, and culturally responsive practices. She is actively involved in professional organizations and is committed to advancing the field of school psychology through research, teaching, and service, with a focus on promoting equitable and effective educational practices for all students.

Brittany St. Jean, is a licensed Clinical and School Psychologist in New Hampshire and serves as Director of Clinical Training at White Birch Educational Services (WBES). Dr. St. Jean recently established a school-based doctoral training fellowship program through her organization's membership with the Association of Psychology Postdoctoral and Internship Centers (APPIC). She currently holds the position of President of the New Hampshire Psychological Association (NHPA) and was recently recognized as a member of the New Hampshire Union Leader's 2024 class of "40 Under 40." Dr. St. Jean's work bridges the fields of clinical psychology and education, with a particular expertise in developing training programs that prepare future psychologists for school-based practice while maintaining cultural responsiveness in therapeutic and consultative approaches.

Marie L. Tanaka, (she/her/ella), PhD, NCSP, HSP, is an adjunct lecturer in San Diego State University's school psychology program. Dr. Tanaka earned her doctorate from the University of Arizona's school psychology program, where she minored in Social, Cultural, Critical Theory. She has several years of experience instructing newcomer immigrant middle school students and has taught adolescents abroad as part of a Fulbright scholarship. Dr. Tanaka's research has covered various topics including the examination of (1) how middle school teachers both support and unknowingly undermine racially/ethnically minoritized newcomer immigrant student growth, (2) experiences of Black Indigenous Women of Color graduate students in school psychology doctoral programs, and (3) school psychology graduate program climates.

Juanita Torres, (she/her/ella) is a bilingual Trauma Psychologist at Reaching HOPE in Colorado. She attended the University of Florida for her B.S. degree in psychology and earned a Psy.D. in clinical psychology from Pacific University's School of Graduate Psychology, where she specialized in working with children and adolescents and Latine mental health. Dr. Torres is passionate about serving Latine children and families with complex trauma and has practiced in a variety of settings, including schools, residential treatment centers, hospitals, community mental health centers, and nonprofits. Dr. Torres is licensed to practice as a psychologist in Colorado.

Natalie Vallarta, M.Ed., is a doctoral student in the School Psychology program at Texas A&M University. She earned her B.A. in Psychology from UCLA and an M.Ed. in Educational Psychology from Texas A&M University. Her research focuses on supporting Spanish-speaking communities, advancing equitable mental health practices, and promoting trauma-informed approaches in schools. She is committed to providing compassionate, culturally and linguistically responsive care to children and families from historically marginalized backgrounds.

Desiree Vega, PhD, LP, NCSP, received her B.A. in Psychology from Binghamton University-State University of New York, and her M.A. and Ph.D. in School Psychology from The Ohio State University. She completed her pre-doctoral internship in the Omaha Public Schools district, where she worked as a bilingual school psychologist from 2010 to 2013. She is a Professor in the School Psychology program at the University of Arizona and previously served as a faculty member at Texas State University. Dr. Vega's research focuses on three primary areas: (1) Understanding bilingual school psychology training and practice; (2) Preparing school psychologists for culturally competent assessment and intervention practice; and (3) Building collaborations to advance college access and persistence. In 2023, she was awarded a Spencer Foundation grant ($49,828) to examine school psychologists' assessment practices with bilingual students within the context of Arizona's restrictive English-only legislation. Dr. Vega is the recipient of numerous awards, including the *Excellence in Graduate Teaching and Mentoring Award* from the Graduate College (2021), the *New Leader Award* from the College of Education and Human Ecology Alumni Office, The Ohio State University (2023), the *Presidential Award for Exceptional Service to Children and School Psychology* from the *National Association of School Psychologists* (2023), the *APA Division 16 Outstanding Contributions to Mentorship Award* (2025), and the *Mentoring Future Scholars Award* (2025).

Jaclyn N. Wolf, Ph.D., is a licensed psychologist and credentialed school psychologist. Dr. Wolf is currently an Assistant Professor (tenure-track) and clinical supervisor in the Psychology Department at San Francisco State University and also works as a testing psychologist at Mind Matters, where she completes psychoeducational evaluations for preschool to college-aged youth. Dr. Wolf earned her bachelor's (psychology with a minor in family studies) and master's degrees (clinical psychology) at California State University, Northridge. She earned her doctoral degree in school psychology at the University of Arizona. Dr. Wolf has provided consultation, therapeutic, and assessment services in several settings, including K-12 schools (public and non-public), hospitals, and residential treatment centers. Dr. Wolf's teaching, research, and clinical practice focus on examining the impact of sociocultural factors on the educational, academic, and mental health outcomes of culturally and linguistically minoritized youth, particularly Spanish-speaking Latine children and adolescents, from a holistic and strengths-based lens. She is also a heritage language learner (Spanish).

Jingyi Yang, is a Ph.D. candidate in School Psychology in the Department of Psychology at the University of South Carolina. Her research interests are resilience-based prevention and intervention, culturally responsive assessments and practices, and school-based mental health. Her ongoing research focuses on health promotions in schools and the identification of autism among culturally and linguistically minoritized populations.

Desiree Vega, PhD, LP, NCSP received her B.A. in Psychology from Binghamton University-State University of New York and her M.A. and Ph.D. in School Psychology from The Ohio State University. She completed her pre-doctoral internship in the Omaha Public Schools district, where she worked as a bilingual school psychologist from 2010 to 2013. She is a Professor in the School Psychology program at the University of Arizona and previously served as a faculty member at Texas State University. Dr. Vega's research focuses on three primary areas: (1) Understanding bilingual school psychology training and practice; (2) Preparing school psychologists for culturally competent assessment and intervention practice; and (3) Building collaborations to advance college access and persistence. In 2023 she was awarded a Spencer Foundation grant ($49,855) to examine school psychologists' assessment practices with bilingual students within the context of Arizona's restrictive English-only legislation. Dr. Vega is the recipient of numerous awards, including the *Excellence in Graduate Teaching and Mentoring Award* from the Graduate College (2021), the *New Faculty Award* from the College of Education and Human Ecology Alumni Office, The Ohio State University (2023), the [illegible] from the [illegible] (2023), the APA Division 16 *Outstanding Contributions to Mentorship Award* (2025) and the *Mentoring Early Scholars Award* (2025).

[illegible] N. Wolf, [illegible] Dr. Wolf is currently an Assistant Professor (tenure track) and [illegible] in the Psychology Department at San Francisco State University and also works as a testing psychologist at Mind Matters, where she completes psychoeducational [illegible] consultation, therapeutic, and assessment services in diverse settings, including K-12 schools (public and non-public), hospitals, and residential treatment centers. Dr. Wolf's teaching, research, and clinical practice focus on examining the impact of sociocultural factors on the educational, academic, and mental health outcomes of culturally and linguistically minoritized youth, particularly Spanish-speaking Latine children and adolescents, from a holistic and strengths-based lens. She is also a heritage language learner (Spanish).

[illegible] Young, [illegible] Ph.D. candidate in School Psychology in the Department of Psychology at the University of South Carolina. Her research interests are evidence-based prevention and intervention, culturally responsive assessments and practices, and school-based mental health. Her ongoing research focuses on health promotions in schools and the identification of autism among culturally and linguistically minoritized populations.

Part I
The Educational Experiences and Needs of Emergent Bilingual Students

Chapter 1
Who Are Emergent Bilingual Students?

Desiree Vega and Jaclyn N. Wolf

In this book, we use “emergent bilinguals” (EBs) to refer to students classified as English language learners (ELLs). The phrase “emergent bilingual” views the development of bilingualism as an asset, whereas the term “English language learner” centers on learning English and ignores these students’ linguistic strengths (García, 2009; Kanno et al., 2024). We also use the term “multilingual learner” to refer to students who speak multiple languages, which emphasizes their linguistic abilities as strengths. There are pros and cons to the various labels (e.g., EB, ELL) used to describe this group of students. For example, no matter how asset-based a label is (e.g., emergent bilingual, multilingual learner), it does not automatically eliminate the inequities these students face (Kanno et al., 2024). Alongside the use of strengths-based terminology, there is work to be done to challenge the system that perpetuates inequities for EB students. For a more in-depth discussion of these issues, we recommend that readers review Kanno et al. (2024).

D. Vega (✉)
Department of Disability & Psychoeducational Studies, University of Arizona, Tucson, AZ, USA
e-mail: dvega2@arizona.edu

J. N. Wolf
Psychology Department, San Francisco State University, San Francisco, CA, USA
e-mail: jaclynwolf@sfsu.edu

D. Vega, J. N. Wolf (eds.), *Culturally and Linguistically Responsive Intervention and Assessment Practices with Emergent Bilingual Students*,
https://doi.org/10.1007/978-3-032-02084-0_1

Demographic Characteristics

EB students represent 10.6% (5.3 million) of US public school students as of fall 2021 (National Center for Education Statistics [NCES], 2024). The rapid growth of this population underscores the need for school personnel to understand the diversity of EB students and address their unique cultural and linguistic needs. While continued population growth is evident, the representation of EB students in states varies (NCES, 2024). States with the highest percentage of EB students include Texas (20.2%), California (18.9%), and New Mexico (18.8%). In contrast, the following states have the lowest percentages of EB students: West Virginia (0.8%), Vermont (2%), and Montana (2.4%). Relatedly, the quality of robust language instruction available to students classified as ELLs differs considerably (Rutherford-Quach et al., 2021). Thus, where an EB student lives may influence the type and quality of language programming they receive and subsequently impact their academic outcomes.

EB students are linguistically and racially diverse (NCES, 2024). EB students speak over 400 different languages (US Department of Education, 2017), with Spanish being the most common language (76.4%), followed by Arabic (2.5%), English (2.2%), Chinese (1.8%), and Vietnamese (1.4%). With respect to racial and ethnic identity, 77.9% of EB students identify as Latinx, followed by 9.7% Asian, 6.1% White, 4.2% Black, 0.8% Multiracial, 0.7% American Indian/Alaska Native, and 0.6% Pacific Islander. It is also important to note that the majority of students classified as ELL students are US-born and not immigrants (Bialik et al., 2018). EB students and their families are diverse in terms of numerous other factors, including country of origin, religion, immigration status, generational status, socioeconomic status, beliefs about disability, values, traditions, and acculturation level. Thus, educators must not treat this group of students as a monolith.

Conversely, the demographics of school psychologists remain predominantly homogeneous, with 86% identifying as White, 87% identifying as female, and 92% identifying as monolingual (Goforth et al., 2021). Similarly, public school teachers are predominantly White (80%) and female (77%; NCES, 2023). Given the racial, gender, and linguistic disparities between students, school psychologists, and teachers, it is more important than ever for educators to acknowledge this diversity when working with EB students and strive to understand their background characteristics and experiences to provide the best support. Moreover, it is critical to remember that cultural differences do not equate to deficits, and perceiving EB students and their families through a deficit lens will only hinder partnerships and advocacy for their needs.

Historical and Legal Context for EB Students

The historical and legal context of schooling for EB students continues to shape their experiences and opportunities. Dating back to the 1800s, the United States has enacted policies aimed at erasing languages other than English (Nieto, 2009). For example, these policies targeted Native Americans, which sent them to boarding schools where speaking their languages was prohibited. Violence was used to ensure Native American children would not speak their native language and instead would learn English, contributing to language loss and cultural genocide (Aguilar et al., 2021; Palmer & Cooke, 1996; Pember, 2007).

In the early 1900s, laws were passed to further promote the exclusive use of English. The Naturalization Act of 1906 mandated that English be the only language taught in schools and required immigrants to be proficient in English to apply for naturalization (Nieto, 2009). The Immigration Act of 1917 also required immigrants to pass literacy tests and banned immigration from Asia. Thus, these Acts highlight the hostile and extreme measures taken to enforce English usage and limit immigration from specific areas, which continue to be perpetuated. The pervasive devaluation of multilingualism and xenophobia is exemplified by the recent designation of English as the official language of the United States (The White House, 2025) and numerous immigration-related executive orders (Chishti & Bush-Joseph, 2025).

School Segregation Cases

Many people are aware of *Brown v. Board of Education* (1954) for its pivotal role in ending racial segregation in schools nationally. However, many may not be aware of how school segregation impacted non-English-speaking students and those with "non-American" last names. In the landmark case of *Mendez v. Westminster* (1946), which led to the end of school segregation in California, Mexican families were denied the opportunity to enroll their children in the neighborhood school, the White school, based on their surnames and skin color. Instead, they were told they had to send their children to an inferior Mexican school. The school district claimed that school separation was necessary to help these students learn English and become familiar with American ways of being. However, the courts stated that segregation prevented Mexican students from interacting with other students, which denied them the opportunity to learn English and adapt to American culture. The court ruled that Mexican students were being discriminated against because their rights were denied under the Fourteenth Amendment (Valencia, 2005). However, it is critical to note that the subtext of this ruling (i.e., being denied the opportunity to learn English and adapt to American culture) continued to prioritize assimilation and the importance of English over the students' native culture and language.

Diana v. State Board of Education (1970) is an important case demonstrating how Spanish-surnamed children were segregated into self-contained special education classrooms to address their supposed severe intellectual disabilities. Testing was conducted in English, which suggested significantly low intellectual ability. However, when the students were reassessed bilingually, the majority of their IQ scores fell within the average range. The ruling ordered students to be assessed in their primary language; Mexican American and Chinese children in those restrictive placements were to be retested; and children wrongly placed in those classrooms were to be assisted to readjust to general education classrooms.

Title VII: Bilingual Education Act (1968)

The goal of Title VII, known as the Bilingual Education Act (BEA) of 1968, under the Elementary and Secondary Education Act, was to support students with limited English proficiency in acquiring English language skills. However, it did not require bilingual education. Instead, the Act provided funding to districts that provided specialized instruction for EB students (García & Kleifgen, 2018; Nieto, 2009). Reauthorizations to the BEA in 1974 and 1978 defined bilingual education and expanded access to EB students from all socioeconomic backgrounds. Subsequent reauthorizations in 1984 and 1988 provided more funding to English-only programs and included a 3-year limit for participation in bilingual programs (García & Kleifgen, 2018). In 1994, the reauthorization supported the use of dual language programs (García & Kleifgen, 2018), demonstrating a promising shift toward the use of evidence-based models of language instruction.

Lau v. Nichols (1974)

In the *Lau v. Nichols* (1974) case, Chinese American parents sued the San Francisco Unified School District due to a lack of programming and instruction to address their children's linguistic needs. In 1974, the Supreme Court ruled that under Title VI of the Civil Rights Act of 1964, these students' right to meaningful participation in school was denied. Therefore, the school district needed to take steps to address these inequities (García & Kleifgen, 2018; Nieto, 2009). A limitation of this ruling was that it did not mandate bilingual education, nor did it dictate how the District should provide appropriate instruction to meet the students' language needs.

Plyler v. Doe (1982)

Plyler v. Doe (1982) is not specific to bilingualism; however, it is relevant to advocating for the right to a public education for EB students who may also be undocumented immigrants. A class action suit was brought against Texas to challenge a policy that prohibited the enrollment of undocumented students. The Supreme Court ruled that the existing policy violated the Equal Protection Clause of the Fourteenth Amendment. Additionally, the court stated that educating these youth outweighed the long-term consequences of excluding them from attending school. Thus, undocumented immigrant students, who are likely to be classified as ELL students, cannot be denied a public education.

English-Only Movement (1990s–Present)

Unfortunately, despite some progress made in supporting the educational needs of EB students, the 1990s experienced a shift toward anti-immigrant rhetoric that targeted bilingual education and sought to make English the official language of the United States. Unsubstantiated claims reported that bilingual education delayed English acquisition and assimilation to American culture, so English-only programs would enable EB students to learn English and adapt quicker (Nieto, 2009). These anti-bilingualism efforts led to the banning of bilingual education in three states: California, Massachusetts, and Arizona. In 1998, Proposition 227 was passed by California voters. English-only instruction was mandated for EB students, and they were to receive specialized instruction, structured English immersion (SEI; see Chap. 2 for discussion), for 1 year before being moved to mainstream classrooms. Similarly, Proposition 203 (2000) was passed in Arizona, followed by Massachusetts Question 2 (2002), which both banned bilingual instruction and mandated SEI instruction.

Proposition 227 (CA, 1998) was overturned by voters in 2016, and Massachusetts Question 2 (2002) was overturned by voters in 2017. However, Arizona's Proposition 203 (2000) remains in place. Despite promises that bilingual education bans would close educational gaps for EB students, the detrimental impact of these bans on the social–emotional and academic outcomes of EB students has been well-documented (e.g., Lillie et al., 2012; Menken, 2013; Parra et al., 2014). Moreover, Arizona continues to exhibit poor graduation rates among EB students. In the 2019–2020 school year, the high school graduation rate for EB students was 55%, the fourth lowest in the nation, compared to a median state-level graduation rate of 69% and a national average of 71% for EB students and 86% for all students (Office of English Language Acquisition [OELA], 2023). Research has extensively documented the benefits of bilingual education models and the advantages of bilingualism and multilingualism; yet, non-evidence-based instructional models continue to be utilized, causing harm to EB students (Bialystok, 2018; Chamorro & Janke, 2022).

Classification as an English Language Learner

EB students are classified as ELLs upon enrolling in school. The US Department of Justice and US Department of Education (2015) published guidance to ensure that schools provide meaningful participation in education for ELL students. In the fact sheet, they outline the process for classifying and placing ELLs in English Language Development (ELD) instruction, as well as monitoring and exiting these students from ELD programming. Families must complete enrollment packets that include a home language survey, which asks them to report the language(s) spoken at home. If a language other than English is specified, the student must take an English language proficiency assessment in the areas of listening, reading, speaking, and writing (e.g., state test, WIDA Screener) to determine their English language proficiency (Huenergarde & Floyd, 2025).

If a student does not demonstrate English fluency at the predetermined cutoff scores, they will be designated as an ELL student and be eligible to receive ELD services. They will also need to participate in annual testing to monitor their English language development. The types of ELD instructional services available to EB students differ and are discussed in Chap. 2. ELL students are generally reclassified as English proficient once they pass a standardized test (e.g., state test, ACCESS). The test used differs by state, which can result in an individual being classified or reclassified as an ELL in one state but not another (García & Kleifgen, 2018; Huenergarde & Floyd, 2025; National Research Council et al., 2011). School psychologists must understand how English language proficiency is assessed in EB students and what criteria must be met to be reclassified as fluent in English. For an in-depth discussion of classification processes, please see Huenergarde and Floyd (2025).

Reclassification

ELL students who meet the criteria for English proficiency on the language proficiency test are reclassified as English proficient, so they are no longer classified as ELL students. However, their academic performance is generally monitored for at least 2 years after they have been exited from ELD services to ensure they are making adequate progress and were not exited too early (US Department of Justice & US Department of Education, 2015). Thus, the language proficiency of formerly identified ELL students will be retested to determine if there is a need for language support, and subsequent reclassification as an ELL student can occur (US Department of Education, 2016).

Huenergarde and Floyd (2025) examined the classification and reclassification processes for ELL students across all states. They found that all states use identical processes for classification and reclassification (i.e., home language survey and language proficiency testing). They emphasized the need for using multiple sources of data and collaboration with educators, students, and caregivers for reclassification. A small number of states employ multiple methods, such as observations, grades, progress monitoring measures, interviews, and recommendations from a team of educators to determine reclassification. Utilizing a holistic approach to reclassification can reduce the reliance on strict cut scores from standardized tests and allow ELL students to demonstrate their language and literacy skills in ways that are not accurately captured by language proficiency tests (Huenergarde & Floyd, 2025).

Long-Term English Learners

Students who remain classified as ELL students for more than 6 years are referred to as long-term English learners (LTELs; Menken & Kleyn, 2010; Rhinehart et al., 2024). LTEL is not a formal designation, but it represents a unique subset of EB students who have not been deemed English proficient to exit ELD services (Umansky & Avelar, 2023). Given the transitional nature of ELD instruction, there is reason to be concerned when EB students remain classified as ELLs for the majority or all of their schooling experience. The longevity associated with being labeled an ELL student implies that ELD instruction is not meeting their educational needs (Rhinehart et al., 2024). Additionally, these students are generally enrolled in less rigorous courses, which limits their exposure to advanced curricula and opportunities to learn content that will help them achieve reclassification criteria (Umansky & Reardon, 2014).

Being an LTEL positions these students as deficient because of their inability to pass language proficiency tests. However, many LTELs are English-dominant and effectively utilize the English language to meet their course competencies and standards in ways that are similar to their monolingual English-speaking peers (Brooks, 2019; Cushing-Leibner & King, 2015; Menken et al., 2012; Shin, 2020; Umansky & Avelar, 2023). The use of language proficiency tests for reclassification also suggests that language can be standardized and quantified neutrally and objectively (Flores, 2021). Yet, the language proficiency of monolingual English-speaking students is not assessed and is instead assumed to be good enough. A study by the California Department of Education (2011) found that monolingual English-speaking students were unable to meet the English proficiency standards mandated for ELL students. These findings beg the question of whether reclassification criteria need to be reevaluated as EB students are being held to seemingly higher standards based on test scores (Estrada & Wang, 2018).

Being an LTEL can have a detrimental impact on the educational experiences of EB students. Some identified outcomes include limited access to advanced curricular opportunities, an increased risk of dropout, and lower graduation rates (Huang et al., 2016; Menken & Kleyn, 2010; Umansky & Avelar, 2023). Moreover, LTEL status is associated with a higher likelihood of eligibility for special education services due to the presence of a disability (Rhinehart et al., 2024; Sahakyan & Ryan, 2018). Therefore, some EB students may be unable to be reclassified as English proficient due to the presence of a disability, which may make it more challenging for them to pass these tests. As mentioned earlier, a holistic approach to examining language proficiency and reclassification is needed to better address EB students' educational needs.

Special Education Placement and EB Students

There is relatively little data available on special education placement among EB students; however, some federally collected data demonstrate disparities when compared to non-EB students. The Office of English Language Acquisition's (OELA) fact sheet on ELLs with disabilities (2020) provides insights into special education trends. Reported as percentage point differences between EB youth and their monolingual peers, it shows that during the 2017–2018 school year, EBs were most likely to be identified for services more than non-EB learners in the following locations: Illinois (+8.2%), Montana (+9%), New Mexico (+9.2%), and Puerto Rico (+12.9%). Conversely, EBs were least likely to be identified for services compared to their non-EB peers in New Jersey (−9.0%), New Hampshire (−6.7%), and Nebraska (−5.3%). Specific to disability areas under IDEA, in the 2018–2019 school year, the percentage point disparity between EB students and non-EB students was highest in the following disability categories: specific learning disability (+12.3%), speech-language impairment (+2%), and intellectual disability (+0.5%). While disproportionality is not as pervasive for EB students compared to other groups, these data suggest the need to examine patterns on local levels (e.g., state, district, school) to determine the existence of disparities and identify ways to solve them.

When placed in special education, students tend to remain for the duration of their educational career. An examination of the exit reasons for special education shows that in the 2020–2021 school year, only 7.6% of all students with disabilities transferred to general education (US Department of Education, 2024). The most recent data for EB students show that, compared to non-EB students, in the 2017–2018 school year, EB students were 2.2% more likely to exit special education due to dropping out of school, 3.8% due to moving, and 1.3% due to receiving a certificate (OELA, 2020). EBs were also 6.3% less likely to graduate with a regular high school diploma. These disparities are concerning because EB students are not exiting special education due to the fact that they no longer require special education services. Moreover, continued enrollment in special education, dropping out, and receiving a certificate instead of a diploma are likely to have long-term consequences, including limited employment opportunities and a reduced likelihood of postsecondary attendance.

Educators must consider these factors when making initial and continued special education eligibility decisions at Individual Education Program (IEP) meetings for ELL students with disabilities, and develop goals and objectives to promote ELL students' persistence to graduation and knowledge and preparation for postsecondary opportunities. Transition planning, by age 16 at the latest, is a process mandated by IDEA (2004) for all students with an IEP. The focus of transition planning is to prepare youth for college and career readiness as they exit the K-12 system (Sawyer, 2020). For many of the reasons already outlined, dually identified EB students (i.e., students with both an IEP and an ELL designation) face additional challenges within this process.

For example, in a national longitudinal study of these students' transition planning experiences, Trainor et al. (2019) found that the transition component of their IEP was most likely to be developed by school personnel with little input from students and families. This is important as other research (e.g., Romano et al., 2023) has shown that teachers tend to have lower transition expectations for dually identified youth, which can negatively impact how these students perceive their abilities and prospects for future success. This implicit bias can also result in ELL youth taking a more passive role within transition planning meetings compared to their non-ELL peers (Romano et al., 2023; Wu et al., 2023). For dually identified youth, transition planning is most effective when it is a collaborative, personalized, and strengths-based process involving the youth, their caregivers, and teachers (Romano et al., 2023). Ensuring this is the case requires a holistic and culturally and linguistically centered approach that recognizes the additional burdens and barriers placed upon dually identified youth both in their K-12 journey and beyond.

Access to Advanced Educational Programming

Academic outcomes among EB students often lag behind those of their monolingual English-speaking peers. Unfortunately, the school system is unprepared to meet their educational needs, and as a result, they continue to experience academic challenges. Grade retention among EB students is particularly problematic, as they are overrepresented among students who are retained. More specifically, EB students made up 10% of the public school enrollment in the 2017–2018 school year; yet, 14.3% of EB students experienced grade retention (OELA, 2021a). Grade retention is a common practice, although it lacks research to support its efficacy and is associated with adverse long-term effects, including dropout and lower college enrollment rates (Buckmaster et al., 2024). Educators must understand the consequences of retention and identify alternate ways to support the educational needs of EB students.

EB students are underrepresented in advanced educational opportunities, including advanced placement (AP), gifted, and dual enrollment courses (OELA, 2021b, 2022). Not only do they largely attend schools that do not offer AP courses but they are also less likely to enroll in these courses compared to non-EB students (OELA, 2021b). EBs represented only 2% of students enrolled in AP courses in the 2017–2018 school year. They represented 1.5% of students in gifted and talented programs compared to 7.2% of non-EB students (OELA, 2021c). This exclusion from advanced educational programming opportunities severely limits the college and career readiness of EB students, increasing the risk of adverse long-term outcomes (e.g., dropout; Vega, 2023).

Overview of the Book

Given what is known about the educational landscape for EB students, school psychologists and educators alike can play a significant role in advocating for and implementing equitable services that meet their unique cultural and linguistic needs. EBs deserve an educational experience that affirms their identities and provides them with opportunities to succeed; instead, they are blamed for their challenges when the system is failing them. Therefore, educators must consider the contextual factors (e.g., poverty, homelessness, quality of instruction received, language proficiency levels, exposure to trauma) that affect the performance and outcomes of EB students and work together to identify and employ culturally responsive practices (Goforth & Pham, 2023; Ortiz, 2023).

Through the use of culturally responsive intervention and assessment practices, as discussed in this book, school psychologists and other school personnel can collaborate to ensure that EB students receive supports that align with their cultural and linguistic backgrounds. In this book, our contributors address timely topics to help school-based practitioners effectively and equitably support EB students. The first few chapters provide the foundation for the remainder of the book by outlining who EB students are and the experiences they encounter in their schooling. Subsequent chapters outline the advantages and disadvantages of instructional programs available to EBs, along with a discussion of the impact of acculturation on education and outcomes, and considerations when implementing interventions and conducting assessments.

The second section of the book focuses on implementing a multi-tiered system of supports (MTSS) for EB students. The five chapters in this area present a culturally and linguistically responsive (CLR) MTSS approach, discuss how to develop family-school partnerships within the context of an MTSS model, and explore culturally adapted and culturally and linguistically responsive MTSS approaches to support social–emotional and behavioral, language and literacy, and math needs. It also discusses best practices when collaborating with interpreters throughout the intervention process.

The book culminates with a focus on using culturally responsive assessment practices when evaluating EB students for different disability categories and areas of concern, including specific learning disability, social–emotional concerns, intellectual disability, speech-language impairments, autism, and dyslexia. It also discusses key collaborations with speech-language pathologists throughout the assessment process. The book provides practical recommendations that are culturally responsive for educators to support EB students.

References

Aguilar, L. N., Shearin, J., Wamnuga-Win, S. K., & Mojica, K. (2021). Indigenous youth in schools: Consequences of colonialism and advocating for a better future. *Communiqué, 50*(1), 1.

Bialik, K., Scheller, A., & Walker, K. (2018). *6 Facts about English language learners in U.S. public schools*. Pew Research Center. https://www.pewresearch.org/short-reads/2018/10/25/6-facts-about-english-language-learners-in-u-s-public-schools/

Bialystok, E. (2018). Bilingual education for young children: Review of the effects and consequences. *International Journal of Bilingual Education and Bilingualism, 21*(6), 666–679.

Brooks, M. D. (2019). *Transforming literacy education for long-term English learners: Recognizing brilliance in the undervalued*. Routledge.

Buckmaster, J. L., Urick, A., & Ford, T. G. (2024). A quasi-experimental, longitudinal study of grade retention on language outcomes for English Language Learners. *Journal of Education for Students Placed at Risk (JESPAR), 29*(4), 332–362.

California Department of Education. (2011). *A comparison study of kindergarten and grade 1 English-fluent students and English learners on the 2010–11 edition of the CELDT*. Author.

Chamorro, G., & Janke, V. (2022). Investigating the bilingual advantage: The impact of L2 exposure on the social and cognitive skills of monolingually-raised children in bilingual education. *International Journal of Bilingual Education and Bilingualism, 25*(5), 1765–1781.

Chishti, M., & Bush-Joseph, K. (2025). *In first 100 days, Trump 2.0 has dramatically reshaped the U.S. immigration system, but is not meeting mass deportation aims*. Migration Information Source. https://www.migrationpolicy.org/article/trump-2-immigration-first-100-days

Cushing-Leubner, J., & King, K. A. (2015). Long-term English learners and language education policy. In A. Yiakoumetti (Ed.), *Multilingualism and language in education: Current sociolinguistic and pedagogical perspectives from Commonwealth countries* (pp. 199–220). Cambridge University Press.

Estrada, P., & Wang, H. (2018). Making English learner reclassification to fluent English proficient attainable or elusive: When meeting criteria is and is not enough. *American Educational Research Journal, 55*(2), 207–242.

Flores, N. (2021). A raciolinguistic perspective on standardized literacy assessments. *Linguistics and Education, 64*, 100868. https://doi.org/10.1016/j.linged.2020.100868

García, O. (2009). Emergent bilinguals and TESOL: What's in a name? *TESOL Quarterly, 43*(2), 322–326.

García, O., & Kleifgen, J. A. (2018). *Educating emergent bilinguals: Policies, programs, and practices for English learners*. Teachers College Press.

Goforth, A. N., Farmer, R. L., Kim, S. Y., Naser, S. C., Lockwood, A. B., & Affrunti, N. W. (2021). Status of school psychology in 2020: Part 1, demographics of the NASP membership survey. *NASP Research Reports, 5*(2), 1–17.

Goforth, A. N., & Pham, A. V. (2023). *Culturally responsive school-based practices: Supporting mental health and learning of diverse students*. Oxford University Press.

Huang, M., Haas, E., Zhu, N., & Tran, L. (2016). *High school graduation rates across English learner student subgroups in Arizona (REL 2017–205)*. U.S. Department of Education, Institute of Education Sciences, National Center for Education Evaluation and Regional Assistance, Regional Educational Laboratory West. http://ies.ed.gov/ncee/edlabs

Huenergarde, M. C., & Floyd, R. G. (2025). Identification and reclassification criteria for linguistically diverse students with and without disabilities across the United States. *Contemporary School Psychology*, 1–15. https://doi.org/10.1007/s40688-025-00552-9

Individuals with Disabilities Education Improvement Act of 2004, Pub. L. No. 108-446, 118 Stat. 2647 (2004).

Kanno, Y., Rios-Aguilar, C., & Bunch, G. C. (2024). English learners? Emergent bilinguals? Multilingual learners? Goals, contexts, and consequences in labeling students. *TESOL Journal, 15*(3), 1–12.

Lillie, K. E., Markos, A., Arias, M. B., & Wiley, T. G. (2012). Separate and not equal: The Implementation of structured English immersion in Arizona's classrooms. *Teachers College Record, 114*(9), 1–33.

Menken, L. (2013). Restrictive language education policies and emergent bilingual youth: A perfect storm with imperfect outcomes. *Theory Into Practice, 52*(3), 160–168. https://doi.org/10.1080/00405841.2013.804307

Menken, K., & Kleyn, T. (2010). The long-term impact of subtractive schooling in the educational experiences of secondary English language learners. *International Journal of Bilingual Education & Bilingualism, 13*(4), 399–417. https://doi.org/10.1080/13670050903370143

Menken, K., Kleyn, T., & Chae, N. (2012). Spotlight on "long-term English language learners": Characteristics and prior schooling experiences of an invisible population. *International Multilingual Research Journal, 6*(2), 121–142. https://doi.org/10.1080/19313152.2012.665822

National Center for Education Statistics. (2023). *Characteristics of Public School Teachers. Condition of Education*. U.S. Department of Education, Institute of Education Sciences. https://nces.ed.gov/programs/coe/indicator/clr

National Center for Education Statistics. (2024). *English Learners in Public Schools. Condition of Education*. U.S. Department of Education, Institute of Education Sciences. https://nces.ed.gov/programs/coe/indicator/cgf

National Research Council, Division of Behavioral, Social Sciences, Board on Testing, Assessment, Committee on National Statistics, et al. (2011). *Allocating federal funds for state programs for English language learners*. National Academies Press.

Nieto, D. (2009). A brief history of bilingual education in the United States. *Perspectives on Urban Education, 6*(1), 61–83.

Office of English Language Acquisition. (2020). *English learners with disabilities*. https://ncela.ed.gov/sites/default/files/legacy/files/fast_facts/20201216-Del4.4-ELsDisabilities-508-OELA.pdf

Office of English Language Acquisition. (2021a). *English learner absenteeism, suspension, and Retention*. https://ncela.ed.gov/sites/default/files/legacy/files/fast_facts/202109-Del4-4ELAbsenteeismSuspensionandRetention-508.pdf

Office of English Language Acquisition. (2021b). *English learners in advanced placement and international baccalaureate courses*. https://ncela.ed.gov/sites/default/files/legacy/files/fast_facts/20210803-Del4-4EL-AP-IB-FactSheet508.pdf

Office of English Language Acquisition. (2021c). *English learners in gifted and talented programs*. https://ncela.ed.gov/sites/default/files/legacy/files/fast_facts/Del4-4GiftedTalented-20210208-508.pdf

Office of English Language Acquisition. (2022). *English learners in college credit-bearing courses*. https://ncela.ed.gov/sites/default/files/2022-09/OELACollegeCreditBearing_09012922_508.pdf

Office of English Language Acquisition. (2023). *High school graduation rates for English learners*. https://ncela.ed.gov/sites/default/files/2023-06/ELGradRates-FS-20230602-508.pdf

Ortiz, S. O. (2023). Best practices in nondiscriminatory assessment. In P. L. Harrison, S. L. Proctor, & A. Thomas (Eds.), *Best practices in school psychology: Vol. 1. Data-based and collaborative decision-making* (pp. 149–161).

Palmer, S., & Cooke, W. (1996). Understanding and countering racism with First Nations children in out-of-home care. *Child Welfare, 75*(6), 709–725.

Parra, E. B., Evans, C. A., Fletcher, T., & Combs, M. C. (2014). The psychological impact of English language immersion on elementary age English language learners. *Journal of Multilingual Education Research, 5*(1), 33–65.

Pember, M. A. (2007). A painful remembrance. *Diverse: Issues in Higher Education, 24*, 24–27.

Rhinehart, L. V., Bailey, A. L., & Haager, D. (2024). Long-term English learners: Untangling language acquisition and learning disabilities. *Contemporary School Psychology, 28*(2), 173–185.

Romano, L. E., Trainor, A. A., & Newman, L. A. (2023). Triad transition planning for students receiving special education and English learner services, families, and teachers. *Career*

Development and Transition for Exceptional Individuals, 46(4), 211–222. https://doi.org/10.1177/21651434221143514

Rutherford-Quach, S., Gibney, D. T., Kelly, H., Riccards, J. B., Garcia, E., Hsiao, M., et al. (2021). *Bilingual education across the United States*. CCNetwork.

Sahakyan, N., & Ryan, S. (2018). *Exploring the long-term English learner population across 15 WIDA states*. Wisconsin Center for Education Research, University of Wisconsin–Madison. https://wida.wisc.edu/resources/exploring-long-term-english-learner-population-across-15-wida-states

Sawyer, S. (2020). *Secondary transition planning: The basics*. CA Transition Alliance. https://6abb391c-dbc9-4e2e-9cd4-f10c9c4bb967.filesusr.com/ugd/c055a4_f1b186d9a-b24411eb8971d6583e849b5.pdf

Shin, N. (2020). Stuck in the middle: Examination of long-term English learners. *International Multilingual Research Journal, 14*(3), 181–205. https://doi.org/10.1080/19313152.2019.1681614

The White House. (2025). *Designating English as the official language of the United States*. https://www.whitehouse.gov/presidential-actions/2025/03/designating-english-as-the-official-language-of-the-united-states/

Trainor, A. A., Newman, L., Garcia, E., Woodley, H. H., Traxler, R. E., & Deschene, D. N. (2019). Postsecondary education-focused transition planning experiences of English learners with disabilities. *Career Development and Transition for Exceptional Individuals, 42*(1), 43–55. https://doi.org/10.1177/2165143418811830

Umansky, I. M., & Avelar, J. D. (2023). Canaried in the coal mine: What the experiences and outcomes of students considered long-term English learners teach us about pitfalls in English learner education… and what we can do about it. *Journal of Education for Students Placed at Risk (JESPAR), 28*(1), 122–147.

Umansky, I. M., & Reardon, S. F. (2014). Reclassification patterns among Latino English learner students in bilingual, dual immersion, and English immersion classrooms. *American Educational Research Journal, 51*(5), 879–912. https://doi.org/10.3102/0002831214545110

U.S. Department of Education. (2024). *U.S. Department of Education, Office of Special Education and Rehabilitative Services, Office of Special Education Programs, 45th Annual Report to Congress on the Implementation of the Individuals with Disabilities Education Act, 2023*. https://sites.ed.gov/idea/files/45th-arc-for-idea.pdf

U.S. Department of Education. (2016). *Tools and resources for monitoring and exiting English learners from EL programs and services*. https://www.ed.gov/sites/ed/files/about/offices/list/oela/english-learner-toolkit/chap8.pdf

U.S. Department of Education. (2017). *U.S. Department of Education, EDFacts Data Warehouse (EDW), 2014–15*. SEA File C141, LEP Enrolled. Extracted April 3, 2017. https://web.archive.org/web/20240725005209/https://www.ed.gov/datastory/el-characteristics/index.html#one

U.S. Department of Justice, & U.S. Department of Education. (2015). *Ensuring English learner students can participate meaningfully and equally in educational programs*. https://www.ed.gov/media/document/dcl-factsheet-el-students-201501pdf-21469.pdf

Valencia, R. R. (2005). The Mexican American struggle for equal educational opportunity in Mendez v. Westminster: Helping to pave the way for Brown v. Board of Education. *Teachers College Record, 107*(3), 389–423.

Vega, D. (2023). Exceptionalities. In P. A. Schutz & K. R. Muis (Eds.), *Handbook of educational psychology* (pp. 335–358). Routledge.

Wu, Y., Thurlow, M., & Johnson, D. (2023). A national view of transition planning participation and post-school goals for English learners with disabilities. *Exceptionality, 31*(1), 18–35. https://doi.org/10.1080/09362835.2021.1938060

Chapter 2
Instructional Programming for Emergent Bilingual Students

Patricia Sánchez Lizardi, Marie L. Tanaka, and Alexandro Ornelas

Public schools in the United States are seeing an increase in emergent bilingual (EB) students. This population grew from 4.6 million students (9.4%) in the fall of 2011 to 5.3 million students (10.6%) in the fall of 2021 (National Center for Education Statistics [NCES], 2024). This context calls for intentional efforts to develop or support programs that best meet their educational needs. This chapter presents the different types of instructional programs for EB students (also referred to as multilingual learners, English language learners, dual language learners, and English as a second language learners) within the K-12 education system. Language acquisition and instructional programming models, including English as a second language, sheltered/structured English immersion, transitional bilingual, and dual language models, will be discussed. The chapter begins with an overview of language and second language acquisition and the policies that impact the education of EB students, followed by descriptions of instructional models and their outcomes, concluding with implications and recommendations.

We have no conflicts of interest to disclose. Correspondence concerning this chapter should be addressed to Patricia Sánchez Lizardi, Department of Counseling and School Psychology, San Diego State University, 5500 Campanile Drive, San Diego, CA 92182-8080. Email: plizardi@sdsu.edu

P. Sánchez Lizardi (✉) · M. L. Tanaka · A. Ornelas
Department of Counseling and School Psychology, San Diego State University,
San Diego, CA, USA
e-mail: plizardi@sdsu.edu; mltanaka@sdsu.edu

D. Vega, J. N. Wolf (eds.), *Culturally and Linguistically Responsive Intervention and Assessment Practices with Emergent Bilingual Students*,
https://doi.org/10.1007/978-3-032-02084-0_2

Language Development and Second Language Acquisition

Understanding language development and second language acquisition in the context of instruction for EB students is a first step to developing programs that teach English without detriment to the EB students' first language. Cognitivist perspectives suggest that first language acquisition is a universal and relatively effortless process that every human goes through as part of typical development, implying that children will speak the language of their community without much explicit instruction because they are preprogrammed to acquire the abstract linguistic system of their first language (Kuhl, 2004; Valdés et al., 2015). By extension, multiple language acquisition would occur when the child internalizes the language system of the new language. This would usually happen through a more explicit and intentional manner, such as learning new vocabulary, phonological and grammatical components, writing structures, and social usage for communication (Valdés et al., 2015). However, the cognitivist perspective has been challenged as newer explanations about second language acquisition emerge (Caldwell-Harris & MacWhinney, 2023) and defining who is bilingual or multilingual and to what degree is not a simple task. Second language acquisition is a complex process that draws on research from linguistics, psychology, sociology, and education.

Various diverging theories of language acquisition have been proposed detailing how a second language is acquired (VanPatten et al., 2020). A distinction relevant to educating EB students refers to simultaneous and sequential bilingualism. Simultaneous bilingualism is when a child learns two languages from birth, and sequential bilingualism occurs when a child begins to learn a second language after about 3 years of age, usually by going to daycare or elementary school (Baker & Wright, 2021). Within the field of education and teaching English as a second language, theories such as *Five Hypotheses* (Krashen, 1982), *Basic Interpersonal Communication Skills* (BICS) and *Cognitive Academic Language Proficiency* (CALP; Cummins, 2008), and the *Cognitive Academic Language Learning Approach* (CALLA; Chamot & O'Malley, 1994) have been used to understand children's second language development and have served as a foundation for instructional programs addressing the needs of EB students. Furthermore, contrary to popular belief, bilingualism does not interfere with English language acquisition and proficiency (D'Souza et al., 2020).

Stages of Second Language Acquisition

While a detailed description of second language acquisition is beyond the scope of this chapter, it is important to understand this process as it relates to the education of EB students. Most EB students must learn English while simultaneously learning academic content, requiring educators to be knowledgeable and supportive of this process. A student acquiring a second language typically goes through five predictable stages (see Table 1.1; Krashen & Terrell, 1988); however, a specific timeline

Table 1.1 Stages of second language acquisition

Stage	Description
1. Silent/receptive or preproduction	Students are typically silent but observant of others' conversations and attentive to words and their pronunciation. They tend to interact by using gestures and responding to yes/no type questions.
2. Early production	Students begin to use single words or short phrases and receptively comprehend more words (~1000). They may respond to simple questions (e.g., who, what, where, when).
3. Speech emergence	Students ask simple questions and use short phrases as their vocabulary increases (~3000 words), but communicating their ideas is still difficult due to grammar errors and the complexities of language.
4. Intermediate language proficiency	Students' vocabulary increases (~6000 words), they ask more complex questions, make longer statements, and ask for clarification when necessary.
5. Advanced language proficiency	Students use their acquired English to fully participate in their classroom activities. They continue learning new vocabulary and may need occasional support.

Note: According to Krashen and Terrell (1988) and adapted from Klingner and Eppolito (2014)

for each stage has not been established. By knowing this process, educators will be better equipped to differentiate between students' academic challenges due to language acquisition or learning disabilities, thus reducing EB students' referral to and misidentification for special education (Klingner & Eppolito, 2014). In the subsequent sections, we review how second language acquisition and policies related to the education of EB students may be integrated and implemented in everyday classrooms and schools.

Policies Impacting the Education of EB Students

Federal Policies

The first US federal legislation recognizing EB students was the Bilingual Education Act (BEA) of 1968, which was a product of 1960s' Latinx activism striving for self-determination to empower language-minoritized communities (García & Sung, 2018). Though the BEA's original sentiment was to shift policy to celebrate multilingual and multicultural assets of students, its passing was framed around problematizing languages other than English as "handicaps," ultimately resulting in supporting English-only programs (García & Sung, 2018). As states passed anti-bilingual education laws in the late 1990s and early 2000s (e.g., California [since repealed], Arizona, Massachusetts), the BEA was ultimately replaced with Title III of the No Child Left Behind Act (NCLB, 2002). Following NCLB, the word "bilingual," along with the BEA's original intentions, were muffled in the federal vernacular and replaced with "English language acquisition" (García, 2009), further imposing a deficit-based foundation for the education of EB students.

Before NCLB, federal funds were not allocated for EB students' specific instruction, except through competitive grant programs (Williams, 2021). The more recent Every Student Succeeds Act (ESSA, 2015) maintained the funding and began requiring that EB students be held to the same academic standards and outcomes as non-EB students, as measured by statewide assessments in English language proficiency, reading/language arts, and mathematics, except when they are within their first 12 months of attending school in the United States or have a disability. Still, instead of allowing theory and research to guide best practices in bilingual education, federal requirements and policies around accountability may overshadow and further dictate teaching practices to focus on teaching to the test (King & Bigelow, 2018).

Federally, EB students have rights to "equal access" to instructional programming (*Lau v. Nichols*, 1974), which must be based on sound theory, have allocated resources and personnel, and be evaluated to be effective (*Castañeda v. Pickard*, 1981). EB students also may not be segregated from native English-speaking peers (*Keyes v. Denver*, 1973). Though federal policies also require schools to communicate with caregivers in a language they can understand (Title III, 2015), in practice, state education agencies (SEAs), local education agencies (LEAs), districts, and schools may not implement desegregated access to such services (Coady et al., 2022).

Federal regulations discuss the need and expectation for caregivers to be informed in their primary language of why and how their child was assessed, the results, and the kind of instructional programming in which their child will participate. Additionally, caregivers must be informed of how such programming will meet their child's academic needs, the requirements for exiting from that instructional programming, and if the state is not meeting accountability targets with certain instructional programming (Zacarian, 2012).

State Laws and Policies

Instructional models for EB students vary by state and often by districts and schools; they are also dependent on student needs and staffing resources (Rutherford-Quach et al., 2021; Zacarian, 2012). For example, some states (e.g., Wisconsin) may require bilingual education programming only if a certain number of students from the same language group are enrolled (López & Iribarren, 2014; Rutherford-Quach et al., 2021); others may explicitly mandate bilingual education or may leave it up to LEAs to decide how to meet EB student needs (López et al., 2015). States and LEAs also determine how they identify EB students, such as through home language surveys, parent interviews, teacher input, or other assessments. Once their child is identified as an EB student, caregivers have limited time to withdraw their child from language development programming, depending on SEAs/LEAs requirements. These state-mandated requirements often limit what school leaders can implement in their districts and buildings (López & Iribarren, 2014).

Though states and LEAs decide which assessment to use to measure a student's English language ability, report accountability, and provide accommodations for EB students, tests such as the *World-Class Instructional Design and Assessment* (WIDA) or the *Access Placement Test* (W-APT), are often used as high-stakes methods to determine long-term academic trajectories (King & Bigelow, 2018). Further, how students exit English language development (ELD) programming also differs among states; some may require certain scores on annual assessments, often keeping students in ELD programming until they can take the test again in hopes of being reclassified as proficient in English (Florez, 2012). Another major criticism of high-stakes assessments for ELD is how they may not adequately differentiate among students with vastly diverse needs and educational backgrounds, further obscuring their instructional levels and needs (King & Bigelow, 2018).

English-Only Ideology

Although states, LEAs, and districts vary in their assessment, placement, accountability metrics, and educational programming, Arizona is the only state in the United States that explicitly prohibits bilingual education (Proposition 203), implementing its instructional programming in 2 h of ELD per day, a decrease from the original 4 h per day (Kaveh et al., 2022). English-only measures were also previously adopted by California (Proposition 227, 1998) and Massachusetts (Chap. 386, 2002), though they have since been repealed by voters. The roots of these initiatives originated from proponents of making English the official language of the United States (Brown, 2023; Wiley & Wright, 2004).

English-only education may further exacerbate opportunity gaps for positive academic outcomes of EB students (Rumberger & Tran, 2010). Students who participated in English-only education in Massachusetts, for example, described challenges in monolingual settings such as feeling dehumanized, being unable to communicate what they know due to monolingualism, and being ridiculed for their level of English; they all described desiring a more bilingual model for their education (Dort, 2019). Furthermore, despite federal regulations prohibiting segregation, English-only programming's side effect frequently segregates students based on language and race/ethnicity (Tanaka, 2023).

Although most states are overturning explicitly monolingual and restrictive language policies, in practice and everyday use, they may still promote and perpetuate English-only ideals and English hegemony (Chang-Bacon, 2022). Such monolingual, English-first mentalities prioritize learning English over all else, implicating that students' home languages may interfere with or be at the detriment of learning outcomes (i.e., subtractive views; Bernstein et al., 2023). These subtractive views perpetuate messaging that students' linguistic and cultural assets should be seen as deficits or hindrances to their education. Devaluing what EB students may bring to their educational experiences has tangible, negative consequences for students' educational outcomes (Martinez & Martinez, 2017). These English-only or English-first ideals seem to be the unspoken foundation of instructional programming models that mostly hold subtractive views of multilingualism.

Instructional Programming Models

Instructional programs to educate EB students seek to support students in becoming proficient in English and meeting federal/state academic standards; this programming is often referred to as ELD. There are various models of instruction, but they are mainly categorized as those that aim to "immerse" students in the mainstream language and those that aim to bilingualism and biliteracy (Baker & Wright, 2021). There are also variations to each model; in practice, they may look different among school districts (Sugarman, 2018). This section describes English-only models such as English as a second language (ESL) and sheltered/structured English immersion (SEI). We also introduce transitional bilingual (TB) and dual language (DL) models; the latter also aims for EB students to become proficient and meet academic standards in their native language.

English-Only Models

These models aim to improve EB students' English listening, speaking, reading, and writing skills to effectively participate in academic and social settings where English is required. There is no intention to maintain or develop the EB students' first language (Baker & Wright, 2021). In these models, teachers are usually monolingual English speakers, and EB students, who typically speak different languages, receive instruction in English with minimal to no use of their first language. English-only models are sometimes referred to as ESL, English for speakers of other languages (ESOL), and ELD programs.

English as a Second Language

ESL programs offer a specialized instructional approach to help EB students develop proficiency in English. It is commonly used in school districts with a highly diverse language population, as it allows students from various language backgrounds to be in the same class, eliminating the need for teachers to be proficient in students' home languages (Sugarman, 2018). Even though teachers who do not speak the students' home languages teach in ESL programs, bilingual educators tend to display more significant positive attitudes toward EB students (Rader-Brown & Howley, 2014). There are multiple models implemented in ESL programs depending on the student's English proficiency level. ESL instruction is commonly implemented through a push-in or pull-out model (Baecher & Bell, 2017).

Push-in model This model involves an ESL teacher collaborating with the monolingual English teacher to assist EB students. It may include co-teaching alongside the general education teacher, conducting small group sessions, or delivering personalized assistance through targeted intervention to EB students in the classroom

(Ferlazzo & Hull-Sypnieski, 2018; Mofield, 2020). The aim is to offer specific language guidance while ensuring students can fully engage with the general education curriculum. There are several advantages of implementing a push-in ESL model. It fosters integration by ensuring that EB students become part of the general education classroom, promotes social inclusion and a stronger sense of belonging, provides direct access to grade-level content and instruction, and potentially improves students' academic performance (Baecher & Bell, 2017). Moreover, it creates opportunities for language development as learners engage in authentic contexts to practice and refine their language skills.

Despite its advantages, implementing a push-in ESL model also presents some challenges. One significant concern is the limited time available for the ESL teacher to address the diverse needs of each EB student within the classroom setting, potentially impacting their learning outcomes. This limitation may impede personalized attention, disrupt classroom dynamics, and need careful coordination between ESL and monolingual teachers (Whiting, 2017). Furthermore, both ESL and monolingual general education teachers must receive adequate training in collaborative instruction and strategies specifically designed to support EB students for this model to be effective (Baker & Wright, 2021; Olds et al., 2021).

Pull-out model ESL pull-out models consist of removing or "pulling out" EB students from their monolingual classroom to participate in small group-targeted English language instruction with other EB students who are working toward similar English language proficiency goals. These small groups typically last 30–45 min per session and occur during content instruction periods, resulting in EB students missing general education curriculum content (Zacarian & Haynes, 2012). Research suggests that EB students participating in ESL pull-out programs tend to experience greater academic underperformance than their peers in ESL push-in models because ESL instruction through a push-in model is integrated within the general education classroom (Bell & Baecher, 2012; Maxwell, 2014). This means that EB students are exposed to the general curriculum while developing their English skills. Sugarman (2018) states that this integrated push-in model better supports EB students' overall academic progress.

Sheltered English Immersion

Sheltered language instruction was originally designed for teaching minoritized languages and promoting multilingualism but has since been appropriated and transformed into US English language instruction in English-dominant contexts (Chang-Bacon, 2022). Though sheltered English instruction models vary by state and district, the idea behind such an approach is to allow EB students to access general education curricula by teaching them English to develop conceptual understandings in all subject areas (e.g., *Sheltered Instruction Observation Protocol* [SIOP]; Echevarría et al., 2016). These models also differ from bilingual immersion school programs (see dual language model section).

The definition of what is considered "sheltered" has also evolved and differentiated, where it could refer to focusing on content being delivered in comprehensible ways (since native English speakers would typically not be present) or where both content and language are combined in a way that does not occur in general education native English-speaking classrooms (Cassels Johnson et al., 2017). Sheltered models differ in populations served (i.e., EB students only or a mixture of EB and native-English-speaking students) and who is teaching (i.e., specialized bilingual or general education teachers). Even within the same district, sheltered instruction can vastly differ based on how educators interpret policies and the resources afforded to them (e.g., funding for EB-specific training and availability of instructors with such training; see Cassels Johnson et al., 2017 for further origins and history of sheltered English immersion).

Despite the variability, according to The Center on Instruction (Moughamian et al., 2009), sheltered programming is defined as a model that "facilitate[s] student access to content concepts and promote[s] the development of academic English" (p. 6). Teachers may use strategies such as visual aids, focus on vocabulary acquisition, and physical activities in sheltered programming. Sheltered English immersion focuses on instructing academic content through using the English language at a level that matches the students' levels of proficiency in English and includes explicit English language instruction.

Structured English Immersion

Unlike *sheltered* English programs, *structured* programs have the main goal of preparing students to participate in English-only general education classrooms promptly; the primary goal is English language acquisition (Moughamian et al., 2009). Though EB students may find ELD-specific coursework and schedules within structured immersion programs helpful, they may also have less freedom to choose their course schedules due to the often-prescriptive nature of this programming (Lillie, 2016) and the deleterious effects that structured programming may pose to EB students' identities (López, 2010). As such, the longer EB students remain in structured English programming, the less they seem to enjoy it (Lillie, 2016).

Sheltered English immersion is often used interchangeably with *structured* English immersion, the prescriptive instructional model that focuses on content areas and similarly immerses EB students in English language content classrooms. Unfortunately, the confusion and lack of differentiation and definition around these terms make it difficult to implement and understand policy and research (Cassels Johnson et al., 2017). Still, due to the *sheltered* or *structured* nature of programming, EB students are grouped by proficiency, which ignores developmental appropriateness and often grade-level needs (Cruze et al., 2019). More concerningly, EB students are often excluded from monolingual educational experiences or prevented from engaging with peers who are not in ELD programming. Some have even argued that sheltered and structured programs violate *Lau v. Nichols* (1974) because such segregation without proper instructional accommodations does not provide equal educational opportunities to EB students (Cassels Johnson et al., 2017; Cruze et al., 2019; Jiménez-Castellanos et al., 2014).

Bilingual Models

Bilingual–bicultural education refers to a system that uses two languages for instruction, one of them English, to support the academic development of children who are learning English as a second (or additional) language. Baker and Wright (2021) differentiate between weak models of bilingual education, where bilingualism is not the aim (i.e., transitional bilingual models), and strong ones, those whose aim is bilingualism and biliteracy (i.e., dual-language models).

Transitional Bilingual Model

This model may be preferable to English-only models in that EB students are allowed to use their home language, at least temporarily, in the classroom while acquiring oral language and academic proficiency in English (Baker & Wright, 2021). Initially, EB students receive instruction in their first language, and as they increase their English proficiency, their overall academic instruction in English also increases. There are early-transitional bilingual models, where students exit by the end of second or third grade, and late-transitional, where students continue receiving instruction in their first language until fifth or sixth grade. In transitional bilingual programs, the goal is for students to become only English proficient and not bilingual (Polanco & Baker, 2018). Therefore, once students exit the program, most of their academic instruction is in English. While EB students improve their English proficiency under this model, it comes with the cost of lost proficiency in their native language and decreased exposure to their cultural background, thus resulting in subtractive bilingualism (Baker & Wright, 2021).

Dual-Language Models

Dual-language models aim for students to achieve bilingual skills, including academic proficiency in multiple languages (Sugarman, 2018). Therefore, students receive instruction in two languages. In a one-way model, all EB students from the same language group receive English language instruction for part of the day. In two-way programs, groups are ideally formed by 50% EB students and 50% non-EB students. The instructional time in each language varies by program, from 50/50 (i.e., 50% of the time, the instruction is in EB students' first language and 50% of the time it is in English) to models in which the majority of instruction is in the EB students' first language during early elementary years (e.g., 80/20 or 90/10 models) but shifts toward 50/50 as EB students move through grade levels (Moughamian et al., 2009; Polanco & Baker, 2018). Most dual-language programs are offered only in elementary grades, but some school districts offer them at the middle and high school levels. Dual-language models bolster EB students' academic success by allowing them to develop academic and social communication proficiency in two languages (Baker & Wright, 2021). The outcomes of dual-language models are bilingualism and biliteracy. Other names for dual-language programs are developmental bilingual, dual immersion, and dual language immersion.

Instructional Programming Models and Outcomes

According to the US Department of Education (U.S. DOE, 2023), in the 2019–2020 academic year, 71% of EB students graduated high school (compared to 86% of non-EB students) nationwide. Though 4-year graduation rates vary by state (ranging from 39% in NY to 95% in WV; U.S. DOE, 2023), bilingual models using EB students' native language are associated with higher academic achievement (Baker & Wright, 2021), including enrolling in college (Garza-Reyna, 2019), especially in states with high proportions of Latine populations (López et al., 2015). One of the best predictors of EB students dropping out of school has been the involvement in segregated ELD programming, with each year in this type of programming increasing the likelihood of attrition (Cortina, 2009). Segregating EB students by language also leads to segregation by race/ethnicity and socioeconomic status (Gandara & Orfield, 2012).

In the short term, EB students in English-only programming (ESL, SEI) perform better on English language assessments (Colón et al., 2022); however, in the long term, EB students in bilingual programs such as developmental bilingual and transitional bilingual have had significantly higher scores (Baker & Wright, 2021; Umansky & Reardon, 2014; Valentino & Reardon, 2015). Among elementary school EB students reclassified as fluent English proficient, those who received dual-language programming performed better in math, English language arts, and reading than those enrolled in SEI programming (Marquez, 2018). Bilingual models have the most robust evidence for EB students' English proficiency and academic outcomes (Collier & Thomas, 2017). Furthermore, bilingual models have shown effectiveness in developing both Spanish and English in the first 2 years of elementary school, with dual-language models being more effective than transitional ones (Murphy, 2014). Though bilingual education has substantive evidence for developing multilingual capacities (Collier & Thomas, 2017; Colón et al., 2022; Polanco & Baker, 2018), access to these programs has become "gentrified," where it is often offered to and benefitting more privileged students whose primary language is English (but want to become bilingual), at the expense of EB students who need specialized programming to gain English proficiency (Cervantes-Soon et al., 2017; Valdez et al., 2016). This is not surprising given how bilingual education models have been commodified in a way that has systemically ignored historical contexts of bilingual education as forms of activism and empowerment (e.g., BEA; García & Sung, 2018).

Implications on Assessment and Intervention

Delivering effective bilingual instruction to EB students has social justice implications since achieving English proficiency allows for their full participation in all areas of life (e.g., school, work, community) while maintaining their first language and cultural identity. Furthermore, English language proficiency is a factor used to determine the type of academic environment in which EB students will be placed. The English Language Proficiency for the 21st Century (ELPAC21) and ACCESS (WIDA) are assessments used to determine EB students' English proficiency (Umansky & Porter, 2020). Educators are encouraged to plan interventions that consider EB students' English proficiency level. For example, when an EB student is referred for assessment to determine eligibility for special education, determining their English language proficiency is a first step. In doing so, the misidentification of EB students as disabled may be reduced (Klingner & Eppolito, 2014). There is no one-size-fits-all in the assessment of EB students; therefore, educators should prepare themselves to not only understand the second language acquisition process but also know about the language and culture of their EB students. These competencies have been identified as critical in preparing bilingual school psychologists (Harris et al., 2021; Ortiz et al., 2023; Sánchez Lizardi et al., 2024; Vega et al., 2019).

Recommendations for Practice

A simple yet important recommendation is to move away from the current deficit-based ideology, pervasive in the literature and praxis about EB students. For example, terms such as ELL and ESL emphasize what students lack rather than acknowledging the many strengths and various home languages that EB students bring to the educational setting. Though the term EB student moves toward a justice-based stand (García et al., 2008; González-Howard & Suárez, 2021), it continues to be somewhat deficit-based given that "emergent" suggests "beginner" or "nascent," prompting to view EB students as always being at an early English level proficiency, impacting how they are perceived in the educational environment, or when to remove such an artificial label to allow full participation in monolingual settings. The authors propose using multilingual learners (MLs) to further emphasize students' language assets. Utilizing EB students' native languages and cultural backgrounds as assets has improved academic development (Scanlan & López, 2012). Additionally, educators' vernacular when referring to and discussing EB students may impact the opportunities they provide their students, whether they are aware of it or not (Umansky et al., 2020; Tanaka & Vega, 2024). Though challenging the notions of English hegemony will be an "uphill battle" to unpack monolingualism (Chang-Bacon, 2022), critical examination of where policies are coming from and why will help establish a more equitable translation among research, policy, and practice.

At the classroom level, teachers must be knowledgeable of second language acquisition to further promote EB students' learning. Because knowledge of content and curricula alone does not guarantee EB student engagement, fostering a sense of belonging and incorporating instructional activities that directly draw from EB students' own linguistic and cultural experiences is crucial in furthering EB students' self-efficacy and their academic development (Antrop-Gonzalez et al., 2005; López & Iribarren, 2014). For example, using a systemic perspective, Aganza et al. (2015) developed a survey to identify EB students' cultural assets that could be included during academic instruction and assessment to support their educational experience and to promote their sense of school belonging.

Data-Based Decision-Making

While a sizable body of research exists comparing the effectiveness of instructional programming for EB students (Baker & Wright, 2021), outcome measures usually center around academic performance (i.e., high-stakes assessment scores) and high school graduation rates. Similarly, EB students tend to be grouped into a monolith, further obscuring differential needs. Accuracy in data collection and critically examining how instructional outcomes are reported is key in further evaluating the outcomes for EB students receiving varying instructional programming across the country. Beyond the minimum federal requirements, educators could reflect on local EB populations and patterns to better cater to their students and families. For example, gathering data to illustrate the need for resources for a specific population could assist schools in advocating for school-family liaisons or consultants to implement certain models of instruction. Rather than a one-size-fits-all model, schools and districts could collect and analyze disaggregated data such as students' prior educational history or ethnicity within a country of origin. Additionally, practitioners could collect data to include long-term outcomes on social–emotional well-being, career paths, employment, or socioeconomic status that may shed light on the benefits of having a multilingual society, which begins by supporting strong bilingual models of instruction.

Advocacy

Though allocating funds through policy has been a step forward in educating EB students, they are inadequate for alleviating the current shortage of educators with backgrounds and specializations in multiple language acquisition. They are also insufficient for providing training and quality professional development required to sustain educational professionals presently serving EB students (e.g., Cassels Johnson et al., 2017). Advocating for more funds for Title III and research to examine outcomes of different programming will ensure that policies are evidence-based and that teachers receive appropriate support to fully foster EB students' growth.

As school leaders and districts are bound by state-level policies, educators must become active advocates for determining curricula and educational practices that ensure EB students have equitable access to quality education. For example, despite the ample evidence for the benefits of bilingual programming incorporating EB students' native language (Umansky & Reardon, 2014), such practices are not consistently implemented. At the school level, educators could examine their placement practices to avoid unintentional segregation of EB students based on their English language proficiency. By promoting integration and building EB students' social capital, school leaders can lessen the likelihood that EB students will become disengaged and ultimately drop out (Lillie, 2016). Schools could also create partnerships with local universities and colleges to further leverage resources and continuously monitor and evaluate EB student outcomes based on evidence-based practices (López & Iribarren, 2014). Even with partnerships and programming, one crucial practice would be to move toward more critically conscious practice in uplifting the most marginalized of voices (Cervantes-Soon et al., 2017).

Conclusion

This chapter has presented how education programming for EB students is filled with controversies associated with diverging theories about second language acquisition, state and federal policies regulating bilingual education, and systemic educational practices that have been discriminatory. As US schools continue to grow more diverse, multilingualism is no longer an option but a reality. Dual-language models, whose outcomes are bilingualism, should be supported from the perspective of EB students rather than at the sole or express benefit of monolingual English students. We have highlighted the evidence supporting the effectiveness of dual language models for EB students in the academic and social–emotional domains. In the day-to-day, educators need to be knowledgeable about the benefits of bilingual instructional programs and receive the necessary professional development. This chapter serves as a contextual backdrop for beginning to engage in more critically conscious reflections on the educational models for EB students. It will be the responsibility of educators, districts, and policymakers to heed research-based recommendations and nuanced historical realities that have privileged monolingualism and commodified bilingualism.

References

Aganza, J. S., Godinez, A., Smith, D., Gonzalez, L., & Robinson-Zañartu, C. (2015). Using cultural assets to enhance assessment of Latino students. *Contemporary School Psychology, 19*, 30–45. https://doi.org/10.1007/s40688-014-0041-7

Antrop-González, R., Vélez, W., & Garrett, T. (2005). Dónde están los estudiantes Puertorriqueños/os exitosos? [Where are the academically successful Puerto Rican students?]: Success factors of high-achieving Puerto Rican high school students. *Journal of Latinos and Education, 4*(2), 77–94. https://doi.org/10.1207/s1532771xjle0402_2

Baker, C., & Wright, W. E. (2021). *Foundations of bilingual education and bilingualism* (7th ed.). Channel View Publications. https://doi.org/10.21832/BAKER9899

Baecher, L., & Bell, A. B. (2017). Opportunity to teach: Push-in and pull-out models of English learner instruction. *Journal of Education and Culture Studies, 1*(1), 53. https://doi.org/10.22158/jecs.v1n1p53

Bell, A. B., & Baecher, L. (2012). Points on a continuum: ESL teachers reporting on collaboration. *TESOL Journal, 3*, 488–515. https://doi-org.ezproxy4.library.arizona.edu/10.1002/tesj.28

Bernstein, K. A., Anderson, K. T., Close, K., & Rodriguez Martinez, S. (2023). Teacher beliefs about multilingual learners: How language ideologies shape teachers' hypothetical policy-making. *International Multilingual Research Journal, 17*(3), 191–219. https://doi.org/10.1080/19313152.2023.2182094

Brown, L. (2023). The (il)legitimacy of Arizona's English-only language policy: An analysis of legitimacy in language policy discourse. https://doi.org/10.31235/osf.io/e94su

Caldwell-Harris, C. L., & MacWhinney, B. (2023). Age effects in second language acquisition: Expanding the emergentist account. *Brain & Language, 241*, Article e105269. https://doi.org/10.1016/j.bandl.2023.105269

Cassels Johnson, D., Stephens, C., Nelson, J. J., & Johnson, E. J. (2017). Violating Lau: Sheltered English instruction programs and equal educational opportunity. *Journal of Education Policy, 33*(4), 488–509. https://doi.org/10.1080/02680939.2017.1380847

Castañeda v. Pickard, 648 F.2d 989 (5th Cir. 1981). https://web.stanford.edu/~hakuta/www/LAU/IAPolicy/IA1bCastanedaFullText.htm

Cervantes-Soon, C. G., Dorner, L., Palmer, D., Heiman, D., Schwerdtfeger, R., & Choi, J. (2017). Combating inequalities in two-way language immersion programs: Toward critical consciousness in bilingual education spaces. *Review of Research in Education, 41*(1), 403–427. https://doi.org/10.3102/0091732X17690120

Chamot, A. U., & O'Malley, J. M. (1994). *The CALLA handbook: Implementing the cognitive academic language learning approach*. Addison-Wesley.

Chang-Bacon, C. K. (2022). Who's being 'sheltered?': How monolingual language ideologies are produced within education policy discourse and sheltered English immersion. *Critical Studies in Education, 63*(2), 212–228. https://doi.org/10.1080/17508487.2020.1720259

Coady, M. R., Ankeny, B., & Ankeny, R. (2022). Is language a 'right' in U.S. education?: Unpacking *Castañeda's* reach across federal, state, and district lines. *Language Policy, 21*, 305–329. https://doi.org/10.1007/s10993-021-09604-1

Collier, V. P., & Thomas, W. P. (2017). Validating the power of bilingual schooling: Thirty-two years of large-scale, longitudinal research. *Annual Review of Applied Linguistics, 37*, 203–217. https://doi.org/10.1017/s0267190517000034

Colón, V., Szabo, S., & Riley, J. (2022). The effects of transitional bilingual education vs. dual language immersion on English language learners' reading assessment scores. In I. Management Association (Ed.), *Research anthology on bilingual and multilingual education* (pp. 1396–1410). IGI Global. https://doi.org/10.4018/978-1-6684-3690-5.ch070

Cortina, R. (2009). Immigrant youth in High School: Understanding educational outcomes for students of Mexican origin. In T. G. Wiley, J. S. Lee, & R. W. Rumberger (Eds.), *The education of language minority immigrants in the United States* (pp. 113–135). Multilingual Matters.

Cruze, A., Cota, A., & López, F. (2019). A decade after institutionalization: Educators' perspective of structured English immersion. *Language Policy, 18*, 431–453. https://doi.org/10.1007/s10993-018-9495-1

Cummins, J. (2008). BICS and CALP: Empirical and theoretical status of the distinction. In N. H. Hornberger (Ed.), *Encyclopedia of language and education* (pp. 487–499). Springer. https://doi.org/10.1007/978-0-387-30424-3_36

Dort, R. (2019). *English language learners: Students reflect on their high school monolingual experiences*. [Doctoral dissertation, Northeastern University College of Professional Studies].

D'Souza, D., Brady, D., Haensel, J. X., & D'Souza, H. (2020). Is mere exposure enough? The effects of bilingual environments on infant cognitive development. *Royal Society Open Science, 7*, Article 180191. https://doi.org/10.1098/rsos.180191

Echevarría, J., Vogt, M., & Short, D. (2016). *Making content comprehensible for English learners: The SIOP model* (5th ed.). Pearson.

Every Student Succeeds Act. 20 U.S.C. 6301 (2015). https://www.congress.gov/bill/114th-congress/senate-bill/1177/text

Ferlazzo, L., & Hull-Sypnieski, K. (2018). *The ell teacher's toolbox: Hundreds of practical ideas to support your students*. Jossey-Bass.

Florez, I. R. (2012). Examining the validity of the Arizona English language learners assessment cut scores. *Language Policy, 11*, 33–45. https://doi.org/10.1007/s10993-011-9225-4

Gandara, P., & Orfield, G. (2012). Segregating Arizona's English learners: A return to the "Mexican Room"? *Teacher College Record, 114*, 1–27.

García, O. (2009). *Bilingual education in the 21st century: A global perspective*. Wiley-Blackwell.

García, O., Kleifgen, J. A., & Falchi, L. (2008). *From English language learners to emergent bilinguals*. Equity Matters: Research Review No. 1. The Campaign for Educational Equity. Teachers College, Columbia University.

García, O., & Sung, K. K. (2018). Critically assessing the 1968 bilingual education act at 50 years: Taming tongues and Latinx communities. *Bilingual Research Journal, 41*(4), 318–333. https://doi.org/10.1080/15235882.2018.1529642

Garza-Reyna, G. L. (2019). The academic preparedness of Latino students in dual language and transitional bilingual education programs. *Journal of Latinos and Education, 18*(4), 340–348. https://doi.org/10.1080/15348431.2017.1394858

González-Howard, M., & Suárez, E. (2021). Retiring the term English language learners: Moving toward linguistic justice through asset-oriented framing. *Journal of Research in Science Teaching*, 1–4. https://doi.org/10.1002/tea.21684

Harris, B., Vega, D., Peterson, L. S., & Newell, K. W. (2021). Critical issues in the training of bilingual school psychologists. *Contemporary School Psychology, 25*(3), 273–287. https://doi.org/10.1007/s40688-020-00340-7

Jiménez-Castellanos, O., Blanchard, J., Atwill, K., & Jiménez-Silva, M. (2014). Beginning English literacy development and achievement among Spanish-speaking children in Arizona's English-only classrooms: A four-year two-cohort longitudinal study. *International Multilingual Research Journal, 8*(2), 104–123. https://doi.org/10.1080/19313152.2013.875812

Kaveh, Y. M., Bernstein, K. A., Cervantes-Soon, C., Rodriguez-Martinez, S., & Mohamed, M. (2022). Moving away from the 4-hour block: Arizona's distinctive path to reversing its restrictive language policies. *International Multilingual Research Journal, 16*(2), 113–135. https://doi.org/10.1080/19313152.2021.1973261

Keyes v. School District No. 1, Denver, 413 U.S. 189 (1973). https://supreme.justia.com/cases/federal/us/413/189/

King, K., & Bigelow, M. (2018). The language policy of placement tests for newcomer English learners. *Educational Policy, 32*(7), 936–968. https://doi.org/10.1177/0895904816681527

Klingner, J., & Eppolito, A. M. (2014). *English language learners: Differentiating between language acquisition and learning disabilities*. Council for Exceptional Children.

Krashen, S. (1982). *Principles and practice in second language acquisition*. Pergamon.

Krashen, S. D., & Terrell, T. D. (1988). *The natural approach: Language acquisition in the classroom*. Prentice Hall International.

Kuhl, P. (2004). Early language acquisition: Cracking the speech code. *Nature Reviews Neuroscience, 5*, 831–843. https://doi.org/10.1038/nrn1533

Lau v. Nichols, 414 U.S. 563 (1974). https://www2.ed.gov/about/offices/list/ocr/ell/lau.html

Lillie, K. E. (2016). The lost generation: Students of Arizona's structured English immersion. *International Journal of Bilingual Education and Bilingualism, 19*(4), 408–425. https://doi.org/10.1080/13670050.2015.1006162

López, F. A. (2010). Identity and motivation among Hispanic ells. *Education Policy Analysis Archives, 18*, 16–49. https://doi.org/10.14507/epaa.v18n16.2010

López, F., McEneaney, E., & Nieswandt, M. (2015). Language instruction educational programs and academic achievement of Latino English learners: Considerations for states with changing demographics. *American Journal of Education, 121*, 417–450. https://doi.org/10.1086/680410

López, F., & Iribarren, J. (2014). Creating and sustaining inclusive instructional settings for English language learners: Why, what, and how. *Theory Into Practice, 53*(2), 106–114. https://doi.org/10.1080/00405841.2014.885810

Marquez, C. C. (2018). *Differences in reclassified fluent English proficient students' academic achievement between dual language and structured English immersion program.* [Doctoral dissertation, Northcentral University School of Education].

Martinez, D., & Martínez, R. (2017). Researching the language of race and racism in education. In K. King et al. (Eds.), *Research methods in language and education. Encyclopedia of language and education* (3rd ed., pp. 503–516). Springer.

Maxwell, L. A. (2014). ESL and classroom teachers team up to teach common core. *The Education Digest, 79*(5), 4–9.

Mofield, E. L. (2020). Benefits and barriers to collaboration and co-teaching: Examining perspectives of gifted education teachers and general education teachers. *Gifted Child Today, 43*(1), 20–33. https://doi.org/10.1177/1076217519880588

Moughamian, A. C., Rivera, M. O., & Francis, D. J. (2009). *Instructional models and strategies for teaching English language learners*. RMC Research Corporation, Center on Instruction. https://eric.ed.gov/?id=ED517794

Murphy, A. F. (2014). The effect of dual-language and transitional-bilingual education instructional models on Spanish proficiency for English language learners. *Bilingual Research Journal, 37*(2), 182–194. https://doi.org/10.1080/15235882.2014.934971

National Center for Education Statistics. (2024). *English learners in public schools. Condition of education*. U.S. Department of Education, Institute of Education Sciences. Retrieved July 12, 2024, from https://nces.ed.gov/programs/coe/indicator/cgf

No Child Left Behind Act – English language acquisition, language enhancement, and academic achievement act. 20 U.S.C. § 6801 et seq. (2002). https://www.congress.gov/bill/107th-congress/house-bill/1

Olds, J., McCraney, M., Panesar-Aguilar, S., & Cale, C. (2021). Adopting instructional strategies for English language learners in elementary classrooms. *World Journal of Education, 11*(3), 18. https://doi.org/10.5430/wje.v11n3p18

Ortiz, A., Sánchez Lizardi, P., Calvillo, O., D'Costa, S., Anguiano, R., Robinson-Zañartu, C., Ni, H., Jimerson, S. R., & Laija-Rodriguez, W. (2023). A collaborative journey to inform the development of Bilingual school psychology competencies in California. *Communiqué, 51*(5), 21–24.

Polanco, P., & Baker, D. L. (2018). Transitional bilingual education and two-way immersion programs: Comparison of reading outcomes for English learners in the United States. *Athens Journal of Education, 5*(4), 423–444. https://doi.org/10.30958/aje.5-4-5

Rader-Brown, L., & Howley, A. (2014). Predictors of the instructional strategies that elementary school teachers use with English language learners. *Teachers College Record: The Voice of Scholarship in Education, 116*(4), 1–34. https://doi.org/10.1177/016146811411600406

Rumberger, R. W., & Tran, L. (2010). State language policies, school language practices, and the English Learner achievement gap. In P. Gándara & M. Hopkins (Eds.), *Forbidden language: English learners and restrictive language policies* (pp. 195–215). Teachers College Press.

Rutherford-Quach, S., Torre Gibney, D., Kelly, H., Ballen Riccards, J., Garcia, E., Hsiao, M., Pellerin, E., & Parker, C. (2021). *Bilingual education across the United States*. CCNetwork.

Sánchez Lizardi, P., Anguiano, R., D'Costa, S., Ortiz, A., Robinson-Zañartu, C., Laija-Rodriguez, W., et al. (2024). Toward certification of bilingual school psychologists: Process, competencies, and visions. *School Psychology Review*, 1–17. https://doi.org/10.1080/2372966X.2024.2388020

Scanlan, M., & López, F. (2012). ¡Vamos! How school leaders promote equity and excellence for culturally and linguistically diverse students. *Educational Administration Quarterly, 48*, 583–625. https://doi.org/10.1177/0013161X11436270

Sugarman, J. (2018, June). *A matter of design: English learner program models in K-12 education*. Policy Briefs. Migration Policy Institute. https://www.migrationpolicy.org/research/english-learner-program-models-k-12-education

Tanaka, M. L. (2023). *Rotten soil: Positioning middle school teachers of minoritized adolescent newcomers*. [Doctoral dissertation, University of Arizona]. University of Arizona Repository. https://repository.arizona.edu/bitstream/handle/10150/669742/azu_etd_19745_sip1_m.pdf?sequence=1

Tanaka, M. L., & Vega, D. (2024). Beyond asset-based frameworks: Middle school teachers perpetuating raciolinguistic paradigms. *School Psychology Review*, 1–12. https://doi.org/10.1080/2372966X.2024.2361625

Title III – Language instruction for English learners and immigrant students. 20 U.S.C. § 6801 *et seq.* (2015). https://oese.ed.gov/offices/office-of-formula-grants/school-support-and-accountability/essa-legislation-table-contents/title-iii-part-a/#TITLE-III-PART-A

Umansky, I. M., Callahan, R. M., & Lee, J. C. (2020). Making the invisible visible: Identifying and interrogating ethnic differences in English learner reclassification. *American Journal of Education, 126*(3), 335–388. https://doi.org/10.1086/708250

Umansky, I. M., & Porter, L. (2020). State English learner education policy: A conceptual framework to guide comprehensive policy action. *Education Policy Analysis Archives, 28*(17). https://doi.org/10.14507/epaa.28.4594

Umansky, I. M., & Reardon, S. F. (2014). Reclassification patterns among Latino English learner students in bilingual, dual immersion, and English immersion classrooms. *American Educational Research Journal, 51*, 879–912. https://doi.org/10.3102/0002831214545110

United States Department of Education. (2023, June). *High school graduation rates for English learners*. Office of English Language Acquisition. https://files.eric.ed.gov/fulltext/ED628866.pdf

Valdés, G., Poza, L., & Brooks, M. D. (2015). Language acquisition in bilingual education. In W. E. Wright, S. Boun, & O. García (Eds.), *The handbook of bilingual and multilingual education* (pp. 56–74). Wiley.

Valdez, V. E., Freire, J. A., & Delavan, M. G. (2016). The gentrification of dual language education. *Urban Review, 48*, 601–627. https://doi.org/10.1007/s11256-016-0370-0

Valentino, R. A., & Reardon, S. F. (2015). Effectiveness of four instructional programs designed to serve English learners: Variation by ethnicity and initial English proficiency. *Educational Evaluation and Policy Analysis, 37*(4), 612–637. https://doi.org/10.3102/0162373715573310

VanPatten, B., Keating, G. D., & Wulff, S. (Eds.). (2020). *Theories in second language acquisition: An introduction* (3rd ed.). Routledge.

Vega, D., Wolf, J. N., Barton, D. O., Stathatos, M., Iurino, C., & Hammer, L. (2019). Identifying the training experiences and needs of bilingual school psychologists. *Psychology in the Schools, 56*(10), 1687–1699. https://doi.org/10.1002/pits.22288

Whiting, J. (2017). Caught between the push and the pull: ELL teachers' perceptions of mainstreaming and ESOL classroom teaching. *NABE Journal of Research and Practice, 8*(1), 9–27. https://doi.org/10.1080/26390043.2017.12067793

Wiley, T. G., & Wright, W. E. (2004). Against the undertow: Language-minority education policy and politics in the "age of accountability". *Educational Policy, 18*(1), 142–168. https://doi.org/10.1177/0895904803260030

Williams, C. P. (2021, December 8). *A new federal equity agenda for dual language learners and English learners*. The Century Foundation. https://tcf.org/content/report/new-federal-equity-agenda-dual-language-learners-english-learners/

Zacarian, D. (2012). *Serving English learners: Laws, policies, and regulations*. Colorín Colorado. https://www.colorincolorado.org/sites/default/files/Policy_Guide_Final.pdf

Zacarian, D., & Haynes, J. (2012). *The essential guide for educating beginning English learners*. Corwin.

Chapter 3
Acculturation Considerations in the Pre-referral and Assessment Process

Fedra A. Calderón

Why Is Understanding Acculturation Critical?

In school psychology, social justice refers to efforts to dismantle barriers that lead to educational and psychological inequalities among various social identities, such as race, ethnicity, gender, and socioeconomic status (NASP, 2020). Nevertheless, there is a pressing need for increased discussions about social justice, particularly concerning acculturation, due to the persistent educational inequities experienced by culturally and linguistically minoritized (CLM) students (Sabnis & Proctor, 2021; Watts, 2021). According to the National Center for Education Statistics (NCES, 2024), public school diversity has steadily increased, with more than 5 million students, or 10%, identified as emergent bilinguals, reflecting the growing number of multicultural families. This demographic shift highlights CLM children's specific challenges, especially during the acculturation process, where they navigate to find a balance between adapting to mainstream cultural norms and retaining their cultural identity. Schools, which often serve as children's initial exposure to the dominant culture, play a pivotal role in this journey. Thus, practitioners must deepen their understanding of CLM students' experiences to promote their academic and social–emotional integration. This chapter emphasizes the importance of culturally responsive practices, particularly in the roles of school psychologists in supporting CLM students. It explores the concept of acculturation, especially during the pre-referral and evaluation phases, to promote an inclusive and equitable educational environment that benefits all students, regardless of their linguistic and cultural backgrounds.

F. A. Calderón (✉)
Department of Disability and Psychoeducational Studies, University of Arizona, Tucson, AZ, USA
e-mail: facalderon@arizona.edu

D. Vega, J. N. Wolf (eds.), *Culturally and Linguistically Responsive Intervention and Assessment Practices with Emergent Bilingual Students*,
https://doi.org/10.1007/978-3-032-02084-0_3

Acculturation as a Process

Culture

Understanding acculturation involves examining the dynamic and complex nature of culture. Culture shapes identities, influences interactions, and plays a key role in the ongoing process of meaning-making. Rather than being static, culture exists as a contested arena where power dynamics shape interpretations and perceptions, which can lead to divisions, conflicts, cultural trauma, disruptions, and social disintegration (Anderson-Levitt, 2012; Greenberg et al., 2020). Immigrants face intensified challenges when adapting to a dominant culture due to the complexities within cultural systems, including various subgroups with unique relationships to the dominant culture (Hod & Sagy, 2022). This highlights the significance of acculturation in understanding how individuals and groups adapt, particularly as diverse students navigate educational settings. They strive to maintain their cultural identities while integrating into prevailing cultural norms. Thus, understanding culture and acculturation is crucial in educational contexts, as it helps practitioners create inclusive environments and address the specific needs of CLM students.

Defining Acculturation

Acculturation, viewed through a simple lens, refers to the cultural and psychological transformations that occur when individuals or groups from diverse cultural backgrounds interact with one another (Berry & Sam, 2016; van der Zee & Oudenhoven, 2022). This process is multi-dimensional, impacting individuals' emotional, cognitive, and behavioral functioning. It may involve accepting aspects of a new culture while also allowing the rejection of such influences (Berry & Sam, 2016; Bornstein et al., 2019). Although the term is often linked to immigrants and refugees, the experiences of acculturation pertain to various groups, including ethnic majorities, minorities, and Indigenous populations (Ward & Geeraert, 2016).

It is crucial to distinguish acculturation from assimilation, which is often misconstrued as a synonym. Assimilation implies a one-dimensional process of conforming to the dominant culture, overlooking the complexities of adaptation and integration (Calderon-Berumen, 2019). This notion suggests a disconnection from one's home culture, which is linked to negative well-being outcomes. In contrast, acculturation acknowledges the mutual influences among cultural groups and the diverse responses individuals and communities demonstrate while navigating their cultural experiences. Grasping these distinctions is crucial for a deeper understanding of cultural dynamics and enhancing acculturation discourse.

Acculturation Frameworks: Challenges and Nuances

While several acculturation models have been proposed, Berry's 1980 two-dimensional model has been influential in subsequent research (e.g., Arends-Tóth & van de Vijver, 2006; Bornstein, 2017; Ward & Geeraert, 2016). This model emphasizes the desire to maintain one's ethnic culture while engaging with the dominant culture. However, it has faced criticism for potentially oversimplifying the complexities of modern demographics and technology, challenging traditional acculturation models, and highlighting the need for mutual adjustment between immigrants and non-immigrants (van der Zee & Oudenhoven, 2022).

Acculturation occurs at both individual and group levels. Group-level changes can impact social structures, politics, economics, and culture, while individual-level changes influence behavior, identity, values, and attitudes (Berry, 1990). These changes result in a range of adaptation experiences as people and communities adjust to new cultural environments. Ward's (2001) ABCs, and now ABCD, model of acculturation highlights the affective, behavioral, cognitive, and developmental aspects of this journey (Ward & Szabo, 2019). Additionally, Van der Zee and Oudenhoven (2022) propose a dynamic view of acculturation that applies to both immigrants and non-immigrants, addressing today's diverse and global society. Their model outlines five key skills for effective intercultural interactions: (1) cultural empathy, (2) open-mindedness, (3) emotional stability, (4) flexibility, and (5) social initiative. These competencies promote positive intergroup relations and improve cross-cultural understanding. Regardless of the reasons for migration, families from various backgrounds inevitably undergo changes that offer opportunities for growth and skill development while also posing risks of marginalization and exclusion (Juang & Syed, 2019).

Understanding the development of acculturation helps us recognize it as an integral part of the lifespan, highlighting the impact of multiple systemic levels on a child's growth. It is advisable to consider individual experiences and contexts when examining acculturation, rather than relying on broad, one-size-fits-all models. During childhood, when acculturation occurs, children may adopt new cultural practices while letting go of those from their culture of origin (Schwartz et al., 2010). However, these models challenge this idea by suggesting that children navigate their experiences through interactions with both cultural domains, necessitating flexibility in adapting to various expectations and social norms, which can differ significantly among individuals and depend greatly on age and context (Bornstein, 2017; Oppedal & Toppelberg, 2016). As a result, school psychologists should evaluate the sociocultural environments, including family dynamics, peer interactions, and educational settings, to understand how these factors can enhance or hinder children's development of cultural competence and integration.

Cultural Diversity Within the School Context

As families navigate the demands of the dominant culture when children enter school, educational institutions become crucial in shaping the acculturation experience. From an ecological perspective, the context of both family and school is vital to understanding how acculturation unfolds, illustrating the interconnectedness of various environments that impact a child's social and educational journey (Makarova, 2019; Ward & Geeraert, 2016). The subsequent sections will explore the effects of acculturation, enculturation, and psychological adjustment, as well as the challenges faced by schools and practitioners when diverse students enroll in the US public school system.

Acculturation and Enculturation in Schools

As CLM students enter the education system in the United States, they experience *acculturation*, as well as *enculturation*. Enculturation is the process through which individuals learn and internalize the values, norms, and practices of their own culture, which can be especially significant for students from CLM backgrounds (Goforth & Pham, 2023; Hod & Sagy, 2022; Vedder & Motti-Stefanidi, 2016). On the other hand, acculturation involves adapting and learning a new culture's behaviors, customs, norms, language, and values (Goforth & Pham, 2023; Romero & Piña-Watson, 2017; Vedder & Motti-Stefanidi, 2016). In the school context, these processes can facilitate cultural integration and also lead to complex dynamics where students may feel pressured to conform to the dominant culture while simultaneously striving to maintain their cultural identity, leading to challenges in academic performance and psychological adjustment in CLM students (Makarova, 2019; Schultz, 2016; Vedder & Motti-Stefanidi, 2016).

Schools prioritize supporting the enculturation process that aligns with the cultural norms and values of most of their students and staff and expect CLM students to adapt to the dominant culture through acculturation (Vedder & Motti-Stefanidi, 2016). This might be due to schools finding it more accessible to support CLM students' integration into the dominant culture than to understand the social norms and behaviors that diverse students bring to school from home. As a result, this response to diversity fails to acknowledge the cultural aspects that CLM children bring to schools, which may lead school staff to create expectations in behavior and social norms that CLM students may not even be aware of yet (Goforth & Pham, 2023), potentially causing unjust disciplinary referrals. Additionally, some have argued that historically, schools and educational policies were designed to enculturate students into the dominant standards and marginalize non-Westernized perspectives targeting specific groups, such as Japanese, Indigenous, and Mexican individuals (Schultz, 2016).

Practitioners' limited awareness of the acculturation and enculturation process experienced by CLM families can perpetuate the deficit discourse and exacerbate disparities and inconsistencies that can impact practice and advocacy (Goforth & Pham, 2023). These biases may obstruct the development of inclusive and informed worldviews, ultimately shaping how practitioners perceive and interact with CLM students whose behaviors and intersectional identities differ. Therefore, educators must enhance their understanding of how cultural backgrounds influence students' learning experiences and self-perceptions while advocating for culturally responsive practices that promote CLM's academic and psychosocial development.

Academic and Psychological Outcomes

Acculturation and enculturation are two-way processes, requiring not only that CLM students adapt but also that the school culture collaborates on accepting and accommodating these students' identities (Goforth et al., 2017; Goforth & Pham, 2023; Hod & Sagy, 2022). CLM students may encounter numerous challenges, including adapting to new teachers, classroom expectations, learning a curriculum in a different language or alphabet, adjusting to unfamiliar teaching methods, understanding a new grading system, and using technological devices to access educational content. Unfortunately, schools are often inadequately equipped to support the acculturation needs of minoritized students, which can lead to a more significant adjustment challenge for them than for their non-diverse students (Vedder & Motti-Stefanidi, 2016). These combined pressures of acculturation and enculturation can be confusing and may impact CLM students' academic success and overall well-being (Goforth et al., 2017; Vedder & Motti-Stefanidi, 2016).

With such demands, CLM students can develop acculturation stress, which manifests as uncertainty, anxiety, and depression, leading to poor mental and physical health (Sam & Berry, 2010; Romero & Branscome, 2014). Acculturative stress refers to the challenges experienced during the process of adapting to a new culture, including identity questioning and discrimination (Goforth et al., 2015). Acculturation stress can manifest in a variety of ways. For example, a CLM student might be able to perform and follow along with school expectations and daily life activities while still experiencing symptoms similar to psychological disorders (e.g., major depressive disorder; Romero & Branscome, 2014). Consequently, CLM students who display higher levels of anxiety or stress, a confused locus of control, or lack of responsiveness are often referred to evaluations or interventions. Practitioners and school staff need to understand how the acculturation process may impact the social–emotional functioning of CLM students (Collier et al., 2007).

Romero and Piña-Watson (2017) identified the primary sources of acculturative stress, including intergroup discrimination, intragroup marginalization, and family cultural conflict. Intergroup discrimination refers to unjust treatment, biases, and prejudices related to ethnicity or language skills, often resulting in academic challenges and reduced educational opportunities. For instance, some states often discourage bilingual education and perpetuate segregation, impacting CLM's educational success (Wood, 2008). Intragroup marginalization occurs when members of an ethnic group face pressure to fit an idealized representation of their culture, influencing family dynamics, friendships, and other life aspects. Family cultural conflict arises from differences in acculturation levels among family members (i.e., acculturation gap) when parents and children experience differing levels of cultural adaptation (Goforth et al., 2015). Higher levels of acculturative stress have been associated with increased behavioral problems and decreased academic grades (Schwartz et al., 2007), while the acculturation gap significantly predicts behavioral issues in adolescence (Goforth et al., 2015).

The immigrant paradox arises when newer immigrants to the U.S. often demonstrate better developmental outcomes, such as academic achievement and behavioral health, than their US-born peers or those who have been in the country longer, despite facing socioeconomic disadvantages (Marks et al., 2014). However, as newer immigrants acculturate, their academic performance and mental health can decline, potentially due to the loss of cultural values emphasizing education, challenges with discrimination, feelings of isolation, language barriers, and lack of culturally relevant curriculum impacting their academic success and behavioral health, and limited access to mental health services (d'Abreu et al., 2019; Marks et al., 2014; Pham et al., 2017). The phenomenon reflects a complex interplay where some students thrive despite experiencing acculturative stressors that typically hinder their academic success, arising from risk factors such as erosion of family closeness and negative peer influence, alongside protective factors present in newcomer families, including strong cultural values and fewer risky behaviors (Marks et al., 2014); thus, understanding these dynamics is crucial to promote positive development for all CLM youth by acknowledging both the strengths and vulnerabilities of immigrant youth, promoting practices that foster academic success and psychological outcomes while preserving cultural identity.

School Response to Alleviate the Acculturation and Enculturation Processes

The educational system, curriculum, and pedagogy are interrelated and collectively influence the adaptation experiences of CLM students in multicultural societies (Makarova & Birman, 2016). Enculturation can be implemented in schools by adopting curriculum content that teaches students about their and others' cultural heritage and language instruction that continues to foster their native language. Socially, students may gravitate toward peers and staff from similar cultural backgrounds, which reinforces their cultural norms and values. When diverse children learn and maintain both cultures, they demonstrate better development and psychological well-being (Vedder & Motti-Stefanidi, 2016; Pham et al., 2017). Therefore, support programs that promote both cultural heritage and integration into the mainstream culture can help CLM students navigate their multicultural identities (Goforth et al., 2015).

Awareness of individual backgrounds, family dynamics, and community contexts can facilitate the development of tailored interventions for optimal outcomes. Intervention programs should encourage parental involvement and target family structure to address acculturative gaps (d'Abreu et al., 2019; Goforth et al., 2015). Addressing acculturative stress through culturally responsive Social-Emotional Learning (SEL) can improve socio–emotional outcomes and academic success for CLM students (Lau & Shea, 2022). This involves adapting SEL curricula to include culturally relevant examples, integrating students' native languages, and incorporating activities celebrating diverse cultural traditions (Lau & Shea, 2022). Examples can include storytelling circles where students share cultural narratives, cultural celebrations that showcase diverse traditions, and role-playing scenarios that address culturally specific social situations. When students feel a strong sense of belonging in their school, it truly enhances their well-being, motivation, persistence, and openness to feedback (Lokhande & Reichle, 2019). Thus, fostering a culturally responsive educational environment not only enhances the academic and social well-being of CLM students but also plays a vital role in nurturing them to feel valued and connected.

Assessing Acculturation in the Pre-referral and Assessment Process

Assessing acculturation in schools can be intricate and complex (Goforth & Pham, 2023). Yet, it is vital to implement culturally responsive evaluations for CLM students (Vega & Wolf, 2023). Understanding the level of acculturation adds cultural context to a child's development and behavior, illustrating how their culture affects the assessment process (Fuji, 2018). Various methods can be used to collect acculturation data, such as observations, self-reports, record reviews, and interviews (Fuji, 2018; Goforth & Pham, 2023; Romero & Branscome, 2014; Vega & Wolf, 2023). Practitioners need to utilize multiple methods to gather this data, enabling better-informed educational decisions.

Acculturation Measures

Researchers assess acculturation by examining changes in various aspects of an individual's life, such as behaviors (e.g., dress preferences, food choices, language), cultural knowledge (e.g., the history of the new culture), and ethnic identity (e.g., the link between their original culture and the new one; Lechuga, 2008). Consequently, tools designed to evaluate acculturation often contain subscales focusing on these specific areas (Lechuga, 2008). For instance, one subscale may concentrate on language usage, while another might evaluate ethnic identity, providing a more complete understanding of an individual's level of acculturation across diverse life aspects. Although researchers have established operational definitions of acculturation, debates persist regarding the most effective methods for accurately capturing this complex process using psychometric tools. This includes determining which aspects of an individual's life are most influenced by ongoing interaction with another culture and identifying elements of their cultural identity that remain constant (Lechuga, 2008). There is also ambiguity surrounding what should specifically be measured to quantify acculturation effectively. Some argue that focusing on surface changes, such as language, is adequate, while others contend that deeper cultural and psychological factors must also be considered (e.g., Lechuga, 2008). This uncertainty complicates the creation of valid and reliable psychometric instruments to measure acculturation. Therefore, practitioners must consider developmental factors, age differences, psychometric standards, item quantity, and the specific areas of acculturation measured when selecting self-report tools to prevent data misinterpretation (Celenk & Van de Vijver, 2014).

There are a few tools designed to evaluate acculturation within the school system. One available instrument is the Acculturation Quick Screen—Third Edition (AQS III; Collier, 2016). This screener assesses the acculturation levels of K-12 students from CLM backgrounds in public schools in the United States and Canada. It operates on a 48-point scale, categorizing five levels of acculturation: Significantly Less Acculturated, Less Acculturated, In Transition, More Acculturated, and Significantly More Acculturated. Most questions center on language proficiency; thus, practitioners must consider the student's duration in the United States or Canadian school system, any English as a Second Language instruction received, proficiency in both languages, bilingual balance (e.g., equal proficiency and fluency in both languages), cultural identity, and the proportion of ethnic or linguistic peers in the school. The AQS III should be administered at least 4 weeks after enrollment and then annually to monitor the student's progress in acculturation (Collier, 2016).

Typically, students who receive instructional help with adaptation and language transition see a 10% or greater improvement in acculturation progress each year, according to the AQS III (Collier, 2016). Although the AQS III is not an independent predictive tool (Collier, 2016), it can contribute to valuable instructional decisions during the pre-referral and evaluation processes by distinguishing acculturative differences from disability-related issues when CLM students face learning and behavioral challenges (Collier et al., 2007). For example, it can assist in planning interventions for behavioral and learning issues before referring CLM students for evaluations (Collier et al., 2007; Romero & Branscome, 2014). Additionally, it helps school psychologists and evaluation specialists modify testing procedures. For instance, CLM students at lower acculturation levels should not undergo standardized assessments unless those assessments are appropriately adapted for interpretation or administration (Collier et al., 2007).

Another method for assessing acculturation in schools is the Language Acculturation Meter (LAM; Trujillo et al., 2020). This focused self-report tool evaluates language acculturation by considering the educational background and linguistic preferences of CLM students. Targeted at individuals transitioning from Spanish to English, the LAM is available in both languages and can be modified for non-Spanish speakers. It is adaptable for various educational levels, from kindergarten to graduate school, and is typically administered in an interview format, although family involvement is welcomed when needed. The LAM comprises four sections: Background Information (e.g., country of origin), Education History—Part 1 (e.g., years of instruction in English and/or Spanish), Everyday Language Usage—Part 2 (e.g., frequency of English and/or Spanish use), and English Comprehension—Part 3 (e.g., level of understanding of English). Parts 2 and 3 enable respondents to share insights into their language acculturation by rating statements on a nine-point scale, evaluating three areas: Home Environment, Social Interaction, and Academic/Cognitive. By collecting data on the CLM students' background, educational experience, language usage, and self-assessed English comprehension, the LAM establishes a framework that aids evaluators to adopt an ecological perspective, minimizing bias in selecting assessments, interpreting outcomes, and making programming suggestions (Trujillo et al., 2020).

Additionally, other acculturation measures have been developed for younger children and/or adolescents, such as the Children's Acculturation Scale (Franco, 1983); the Children's Hispanic Background Scale (Martinez et al., 1984); the Acculturation Scale for Vietnamese Adolescents (Nguyen & von Eye, 2002); the Acculturation, Habits, and Interests Multicultural Scale for Adolescents (Unger et al., 2002); the Acculturative Stress Inventory for Children (Suarez-Morales et al., 2007); and the Short Acculturation Scale for Hispanic Youth (Barona & Miller, 1994). These measures may provide valuable insights into the acculturation processes experienced by younger populations, allowing a better understanding of their unique challenges.

Qualitative Acculturation Measures

When assessing CLM students, it is essential to gather qualitative data. Given the limitations of norm-referenced scales, which may not accurately reflect students' acculturation, qualitative methods are equally necessary and beneficial for understanding students' acculturation development or status. Methods that can provide insight include practitioners conducting interviews, observations, and/or record reviews. These data can reveal crucial contextual details often overlooked in standardized assessments.

Interviews

Interviews are a powerful tool for assessing acculturation by enabling practitioners to gain a holistic understanding of CLM students and their families (Vega & Wolf, 2023). By conducting interviews in the pre-referral and assessment process, practitioners can build rapport with families and students, gain insights into family dynamics, and deepen their understanding of the student's educational, developmental, and medical history (Hass & Abdou, 2019). Engaging directly with students, families, and teachers allows school psychologists to better comprehend the experiences, strengths, and challenges of CLM students. This process facilitates the collection of vital information, such as developmental history, language usage, family structure, and immigration status, as well as the caregivers' perspectives on their child's educational challenges (Vega & Wolf, 2023). Additionally, interviewing teachers offers valuable insights into students' classroom engagement, instructional methods, and previous interventions.

Establishing trust is particularly critical in the interview process, as it creates a safe environment for families to share sensitive and deeply personal information. When families feel respected and understood, they are more likely to disclose experiences related to trauma, current challenges, family history, and other critical factors that might influence a child's educational performance and overall well-being (Hass & Abdou, 2019). This sensitive information can provide invaluable context for understanding a student's acculturation journey and the broader circumstances impacting their life.

Immigrant families often face unique challenges that shape their educational participation, including systemic, linguistic, and cultural barriers (Hass & Abdou, 2019). Research highlights that these families tend to exhibit lower involvement in education than their English-speaking counterparts, partly due to these obstacles (e.g., Cooper et al., 2010). Practitioners must recognize these challenges and adopt a culturally informed perspective when conducting interviews. Cultural humility is critical as it allows practitioners to understand a family's background and norms before engaging in meaningful dialogue (Hass & Abdou, 2019). This approach ensures that questions are relevant and sensitive, fostering a welcoming and non-threatening environment for families. Employing interpreters skilled in both the language and cultural context can enhance communication by ensuring accuracy and creating space for families to share their stories at their own pace (Francis et al., 2017; Hass & Abdou, 2019).

Through interviews, practitioners can uncover the complexities of individual backgrounds, particularly in bilingual contexts where cultural and linguistic factors intersect (Vega & Wolf, 2023). Open-ended questions encourage detailed responses, providing practitioners with a deeper understanding of the student's acculturation process while supporting family engagement and trust development (Francis et al., 2017; Vega & Wolf, 2023). Collaborating with school and community members familiar with the family's cultural norms further reduces misunderstandings and strengthens relationships between families and professionals (Hass & Abdou, 2019). Ultimately, tailoring communication strategies to each family's unique journey fosters collaboration between educators and families from diverse backgrounds, enhancing the assessment process and promoting positive outcomes for CLM students.

Observations

Classroom observations serve as a valuable tool for assessing a student's acculturation (Asendorpf & Motti-Stefanidi, 2017). Educators can gain valuable insights by systematically monitoring their interactions with peers, engagement in class activities, and responses to the cultural norms of the educational environment. Noting the students' verbal and non-verbal communication can reveal their comfort levels and their ability to navigate between their heritage and mainstream cultures. Furthermore, observing how students integrate into classroom routines, collaborate on tasks, and exhibit behaviors that indicate their understanding or challenges in cultural integration can shed light on their acculturation journey. Gathering feedback from peers and teachers during structured activities can enhance students' knowledge of their social integration and sense of belonging, while also highlighting any barriers they may face. Overall, employing a comprehensive approach with varied observational methods will yield a deeper understanding of the student's acculturation process journey.

Records Review

A review of records can effectively evaluate a student's acculturation by analyzing academic, behavioral, and medical information to gain insights into their integration and well-being. School records, such as attendance, grades, behavioral reports, and participation in after-school programs, can provide insights into the student's engagement and integration within the school community (Vega & Wolf, 2023). Teachers' reports can reveal patterns related to the student's adaptability, interactions with peers, and responsiveness to the curriculum. Furthermore, any assessments related to language proficiency can help gauge a student's level of comfort in navigating the linguistic requirements of the dominant culture (Vega & Wolf, 2023). Moreover, medical records, if available, give important context regarding any health issues, trauma, or mental health challenges that may affect the student's adjustment. Exploring family health practices and access to resources can further illuminate cultural influences on adaptation. By combining academic, behavioral, and medical information, educators can pinpoint challenges and individualize support to facilitate students' successful integration and growth.

Forewarnings to Consider

When practitioners assess acculturation, they must be familiar with the cultural norms, linguistic traits, and educational exceptionalities that their students may exhibit (Fuji, 2018; Romero & Branscome, 2014). For instance, understanding the typical behaviors or ways of expressing emotions across different cultures can make it challenging to accurately assess someone's mental health status, as unusual or unexpected behaviors may be seen as typical in another culture. It is also crucial to recognize that migration can sometimes be linked to stress and an increased risk of mental health issues; therefore, practitioners should be cautious about pathologizing acculturation (Bornstein et al., 2019).

Practitioners must consider how these characteristics interact with the child's cultural and linguistic adaptation and their acculturation processes to ensure appropriate identification, referral, and service decisions for CLM students (Romero & Branscome, 2014). While acculturation measures exist, their applicability may be limited for specific CLM individuals due to a lack of normative data relevant to certain ethnicities and the absence of translations for those who may not understand English (Fuji, 2018). The historical focus on identifying deficiencies in marginalized populations has dominated the research narrative; as a result, assessments often fail to represent these groups' cultures, leading to unreliable findings (Rudmin, 2009). Recognizing that psychometric instruments and standardized tests may harbor cultural biases, school psychologists are encouraged to use a holistic framework combining multiple data sources, including observational narratives and qualitative insights, to inform their understanding of student functioning and address systemic injustices within educational contexts.

Using the ECLECTIC Framework During Evaluations

School psychologists can evaluate acculturation by selecting suitable assessments, interpreting scores more accurately, and providing targeted recommendations. Psychometric tools often display cultural biases that favor or disadvantage students depending on their intersectional identities. This issue contributes to ongoing disproportionality in special education and keeps students of color separate from those belonging to the dominant culture (Sabnis & Proctor, 2021). Therefore, the ECLECTIC framework created by Fuji (2018) may enhance understanding and assessment practices by addressing the multifaceted aspects of culture that influence neuropsychological evaluations, especially for CLM students.

According to Fuji (2018), the ECLECTIC framework is a conceptual model designed to enhance neuropsychological evaluations for culturally diverse clients by considering various cultural dimensions that can impact test performance and interpretation. The acronym ECLECTIC stands for Education (i.e., examining the level and quality of education and literacy), Culture and acculturation (i.e., recognizing the influence of cultural background and the degree of integration into the dominant culture), Language (i.e., assessing proficiency in the language of the evaluation), Economics (i.e., understanding the socioeconomic status and its impact on access to resources), Communication style (i.e., acknowledging different ways cultures interact and express themselves), Testing situation (i.e., ensuring comfort and appropriate motivation during the assessment), Intelligence conceptualization (i.e., recognizing diverse understandings of intelligence across cultures), and Context of immigration (i.e., considering the specific circumstances of the client's immigration experience). By using this framework, practitioners can systematically explore how these factors intersect and affect the validity, accessibility, and fairness of neuropsychological assessments, leading to more culturally informed and ethically responsible evaluation practices.

While school psychologists may not be involved in conducting full neuropsychological assessments, the ECLECTIC framework can be effectively utilized in school psychology. This framework could guide practitioners in conducting culturally responsive assessments and implementing interventions for minoritized student populations. School psychologists can apply the framework's components to understand how students' educational background, cultural identity, language proficiency, socioeconomic status, communication styles, test-taking conditions, cognitive conceptualizations of intelligence, and immigration context influence their academic performance and psychological well-being. By incorporating this framework into evaluations, school psychologists can identify and mitigate potential biases in testing and ensure that the assessments reflect the students' true abilities and experiences. Additionally, the ECLECTIC framework can inform tailored interventions and support strategies that acknowledge the rich cultural contexts of students, fostering an inclusive educational environment that promotes equitable outcomes for all learners.

Brief Case Study: Canela—ECLECTIC Framework in Action

Canela, a 10-year-old fifth grader, moved from México to the United States 4 years ago. She enrolled in a dual language school that supports her bilingualism and biliteracy in both Spanish and English. Canela's teacher noticed she struggled with reading fluency, despite ongoing interventions during the current and previous academic years. These interventions aimed to improve her phonemic awareness and phonics skills, acknowledging the potential for cross-linguistic transfer from Spanish to English (i.e., Chung et al., 2019). The team also emphasized fluency-building activities in English while concurrently assessing her fluency in Spanish. Worried about a potential learning disability, the teacher referred Canela for a psychoeducational evaluation. Ms. Shell, the school psychologist, who is knowledgeable about bilingualism and biliteracy, received the referral. After examining the existing data, Canela's educational team, including the parents, agreed to proceed with the evaluation, and informed consent was obtained. To facilitate the evaluation,

Ms. Shell implemented the ECLECTIC framework to ensure cultural responsiveness, addressing each component systematically as follows:

E: Education: level, quality, and literacy Canela faced limited formal education in México because of socioeconomic challenges. Her preschool and elementary schools, located in rural areas, lacked sufficient resources. Consequently, Ms. Shell prioritized recognizing Canela's existing listening, oracy, writing, and reading skills in both languages over merely identifying deficits. She also considered the disparities in educational opportunities while interpreting standardized test scores and conceptualizing all collected information.

C: Culture and Acculturation Canela's strong ties to her Mexican culture, combined with her limited exposure to Western culture outside of school, influenced her adjustment to the school environment. Ms. Shell recognized the differences between Mexican and US classroom norms and wondered how these cultural expectations could influence Canela's behavior and motivation. As a result, Ms. Shell consulted a colleague familiar with the educational system in México to learn more about the similarities and differences between the two countries. Additionally, Ms. Shell spent time researching the sociocultural environment and personal experiences of children attending rural schools in México (i.e., Bryan & McLaughlin, 2005). Furthermore, Ms. Shell evaluated Canela's level of acculturation through qualitative or standardized methods, acknowledging that high acculturation stress would impact learning and assessment outcomes.

L: Language Spoken and English Proficiency Ms. Shell utilized direct and indirect methods to learn more about Canela's language use and language proficiency in Spanish and English. Indirect methods involved classroom observations to assess Canela's participation and language use during discussions and group activities. Additionally, input from teachers and parents regarding Canela's language use in various settings was utilized, along with a review of records. Direct methods included formal language proficiency tests that assess listening, speaking, reading, and writing skills. These methods also involved structured interviews to evaluate speaking fluency, grammar, and vocabulary. Additionally, listening comprehension tasks utilized video clips or books to gauge understanding through questions and summaries. In choosing standardized assessments and materials, Ms. Shell opted for assessments tailored for Spanish-speaking students in Latinx countries, along with resources reflecting Canela's cultural backgrounds. The combination of direct and indirect methods provided a more comprehensive assessment of language proficiency in both languages.

E: Economics Canela's family encountered significant economic challenges. During the evaluation, Ms. Shell recognized the profound influence of socioeconomic status on language and cognitive development (i.e., Lurie et al., 2021), as well as on learning opportunities and access to essential resources, including healthcare and mental health services.

C: Communication Styles Ms. Shell examined Canela's communication patterns with her family, peers, and teachers to understand her communication style. To collect information in this area, Ms. Shell utilized reports from teachers and parents, observed Canela in various settings, and took the time to get to know Canela and converse with her. Understanding that Mexican culture tends to favor indirect communication, Ms. Shell refrained from asking overly direct questions. Instead, she used open-ended prompts to help Canela share her thoughts more comfortably. She also closely observed Canela's nonverbal signals, such as her facial expressions and body language, recognizing their significance in indirect communication cultures, and modified her own nonverbal cues to be warm and welcoming.

T: Testing Situation: Comfort and Motivation Canela was unfamiliar with standardized assessments and working with a school psychologist and felt nervous. As a response, Ms. Shell showed Canela the testing room, explained the purpose of each test in simple terms beforehand, and shared that the activities were not graded and she was trying to learn more about Canela's strengths. During the assessment, Ms. Shell provided positive reinforcement and clear explanations and avoided any test procedures or items that might be culturally biased.

I: Intelligence Concept of Canela's view of intelligence focused on practical and social abilities, such as helping with daily tasks, understanding social cues, and contributing to her community rather than abstract reasoning. Ms. Shell recognized that this perspective differed from Western notions of intelligence, which often emphasize logical reasoning and academic skills measured by standardized IQ tests. Understanding this, Ms. Shell realized that Western IQ tests may neglect important aspects of intelligence appreciated in Canela's culture. Instead, she observed Canela in real-life situations, such as how she navigated her classroom routines, helped younger students, or solved problems during group activities. She also interviewed Canela's teachers, who described her leadership in class projects, and her family, who shared examples of her helping with family responsibilities and resolving conflicts with peers. This approach helped Ms. Shell form a more complete picture of Canela's strengths through a more culturally responsive lens.

C: Context of Immigration Canela immigrated to the United States at age 6, a formative age for language, identity, and learning. Upon her arrival, she needed to learn a new language and adapt to a new culture, school system, and social expectations. Therefore, understanding her status in México, including the type of school she attended previously, community resources, and socioeconomic status, can help Ms. Shell avoid assumptions based on stereotypes about Mexican immigrants and consider Canela's unique experiences (e.g., reasons for migration, family support). Additionally, although trauma was not evident in Canela's background, Ms. Shell considered the stress of immigration (e.g., separating from extended families, new peer group), which can impact academic performance. Understanding Canela's immigration context strengthened Ms. Shell's interpretation of Canela's academic challenges.

Assessment Outcomes and Conclusions

By implementing the ELECTIC framework, Ms. Shell developed a thorough understanding of Canela's background and experiences, ensuring that educational challenges are not identified as disabilities without exploring alternative explanations. Ms. Shell utilized each component of ELECTIC to evaluate various factors that could enhance her data conceptualization. Analyzing Canela's educational history was vital for understanding her quality of instruction and experiences of interrupted schooling. Additionally, cultural differences and the process of acculturation can significantly influence classroom performance and assessment outcomes, while limited English proficiency should not be misconstrued as a disability.

Economic challenges can hinder cognitive development and distort test results, and varying communication styles may be misinterpreted as learning disabilities. Therefore, creating a fair and comfortable testing environment is essential to mitigate anxiety or biases that could distort the results. Understanding how intelligence is perceived across cultures is crucial in preventing an excessive reliance on Western IQ assessments, which might overlook unique strengths. Moreover, factors related to immigration, such as trauma, can also profoundly impact learning. By addressing each component of the ECLECTIC framework, Ms. Shell conducted a culturally responsive and comprehensive evaluation of Canela, resulting in a more accurate understanding of her learning needs and informing the development of appropriate interventions. While the ECLECTIC framework helps identify relevant data sources and guide their interpretation, clinical judgment remains essential to accurately apply this information when determining eligibility and placement decisions related to the referral question.

Conclusion

The dynamics of acculturation and enculturation are crucial considerations in the pre-referral and assessment processes within school psychology, particularly when supporting CLM students. A deep understanding of a child's cultural identity and their level of integration into the dominant culture provides valuable context for interpreting academic, social–emotional, and behavioral concerns. This insight enables practitioners to determine whether concerns arise from the acculturation process itself or if further evaluation is warranted. As family members and school staff raise concerns about the educational progress of CLM students, practitioners must recognize how cultural adaptation may impact students' functioning. Without this lens, educational decisions are at risk of being misinformed and further perpetuating systemic barriers.

Curricula, standardized assessments, and teaching practices often reflect the dominant culture, which inadvertently marginalizes CLM students. School psychologists must critically assess these tools to prevent reinforcing systemic biases, recognizing that traditional views of objectivity are shaped by the sociocultural power dynamics and biases of the knowledge producer, thus perpetuating existing inequalities (Sabnis & Proctor, 2021). Using culturally responsive practices and frameworks, such as the ECLECTIC model, enables practitioners to transcend traditional data collection frameworks that fail to capture the richness of CLM students' lived experiences. By valuing diverse cultural identities, school psychologists can foster inclusive learning environments that promote equity. These efforts not only support the success of CLM students but also contribute to the broader goal of social justice in education.

References

Anderson-Levitt, K. M. (2012). Complicating the concept of culture. *Comparative Education, 48*(4), 441–454. https://doi.org/10.1080/03050068.2011.634285

Arends-Tóth, J., & van de Vijver, F. J. R. (2006). Assessment of psychological acculturation. In D. L. Sam & J. W. Berry (Eds.), *The Cambridge handbook of acculturation psychology* (pp. 142–160). Cambridge University Press. https://doi.org/10.1017/CBO9780511489891.01

Asendorpf, J. B., & Motti-Stefanidi, F. (2017). A longitudinal study of immigrants' peer acceptance and rejection: Immigrant status, immigrant composition of the classroom, and acculturation. *Cultural Diversity & Ethnic Minority Psychology, 23*(4), 486–498. https://doi.org/10.1037/cdp0000155

Barona, A., & Miller, J. A. (1994). Short acculturation scale for Hispanic youth. *PsycTESTS Dataset*. https://doi.org/10.1037/t03843-000

Berry, J. W. (1980). Acculturation as varieties of adaptation A. Padilla (Ed.). Acculturation: Theory, models and some new findings, 9–25. Westview.

Berry, J. W. (1990). Psychology of acculturation. In J. J. Berman (Ed.), *Nebraska symposium on motivation, 1989: Cross-cultural perspectives* (pp. 201–234). University of Nebraska Press.

Berry, J. W., & Sam, D. L. (2016). Theoretical perspectives. In D. L. Sam & J. W. Berry (Eds.), *The Cambridge handbook of acculturation psychology* (pp. 11–29). Cambridge University Press.

Bornstein, M. H. (2017). The specificity principle in acculturation science. *Perspectives on Psychological Science, 12*(1), 3–45. https://doi.org/10.1177/1745691616655997

Bornstein, M. H., Bernhard, J. K., Bradley, R. H., Chen, X., Farver, J. A. M., Gold, S. J., Hernandez, D. J., Spiel, C., van de Vijver, F., & Yoshikawa, H. (2019). Psychological acculturation: Perspectives, principles, processes, and prospects. In *Routledge international handbook of migration studies* (pp. 19–31). Routledge.

Bryan, L. A., & McLaughlin, H. J. (2005). Teaching and learning in rural Mexico: A portrait of student responsibility in Everyday School Life. *Teaching and Teacher Education, 21*(1), 33–48. https://doi.org/10.1016/j.tate.2004.11.004

Calderon-Berumen, F. (2019). Resisting assimilation to the melting pot. *Journal of Culture and Values in Education, 2*(1), 81–95. https://doi.org/10.46303/jcve.02.01.7

Celenk, O., & Van de Vijver, F. J. (2014). Assessment of psychological acculturation and multiculturalism: An overview of measures in the public domain. *The Oxford Handbook of Multicultural Identity* (pp. 205–226). Oxford University Press.

Chung, S. C., Chen, X., & Geva, E. (2019). Deconstructing and reconstructing cross-language transfer in bilingual reading development: An interactive framework. *Journal of Neurolinguistics, 50*, 149–161. https://doi.org/10.1016/j.jneuroling.2018.01.003

Collier, C. (2016). *Acculturation Quick Screen (AQS-III)*. Cross Cultural Developmental Education Services.

Collier, C., Brice, A. E., & Oades-Sese, G. V. (2007). Assessment of acculturation. In E. C. Lopez, S. G. Nahari, G. B. Esquivel, & S. Proctor (Eds.), *Handbook of multicultural school psychology: An interdisciplinary perspective* (pp. 353–380). Routledge. https://doi.org/10.4324/9780203936528.ch17

Cooper, C. W., Riehl, C. J., & Hasan, A. L. (2010). Leading and learning with diverse families in schools: Critical epistemology amid communities of practice. *Journal of School Leadership, 20*(6), 758–788. https://doi.org/10.1177/105268461002000604

d'Abreu, A., Castro-Olivo, S., & Ura, S. K. (2019). Understanding the role of acculturative stress on Refugee Youth Mental Health: A systematic review and ecological approach to assessment and Intervention. *School Psychology International, 40*(2), 107–127. https://doi.org/10.1177/0143034318822688

Franco, J. N. (1983). Children's acculturation scale. *PsycTESTS Dataset.* https://doi.org/10.1037/t03848-000

Francis, G. L., Haines, S. J., & Nagro, S. A. (2017). Developing relationships with immigrant families: Learning by asking the right questions. *TEACHING Exceptional Children, 50*(2), 95–105. https://doi.org/10.1177/0040059917720778

Fuji, D. E. (2018). Developing a cultural context for conducting a neuropsychological evaluation with a culturally diverse client: The Eclectic framework. *The Clinical Neuropsychologist, 32*(8), 1356–1392. https://doi.org/10.1080/13854046.2018.1435826

Goforth, A. N., & Pham, A. V. (2023). Literacy, language, and acculturation of diverse students. In *Culturally responsive school-based practices: Supporting mental health and learning of diverse students* (pp. 103–135). Oxford University Press. https://doi.org/10.1093/med-psych/9780197516928.003.0003

Goforth, A. N., Pham, A. V., Chun, H., & Castro-Olivo, S. (2017). Acculturation and sociocultural factors in children's mental health services: Applying multicultural consultation frameworks. *Journal of Educational and Psychological Consultation, 27*(3), 239–244. https://doi.org/10.1080/10474412.2016.1275650

Goforth, A. N., Pham, A. V., & Oka, E. R. (2015). Parent–child conflict, acculturation gap, acculturative stress, and behavior problems in Arab American adolescents. *Journal of Cross-Cultural Psychology, 46*(6), 821–836. https://doi.org/10.1177/0022022115585140

Greenberg, J., Arndt, T., & M, L. (2020). Fundamentals of social behavior. In *Social psychology: The science of everyday life* (pp. 36–81). Worth Publishers.

Hass, M. R., & Abdou, A. S. (2019). Culturally responsive interviewing practices. *California School Psychologist, 23*(1), 47–56. https://doi.org/10.1007/s40688-018-0204-z

Hod, Y., & Sagy, O. (2022). School enculturation discourse: A meta synthesis from research in the learning sciences. *Information and Learning Sciences, 123*(9/10), 621–641. https://doi.org/10.1108/ils-11-2021-0103

Juang, L. P., & Syed, M. (2019). The evolution of acculturation and development models for understanding immigrant children and youth adjustment. *Child Development Perspectives, 13*(4), 241–246. https://doi.org/10.1111/cdep.12346

Lau, W. S., & Shea, M. (2022). Empowering English learners in the classroom through culturally responsive social-emotional teaching practices. *Journal of Multilingual and Multicultural Development, 45*(7), 2880–2897. https://doi.org/10.1080/01434632.2022.2078337

Lechuga, J. (2008). Is acculturation a dynamic construct?: The influence of method of priming culture on acculturation. *Hispanic Journal of Behavioral Sciences, 30*(3), 324–339. https://doi.org/10.1177/0739986308319570

Lokhande, & Reichle, B. (2019). Acculturation and school adjustment of children and youth from culturally diverse backgrounds: Predictors and interventions for school psychology. *Journal of School Psychology, 75*, 1–7. https://doi.org/10.1016/j.jsp.2019.06.001

Lurie, L. A., Hagen, M. P., McLaughlin, K. A., Sheridan, M. A., Meltzoff, A. N., & Rosen, M. L. (2021). Mechanisms linking socioeconomic status and academic achievement in early childhood: Cognitive stimulation and language. *Cognitive Development, 58*, 101045. https://doi.org/10.1016/j.cogdev.2021.101045

Makarova, E. (2019). Acculturation and school adjustment of minority students: School and family-related factors. *Intercultural Education, 30*(5), 445–447. https://doi.org/10.1080/14675986.2019.1643559

Makarova, E., & Birman, D. (2016). Minority students' psychological adjustment in the School Context: An integrative review of qualitative research on acculturation. *Intercultural Education, 27*(1), 1–21. https://doi.org/10.1080/14675986.2016.1144382

Marks, A. K., Ejesi, K., & García Coll, C. (2014). Understanding the U.S. immigrant paradox in childhood and adolescence. *Child Development Perspectives, 8*(2), 59–64. https://doi.org/10.1111/cdep.12071

Martinez, R., Norman, R. D., & Delaney, H. D. (1984). Children's Hispanic background scale. *PsycTESTS Dataset*. https://doi.org/10.1037/t16792-000

National Association of School Psychologists. (2020). *The Professional Standards of the National Association of School Psychologists*. https://www.nasponline.org/standards-and-certification/nasp-2020-professional-standards-adopted

National Center for Education Statistics. (2024). English Learners in Public Schools. *Condition of Education*. U.S. Department of Education, Institute of Education Sciences. https://nces.ed.gov/programs/coe/indicator/cgf.

Nguyen, H. H., & von Eye, A. (2002). Acculturation scale for Vietnamese adolescents. *PsycTESTS Dataset*. https://doi.org/10.1037/t03837-000

Oppedal, B., & Toppelberg, C. O. (2016). Acculturation development and the acquisition of culture competence. In D. L. Sam & J. W. Berry (Eds.), *The Cambridge handbook of acculturation psychology* (pp. 71–92). Cambridge University Press.

Pham, A. V., Goforth, A. N., Chun, H., Castro-Olivo, S., & Costa, A. (2017). Acculturation and help-seeking behavior in consultation: A sociocultural framework for mental health service. *Journal of Educational and Psychological Consultation, 27*(3), 271–288. https://doi.org/10.1080/10474412.2017.1287574

Romero, A., & Piña-Watson, B. (2017). Acculturative stress and bicultural stress. *Oxford Handbooks Online*. https://doi.org/10.1093/oxfordhb/9780190215217.013.8

Romero, P. A., & Branscome, J. (2014). Acculturation and sociocognitive factors. *Assessing Bilingual Children in Context: An Integrated Approach*, 191–214. https://doi.org/10.1037/14320-009

Rudmin, F. (2009). Constructs, measurements and models of acculturation and acculturative stress. *International Journal of Intercultural Relations, 33*(2), 106–123. https://doi.org/10.1016/j.ijintrel.2008.12.001

Sabnis, S. V., & Proctor, S. L. (2021). Use of critical theory to develop a conceptual framework for critical school psychology. *School Psychology Review, 51*(6), 661–675. https://doi.org/10.1080/2372966x.2021.1949248

Sam, D. L., & Berry, J. W. (2010). Acculturation: When individuals and groups of different cultural backgrounds meet. *Perspectives on Psychological Science, 5*(4), 472–481. https://doi.org/10.1177/1745691610373075

Schultz, L. (2016). Resisting assimilation: Deliberate acculturation by the American English Language Learner. *Multicultural Perspectives, 18*(2), 103–107. https://doi.org/10.1080/15210960.2016.1159100

Schwartz, S. J., Unger, J. B., Zamboanga, B. L., & Szapocznik, J. (2010). Rethinking the concept of acculturation: Implications for theory and research. *American Psychologist, 65*(4), 237–251. https://doi.org/10.1037/a0019330

Schwartz, S. J., Zamboanga, B. L., & Jarvis, L. H. (2007). Ethnic identity and acculturation in Hispanic early adolescents: Mediated relationships to academic grades, prosocial behaviors, and externalizing symptoms. *Cultural Diversity & Ethnic Minority Psychology, 13*(4), 364–373. https://doi.org/10.1037/1099-9809.13.4.364

Suarez-Morales, L., Dillon, F. R., & Szapocznik, J. (2007). Acculturative stress inventory for children. *PsycTESTS Dataset*. https://doi.org/10.1037/t00023-000

Trujillo, S. M., Greene, J. A., & Carrillo, A. (2020). *Introduction to the language acculturation meter for Spanish-speaking English language learners* (White paper). PAR.

Unger, J. B., Gallaher, P., Shakib, S., Ritt-Olson, A., Palmer, P. H., & Johnson, C. A. (2002). Acculturation, habits, and interests multicultural scale for adolescents. *PsycTESTS Dataset*. https://doi.org/10.1037/t03885-000

van der Zee, K., & van Oudenhoven, J. P. (2022). Towards a dynamic approach to acculturation. *International Journal of Intercultural Relations, 88*, 119–124. https://doi.org/10.1016/j.ijintrel.2022.04.004

Vedder, P., & Motti-Stefanidi, F. (2016). Children, families and schools. In D. L. Sam & J. W. Berry (Eds.), *The Cambridge handbook of acculturation psychology* (pp. 464–482). Cambridge University Press.

Vega, D., & Wolf, J. (2023). Best practices in assessment of bilingual learners in schools. In *Best Practices in School Psychology: Vol. 1. Data-Based and Collaborative Decision Making, 7,* 163–173. essay, NASP.

Ward, C. (2001). The ABCs of acculturation. In D. Matsumoto (Ed.), *The handbook of culture and psychology* (pp. 411–445). Oxford University Press.

Ward, C., & Geeraert, N. (2016). Advancing acculturation theory and research: The acculturation process in its ecological context. *Current Opinion in Psychology, 8*, 98–104. https://doi.org/10.1016/j.copsyc.2015.09.021

Ward, C., & Szabó, Á. (2019). Affect, behavior, cognition, and development. *The Handbook of culture and psychology*, 640–692. https://doi.org/10.1093/oso/9780190679743.003.0020

Watts, J. (2021). Teaching English language learners: A reconsideration of assimilation pedagogy in U.S. schools. *Diaspora, Indigenous and Minority Education, 15*(1), 1–9. https://doi.org/10.1080/15595692.2019.1684890

Wood, M. R. (2008). ESL and bilingual education as a proxy for racial and ethnic segregation in U.S. public schools. *The Journal of Gender, Race, and Justice, 11*(3), 279.

Part II
Implementing Multi-tiered System of Supports with Culturally Adapted Interventions

Chapter 4
Culturally and Linguistically Responsive Multi-tiered System of Supports

Sylvia Linan-Thompson and Meagan Dorman

Educational policies and instructional practices continually evolve as educators and researchers gain deeper insight into student learning. This evolution is driven by the aspiration to elevate overall student achievement and minimize disparities among different student groups. A Multitiered System of Supports (MTSS) framework is operationalized as a dynamic and interconnected three-tiered framework that provides a structured approach to improving outcomes for all students (Witzel & Clarke, 2015). It is an umbrella term for frameworks focused on preventing students' learning and behavioral difficulties by intervening early. The components that underpin Response to Intervention (RTI) and Positive Behavior Interventions and Supports (PBIS), two MTSS frameworks, have been researched and implemented since the 1980s (e.g., Fuchs et al., 1983; Marston et al., 1984).

Although some research conducted since the implementation of multi-tiered frameworks has included demographically diverse populations (e.g., students from racially, ethnically, and economically diverse backgrounds), the results are often not disaggregated (e.g., Wanzek & Vaughn, 2011). This lack of disaggregation leaves educators unable to answer the three essential questions posed by Klingner and Edwards (2006) to ensure MTSS practices are equitable for all students: (1) what works with whom? (2) by whom? and (3) in what contexts? Answering these questions requires not only disaggregating data but also considering students' identities when developing, researching, and implementing interventions and assessments. While the essential components of MTSS, screening and progress monitoring, evidence-based instruction, and data-based decision-making, apply to all students, how they are implemented may vary based on the student population and school needs (Sailor et al., 2021; Schiller et al., 2020; Sugai & Horner, 2020).

S. Linan-Thompson (✉) · M. Dorman
Special Education and Clinical Science, University of Oregon, Eugene, OR, USA
e-mail: Sthomps5@uoregon.edu; Mdorman@uoregon.edu

D. Vega, J. N. Wolf (eds.), *Culturally and Linguistically Responsive Intervention and Assessment Practices with Emergent Bilingual Students*,
https://doi.org/10.1007/978-3-032-02084-0_4

Culturally relevant education (CRE) is not just a pedagogical approach but a commitment to systematically advancing equity and social justice in education. It centers on valuing and affirming students' ethno-racial and linguistic identities, employing rigorous and culturally relevant curricula, and fostering strong, positive relationships between students, families, and educators (Ladson-Billings, 2014). Educators who implement CRE challenge and seek to dismantle the historical forms of oppression manifested in educational content, teaching practices, and administrative policies.

In the United States, CRE originated from the desegregation efforts of the 1960s and 1970s, which sought to secure equal and just educational experiences for Black students (Aronson & Laughter, 2016). During this era, the prevalent notion of "cultural diversity" often led to assimilating students of color into an educational system that predominantly reflected white norms (Warikoo & Carter, 2009). This approach tended to overlook or undervalue the rich and diverse experiences of students from various cultural backgrounds (Johnston et al., 2017). CRE emerged to counter this trend of assimilation, intentionally highlighting the culture, knowledge, language, and experiences of students of color and recognizing these as integral to the learning process (Delpit, 1988; Ladson-Billings, 1992) and as legitimate forms of knowledge in schools. Changes in the demographic characteristics of the school-aged population and the shift toward acknowledging and valuing cultural diversity warrant an examination of educational practices.

Recent demographic data show increases in the racial, ethnic, and linguistic diversity of the US population (U.S. Census Bureau, 2020), a trend also evident in public schools. In 2021, over half of the students enrolled in public schools identified as members of diverse ethno-racial groups, and 5.3 million emergent bilingual (EB) students, students who are in the process of learning English, were enrolled in schools (National Center for Education Statistics [NCES], 2024). Of these students, 76.4% speak Spanish as their home language, and the remaining 23.6% speak nearly 400 different languages.

Against this backdrop, integrating MTSS and culturally and linguistically relevant education are necessary for seamless services. Educational systems must address students' academic and behavioral needs, respect them, and incorporate their cultural and linguistic backgrounds. Such an approach would ensure that interventions and other educational supports are not only effective in maximizing student outcomes and reducing disproportionate identification of students for special education services (Sullivan, 2011) but are also culturally sensitive and inclusive.

This chapter will describe how the MTSS framework can be effectively combined with CRE to create a culturally and linguistically responsive MTSS framework (CL-MTSS). This framework should lead to an integrated educational system that is not only academically robust but also deeply rooted in principles of equity and social justice.

Multitiered System of Supports

Currently, MTSS, RTI, and PBIS describe multilevel prevention frameworks implemented in schools nationwide. Although the term RTI is still used to describe academic multi-tiered frameworks in some states, MTSS is increasingly used as an overarching term to describe systems addressing the academic, behavioral, and social–emotional needs of all students (Sailor et al., 2021; Thurlow et al., 2020). This framework evolved to emphasize prevention and inclusion rather than solely identifying and remedying academic and behavioral challenges (Thurlow et al., 2020). The concept of providing differential support to students in targeted areas of need was inspired by the structured, preventative approaches used in public health systems (Gordon, 1983). MTSS employs a tiered model categorizing interventions into primary (Tier 1), secondary (Tier 2), and tertiary (Tier 3) levels aimed at minimizing risk and addressing specific needs (Sugai & Horner, 2009).

RTI emerged as an alternative method for identifying learning disabilities (Fuchs & Fuchs, 1998), addressing dissatisfaction with the IQ-achievement discrepancy (National Association of Special Education Teachers [NASET], 2023) which was problematic for several student groups, including EB students, students from low-income families, and students of color, who were often overidentified for special education (e.g., Carnine, 2003; Thorius & Maxcy, 2015; Willis, 2019; Young et al., 2005). Further, students often had to fail for 3–4 years before they were eligible for special education services. To address these issues, RTI emphasized evidence-based interventions and continuous progress monitoring (Fuchs & Fuchs, 2006) to promote early intervention and equitable instruction, reducing the misidentification of students of color and EB students (Cramer, 2015; O'Connor et al., 2005; Simmons et al., 2008; Vellutino et al., 2008).

In 1996, Walker and colleagues proposed PBIS, a tiered framework to manage and prevent behavioral challenges while enhancing learning environments. A core concept of PBIS is its focus on contextual fit, ensuring cultural responsiveness by aligning with each school community's unique norms and values (Leverson et al., 2021). PBIS' effectiveness and relevance in diverse settings are underscored by its five core components: identity, voice, supportive environment, situational appropriateness, and data for equity (Leverson et al., 2021). Studies, including randomized control trials, have shown that PBIS effectively reduces disruptive behavior and bullying while improving emotional self-control (Horner et al., 2009; Kelm & McIntosh, 2012). The expansion of PBIS implementation in the United States from 7000 schools in 2008 (Kincaid et al., 2007) to over 26,000 schools by 2018 (Sugai & Horner, 2020) demonstrates its adaptability to various school contexts. This trend extends globally, further highlighting PBIS' adaptability (Nylén et al., 2021; Poed & Whitefield, 2020).

MTSS aims to prevent academic difficulties by providing effective interventions early (Linan-Thompson et al., 2022; Orosco & Klinger, 2010). Using assessment data for decision-making and team-based approaches can improve accountability and reduce the disproportionate identification of students of color (Artiles et al., 2005; O'Connor et al., 2013; Rueda & Windmuller, 2006). For EB students, MTSS can help distinguish between language acquisition and disability during data-based decision-making meetings (Hoover & Soltero, 2018). For example, examining progress-monitoring data is particularly useful in determining if a student is likely to be experiencing learning difficulties. EB students who are likely to have a disability tend to demonstrate persistent difficulties despite targeted instruction in decoding, reading fluency, and spelling, along with uneven or no progress (Adelson et al., 2014).

The success of MTSS relies on fidelity in the implementation of each component. The concept of fair and equal opportunity to learn (Every Student Succeeds Act [ESSA], 2015) extends beyond the mere presence of critical resources, which includes competent teachers, sufficient funding, and a curriculum that is both relevant and challenging. It also encompasses elements integral to the educational environment, such as engaging in culturally responsive tasks and refraining from deficit thinking regarding low-income, ethno-racially minoritized students during the referral and placement stages (National Center for Culturally Responsive Educational Systems [NCCRESt], 2005). For learning to be truly effective, it is essential to achieve a seamless integration of these contextual factors by deploying empirically validated instructional approaches across all levels of the MTSS framework.

Actionable Steps and Practical Recommendations

Unlike their monolingual English-speaking peers, EB students are in the process of becoming bilingual and/or achieving English proficiency and may be learning to read in both languages or transitioning from literacy instruction in their first language (i.e., "L1") to instruction in English (i.e., "L2"; Chiappe et al., 2002). During this period, their language and literacy skills will develop and change at different rates and will be impacted by the quality and language of their instruction. Learning and, as a result, literacy are not compartmentalized by language, and even though some abilities transfer, what students *know* and *can* do in each language is not equal (Gort, 2019). Instructional and assessment practices should respond to this reality.

Effective Instructional Practices

EB students can be enrolled in dual language, bilingual, or English-only programs, and the implementation of MTSS can vary in terms of how much instruction students receive in their L1 and L2. Despite these differences, studies that have examined the effect of MTSS components on EB students' academic outcomes have found them to be effective. Whether instruction is in Spanish or English, explicit instruction in skills such as phonological awareness, print awareness, and alphabetic knowledge (Chiappe et al., 2002; Geva et al., 2000; Graves et al., 2004; Lesaux et al., 2007; Vaughn et al., 2005, 2006), oral reading fluency (Baker & Good, 1995; Leafstedt et al., 2004; Wiley & Deno, 2005), and oral language and comprehension is effective in improving student outcomes in both English (Vaughn et al., 2005) and Spanish (Gerber et al., 2004; Vaughn et al., 2006) in Tiers 1 and 2. Another component of MTSS, the provision of small group instruction and an increase in the intensity of instruction in Tier 2, has also been found to be effective (Gunn et al., 2002; Vaughn et al., 2005, 2006).

The studies cited above provide practices that enhance instruction for EB students and increase the likelihood of academic success. Across all tiers, EB students need effective practices (Echevarria et al., 2006; Goldenberg, 2008; Vaughn et al., 2006). As important as foundational skills are in both literacy and numeracy, students need frequent, systematic instruction in vocabulary, academic language, and listening and reading comprehension across all grades (Callahan, 2005; Carlo et al., 2004; Saunders et al., 2006). These skills are indispensable for learning. Using student experiences to scaffold instruction promotes students' understanding of key concepts and fosters a positive, inclusive learning environment for EB students. This approach ensures that education is not just an additive process but a transformative one, where students' inherent strengths and cultural and linguistic backgrounds play a central role in their learning journey.

A second critical practice is the inclusion of strategies to support English language proficiency during instruction to facilitate content-area learning. The Educators Practice Guide from the What Works Clearinghouse (Baker et al., 2014) outlines four evidence-based recommendations for improving English learners' academic content and literacy instruction. These recommendations often emphasize practices such as:

1. Focusing on teaching key content with simplified language structures but grade-appropriate vocabulary to allow students to learn the essentials. This strategy aligns with recommendation two, emphasizing integrating oral and written English language instruction into content-area teaching.
2. Defining both instructional and content vocabulary, which reflects recommendation two's focus on teaching academic vocabulary intensively across several days using various activities.
3. Delivering content in chunks so students can digest content a little at a time and integrate both the language and content is supported by recommendation two.
4. Using advance organizers, graphic organizers, visuals (e.g., pictures and videos), and realia, corresponding with recommendation two, as these tools help integrate language instruction into content learning.
5. Building background knowledge, especially of less common concepts, teaching key vocabulary, and previewing main ideas align with recommendation one.
6. Providing students multiple opportunities to collaborate with native and proficient English speakers and periodic review of important concepts, reflecting recommendation four, which emphasizes small-group instructional interventions to address literacy and language development needs.
7. Providing structured opportunities for students to write about the content they are learning, using sentence frames or guided writing activities, to help them develop both content knowledge and written language skills. This aligns with recommendation three, emphasizing integrating writing practice into content instruction.

Finally, bilingual teachers (general education, special education, or ESL) and those who understand, speak, read, and/or write a language other than English can use the L1 strategically as a resource. For example, they may use the L1 to provide an overview of essential content or to review concepts or skills to ensure students understand the content correctly (Brice & Roseberry-McKibbin, 2001; Dubetz, 2012; Gersten et al., 2007).

Guidance on Language Use and Assessments

One goal of MTSS is to reduce the number of inaccurate referrals of EB students to supplemental interventions and special education programs. To ensure accurate data collection and appropriate support for EB students, the assessment measures and processes utilized must be culturally and linguistically responsive (see Linan-Thompson et al., 2022, for a comprehensive review of practices). Assessments used as part of MTSS provide educators with data to identify students who need early intervention and those who may have a learning disability (Linan-Thompson et al., 2022). Choosing appropriate assessments and interpreting the results in light of students' educational experiences is an essential yet challenging process for educators implementing an MTSS in schools with EBs. There are many ways in which assessment procedures for EBs are similar to those already in use in typical RTI models within MTSS, but there are some critical differences. These are differences in (a) choosing assessment measures, (b) implementation of universal screening and progress monitoring, and (c) assessment of language proficiency.

The language used to assess students can impact who is identified as needing additional support (Linan-Thompson et al., 2022). Chiappe et al. (2002) found that screening EB students in English in first grade usually results in a higher-than-average identification of students for Tier 2 intervention. A similar phenomenon occurs when students in transitional or dual language programs who are typically assessed in Spanish during kindergarten through second grade are evaluated in English (Linan-Thompson et al., 2022). The shift in the language of the assessment tool can also result in an inaccurate assessment of EB students' academic abilities and an overidentification of students for Tier 2 instruction (Linan-Thompson et al., 2022). For example, in a recent study, 29% of third-grade students did not meet the benchmark in oral reading fluency when assessed in their L1. When they were assessed in English, 69% did not meet benchmark (Linan-Thompson et al., 2022). To ensure data is linguistically appropriate, students who receive instruction in English or dual language programs should be assessed in both languages (Linan-Thompson et al., 2022) until it is clear that English assessments accurately measure students' skills. For most students, it is when their scores in English are equal to or better than their scores in their L1.

Types of Assessments in MTSS

A comprehensive MTSS assessment system includes universal screeners and progress monitoring tools, such as CBMs, to determine which students have met benchmarks and who may require additional support (Fuchs et al., 1983). Universal screening, an assessment implemented at the beginning of the school year, is administered to all students beginning in kindergarten. Progress monitoring is used to track student learning over time. The measures used for progress monitoring are often the same as those employed for universal screening, ensuring a consistent and data-driven approach. This ongoing assessment cycle allows educators to gauge the effectiveness of their practices and interventions and make informed decisions about adjusting or intensifying support for individual students (Center on MTSS, 2021).

When selecting measures for EB students, consider the following: (a) assessments should be consistent with the language of instruction; (b) they should be technically adequate; (c) normed on student populations similar to the school's population; and (d) supported by research. Most importantly, the measures used, whether in English or the student's L1, must be valid and reliable for EBs and demonstrate diagnostic accuracy for predicting learning problems.

Further, when assessing EBs, it is important to choose tools that provide accurate data on student growth and development toward biliteracy by measuring EB children's skills in both languages, especially when enrolled in transitional or dual language programs. Tools should be aligned to allow school personnel to track student progress across grades and between languages. For example, select a CBM measure that can be used with students in grades K-6 and, when possible, in both languages (Linan-Thompson et al., 2022). In addition to the assessments typically used, it is important to collect information on cultural and linguistic influence on performance from parents and families, teachers across grades and content areas, and classroom observations of L1 and L2 instruction (Linan-Thompson et al., 2022).

Behavior Assessments

Chafouleas et al. (2010) identified a crucial gap in the MTSS framework: the lack of consensus on the tools used for assessing behavioral skills despite a well-established agreement on tools for academic assessment. This discrepancy calls for a more balanced approach in MTSS that emphasizes and provides clear guidance on behavioral assessments. The importance of incorporating CLR practices within these assessments is also highlighted in the literature (see Artzi et al., 2022; NCCRESt, 2005) and points to the need for tools that are not only effective but also sensitive to diverse student backgrounds. See Chap. 11 in this volume for a more in-depth description of social-emotional and behavior assessments.

Data-Based Decision-Making

The accuracy of assessment data is critical because it is used to make decisions about the type of instruction students will receive. Together, educators analyze student data to group students, design interventions, establish student growth, and adjust instruction and interventions to meet students' needs. Sailor et al. (2021) emphasized the significant enhancement of the MTSS framework through collaboration among teachers, administrators, and support staff. The collective effort is critical for the successful deployment of MTSS practices. Culturally valid data-based decision-making is characterized as a process by which decisions are made considering the cultural factors, language, and sociocultural context when gathering, analyzing, or evaluating student data (Vincent et al., 2011), and in which teachers with expertise, such as the ESL teacher, are included. The collective effort is critical for the successful deployment of MTSS practices.

Despite challenges in implementing MTSS in schools and classrooms that serve EB students, there are examples of educators who implement culturally responsive assessments and instruction across tiers. Implementing culturally and linguistically responsive MTSS requires not only the implementation of each component with fidelity but also teachers who do not hold deficit views about their students. Teachers who validate and acknowledge students' cultures increase cultural relevance through materials that match culture and language (Jackson, 2021). They also recognize that children come to school with different experiences with literacy and numeracy and use those experiences to build their students' skills and knowledge, recognize and acknowledge students' discourse and behavioral styles as differences and not deficits, and recognize bilingualism as an asset. Teachers who engage in these behaviors respect students' values and views (Moll & González, 1994). Building culturally responsive practices can be challenging for teachers who have not received professional development (PD) in integrating students' culture into academic and behavioral evidence-based practices. Rather than expect teachers to acquire these skills and knowledge individually, educators in leadership positions should plan and provide teachers with PD that supports their acquisition of needed skills and develop school-wide systems that support implementing new practices.

Continuing Challenges

Although studies demonstrate that implementing MTSS can be effective for EB students, the disproportionate representation of students from diverse ethno-racial and linguistic backgrounds in special education continues to be an issue (Artiles, 2011; Hosp & Reschly, 2003; Willis, 2019). There are several reasons why implementing MTSS may not lead to improved outcomes and fewer referrals to special education. First, the focus on the child without also examining the context in which EB students learn places the blame for failure to learn on the student (Jackson, 2021; Thorius & Maxcy, 2015). As long as the focus is on the student, the institutional factors that can impact student achievement and behavior are ignored and thus not addressed (Hartlep & Ellis, 2012). Further, an outcome-focused approach may lead many teachers to continue to hold deficit views of students despite the prevention focus of RTI (Solano-Flores, 2008; Orosco & Klingner, 2010; Sabnis et al., 2020). Second, educators' perception that they lack the knowledge needed to implement MTSS successfully points to the need for more consistent and comprehensive training (Castillo et al., 2022; Gulamhussein, 2013; Lesh et al., 2021). Given that 45% of middle and 29% of high schools nationally have adopted MTSS models (Schiller et al., 2020), it is clear that addressing discrepancies in skill perceptions among different educational roles is crucial and emphasizes the importance of equitable training.

The third factor is teachers' lack of understanding of EB students' academic needs. Because they are learning in a second language, teachers need to understand how to implement practices and strategies that support language acquisition (Hoover & Soltero-González, 2018) and the critical role that vocabulary instruction (e.g., Carlo et al., 2004) and academic language (Bailey, 2006; Callahan, 2005; Saunders et al., 2006) play in students' academic growth. The fourth factor is the continued challenge of implementing linguistically appropriate assessment procedures. The main issues are the lack of time to assess students in transitional or dual language programs in more than one language, the lack of normative data that informs typical development when a student is learning a second language, and the lack of assessments in many languages. Last is the extent of variation within MTSS models, leading to diverse implementations of practices (Castillo et al., 2022). Although MTSS being adapted to meet student needs based on contextual factors is advantageous, this very flexibility can pose challenges in offering guidance for tailoring PD and building staff capacity. This aligns with Shapiro's (2014) and Sugai and Horner's (2009) findings on the differences in implementation using standard protocols versus problem-solving approaches within MTSS.

In educational research, there is a pressing need for a comprehensive examination of student and community profiles. This involves considering various factors such as language proficiency, language of instruction, ethnicity, life experiences, and other unique characteristics of the student population. Disaggregating assessment data, or separating by subgroups, is key to understanding the impacts of instruction and interventions on targeted populations. For example, it can show how the same intervention might yield different outcomes for students of different ethnicities or those with varying language proficiency levels.

Conclusion

Integrating MTSS and CRE principles can lead to a transformative approach, promoting early intervention practices that respect and incorporate students' cultural and linguistic identities while targeting the reduction of misidentification in special education (Cramer, 2015; Sailor et al., 2021). This approach not only requires fidelity in the application of its components but also a reimagining of the educator's role in fostering equity. Educators are called upon to employ data-based decision-making that is culturally valid, to dismantle deficit views, and to validate and leverage the cultural and linguistic assets students bring to the learning environment (Jackson, 2021; Moll & González, 1994). Furthermore, evolving demographic data underscore the urgency for an educational paradigm that accommodates and celebrates the linguistic and cultural diversity represented by EB students, thereby enhancing the inclusivity and effectiveness of educational interventions (US Census Bureau, 2020).

The importance of professional development tailored to these ends cannot be overstated, as it ensures that educators are equipped with the necessary skills to implement CLR MTSS effectively (Gulamhussein, 2013). Moreover, the literature suggests that collaboration among teachers, administrators, and support staff is crucial for the successful deployment of MTSS practices (Ronfeldt et al., 2015), highlighting the need for concentrated efforts to promote high-quality collaboration for educators within and outside of their content specialties.

The road to educational equity requires commitment, collaboration, and innovation. Educators, administrators, policymakers, and communities must work together to ensure that these transformative practices are not just ideas but realities in classrooms and schools. Ultimately, the goal of a CL-MTSS model is to build an educational system where every student can thrive and contribute meaningfully to society. It is about creating a future where education is not just a pathway to knowledge but a bridge to equity and understanding.

References

Adelson, V., Geva, E., & Fraser, C. (2014). *Identification, assessment, and instruction of English language learners with learning difficulties in the elementary and intermediate grades.* Ontario Institute for Studies in Education, University of Toronto. https://ctserc.org/documents/resources/ELLs-with-special-needs.pdf

Aronson, B., & Laughter, J. (2016). The theory and practice of culturally relevant education: A synthesis of research across content areas. *Review of Educational Research, 86*(1), 163–206.

Artiles, A. J., Rueda, R., Salazar, J., & Higareda, I. (2005). Within-group diversity in minority disproportionate representation: English language learners in urban school districts. *Exceptional Children, 71*, 283–300.

Artiles, A. J. (2011). Toward an interdisciplinary understanding of educational equity and difference: The case of the racialization of ability. *Educational Researcher, 40*, 431–445. https://doi.org/10.3102/0013189X11429391

Artzi, L., Hsin, L. B., Sanford, A. K., Brown, J. E., & Guin, S. (2022). Meeting the language needs of emergent multilingual students at risk for learning disabilities through multitiered systems of support. *Learning Disabilities Research & Practice, 37*(3), 189–203. https://doi.org/10.1111/ldrp.12288

Bailey, A. (2006). From lambie to lambaste: The conceptualization, operationalization, and use of academic language in assessment of ELL students. In K. Rolstad (Ed.), *Rethinking school language*. Erlbaum.

Baker, S. K., & Good, R. (1995). Curriculum-based measurement of English reading with bilingual Hispanic students: A validation study with second-grade students. *School Psychology Review, 24*, 561–579.

Baker, S., Lesaux, N., Jayanthi, M., Dimino, J., Proctor, C. P., Morris, J., Gersten, R., Haymond, K., Kieffer, M. J., Linan-Thompson, S., & Newman-Gonchar, R. (2014). *Teaching academic content and literacy to English learners in elementary and middle school (NCEE 2014-4012)*. National Center for Education Evaluation and Regional Assistance, Institute of Education Sciences, U.S. Department of Education. https://ies.ed.gov/ncee/wwc/Docs/PracticeGuide/english_learners_pg_040114.pdf

Brice, A., & Roseberry-McKibbin, C. (2001). Choice of languages in instruction: One language or two? *Teaching Exceptional Children, 33*(4), 10–16. https://doi.org/10.1177/004005990103300402

Callahan, R. M. (2005). Tracking and high school English learners: Limiting opportunity to learn. *American Educational Research Journal, 42*(2), 305–328. https://doi.org/10.3102/00028312042002305

Carlo, M. S., August, D., McLaughlin, B., Snow, C. E., Dressler, C., Lippman, D. N., David, N., Teresa, J., & White, C. E. (2004). Closing the gap: Addressing the vocabulary needs of English-language learners in bilingual and mainstream classrooms. *Reading Research Quarterly, 39*, 188–215.

Carnine, D. (2003). *IDEA: Focusing on improving results for children with disabilities. Testimony before the Subcommittee on Education Reform. Hearing before the Subcommittee on Education Reform of the Committee on Education and the Workforce. House of Representatives, One Hundred Eighth Congress, First Session*. https://archive.org/stream/ERIC_ED482635/ERIC_ED482635_djvu.tx

Castillo, J. M., Scheel, N. L., Wolgemuth, J. R., Latimer, J. D., & Green, S. M. (2022). A scoping review of the literature on professional learning for MTSS. *Journal of School Psychology, 92*, 166–187. https://doi.org/10.1016/j.jsp.2022.03.010

Center on MTSS. (2021). *Essential components of MTSS*. https://mtss4success.org/essential-components

Chafouleas, S. M., Volpe, R. J., Gresham, F. M., & Cook, C. R. (2010). School-based behavioral assessment within problem-solving models: Current status and future directions. *School Psychology Review, 39*, 345–349. https://doi.org/10.1080/02796015.2010.12087756

Chiappe, P., Siegel, L., & Wade-Woolley, L. (2002). Linguistic diversity and the development of reading skills: A longitudinal study. *Scientific Studies of Reading, 6*(4), 369–400.

Cramer, L. (2015). Inequities of intervention among culturally and linguistically diverse students. *Penn GSE Perspectives on Urban Education, 12*(1), 14–21.

Delpit, L. (1988). The silenced dialogue. Power and pedagogy in educating other people's children. *Harvard Educational Review, 58*, 280–298.

Dubetz, N. E. (2012). Understanding the language choices of novice bilingual teachers during sheltered English instruction. *Journal of Multilingual Education Research, 3*(4), 43–62.

Echevarria, J., Short, D., & Powers, K. (2006). School reform and standards-based education: An instructional model for English language learners. *Journal of Educational Research, 99*(4), 195–210.

Every Student Succeeds Act (ESSA), Pub. L. 114-95, 20 U.S.C. § 1177 (2015). https://www.congress.gov/114/plaws/publ95/PLAW-114publ95.pdf

Fuchs, L. S., Deno, S. L., & Marston, D. (1983). Improving the reliability of curriculum-based measures of academic skills for psychoeducational decision making. *Assessment For Effective Intervention, 8*, 135–149. https://doi.org/10.1177/073724778300800301

Fuchs, D., & Fuchs, L. S. (1998). Researchers and teachers working together to adapt instruction for diverse learners. *Learning Disabilities Research & Practice, 13*(3), 126–137.

Fuchs, D., & Fuchs, L. S. (2006). Introduction to response to intervention: What, why, and how valid is it? *Reading Research Quarterly, 41*(1), 93–98.

Gerber, M., Jimenez, T., Leafstedt, J., Villaniz, J., Richards, C., & English, J. (2004). English reading effects of small-group intensive intervention in Spanish for K-1 English learners. *Learning Disabilities Research and Practice, 19*, 239–251.

Gersten, R., Baker, S. K., Shanahan, T., Linan-Thompson, S., Chiappe, P., & Scarcella, R. (2007). *Effective literacy and English language instruction for English learners in the elementary grades: A practice guide (NCEE 2007-4011)*. National Center for Education Evaluation and Regional Assistance, Institute of Education Sciences, U.S. Department of Education. http://ies.ed.gov/ncee/wwc/practiceguides

Geva, E., Yaghoub-Zadeh, Z., & Schuster, B. (2000). Part IV: Reading and foreign language learning: Individual differences in word recognition skills of ESL children. *Annals of Dyslexia, 50*, 121–154.

Goldenberg, C. (2008). Teaching English language learners: What the research does—and does not—say. *American Educator, 12*(2), 8–22.

Gordon, R. S. (1983). An operational classification of disease prevention. *Public Health Reports, 98*(2), 107–109.

Gort, M. (2019). Developing bilingualism and biliteracy in early and middle childhood. *Language Arts, 96*(4), 229–243.

Graves, A., Gersten, R., & Haager, D. (2004). Literacy instruction in multiple-language first-grade classrooms: Linking student outcomes to observed instructional practice. *Learning Disabilities Research and Practice, 19*(4), 262–272.

Gulamhussein, A. (2013). *Teaching the teachers: Effective professional development in an era of high stakes accountability*. National School Board Association, Center for Public Education. http://conference.ohioschoolboards.org/2017/wp-content/uploads/sites/17/2016/07/1pm111317A114Job-embedPD.pdf

Gunn, B., Smolkowski, K., Biglan, A., & Black, C. (2002). Supplemental instruction in decoding skills in Hispanic and non-Hispanic students in early elementary school: A follow-up. *Journal of Special Education, 36*, 69–79.

Hartlep, N. D., & Ellis, A. L. (2012). Just what is response to intervention and what's it doing in a nice field like education? A critical race theory examination of response to intervention. *Counterpoints, 425*, 87–108.

Hoover, J. J., & Soltero-González, L. (2018). Educator preparation for developing culturally responsive MTSS in rural community elementary schools. *Teacher Education and Special Education, 41*(3), 188–202.

Horner, R. H., Sugai, G., Smolkowski, K., Eber, L., Nakasato, J., Todd, A. W., & Esperanza, J. (2009). A randomized, waitlist controlled effectiveness trial assessing school-wide positive behavior support in elementary schools. *Journal of Positive Behavior Interventions, 11*(3), 133–144. https://doi.org/10.1177/1098300709332067

Hosp, J. L., & Reschly, D. J. (2003). Referral rates for intervention or assessment: A meta-analysis of racial differences. *The Journal of Special Education, 37*, 67–80. https://doi.org/10.1177/00224669030370020201

Jackson, D. (2021). *Leveraging MTSS to ensure equitable outcomes*. American Institutes for Research. https://mtss4success.org/sites/default/files/2021-07/MTSS_Equity_Brief.pdf

Johnston, E., D'Andrea Montalbano, P., & Kirkland, D. E. (2017). *Culturally responsive education: A primer for policy and practice*. Metropolitan Center for Research on Equity and the Transformation of Schools, New York University. https://docs.steinhardt.nyu.edu/pdfs/metrocenter/atn293/pdf/CRE_Brief_2017_PrintBooklet_170817.pdf

Kelm, J. L., & McIntosh, K. (2012). Effects of school-wide positive behavior support on teacher self-efficacy. *Psychology in the Schools, 49*(2), 137–147. https://doi.org/10.1002/pits.20624

Kincaid, D., Childs, K., Blase, K. A., & Wallace, F. (2007). Identifying barriers and facilitators in implementing schoolwide positive behavior support. *Journal of Positive Behavior Interventions, 9*(3), 174–184. https://doi.org/10.1177/10983007070090030501

Klingner, J. K., & Edwards, P. A. (2006). Cultural considerations with response to intervention models. *Reading Research Quarterly, 41*(1), 108–117. https://doi.org/10.1598/RRQ.41.1.6

Ladson-Billings, G. (1992). Culturally relevant teaching: The key to making multicultural education work. In C. A. Grant (Ed.), *Research and multicultural education* (pp. 106–121). Falmer Press.

Ladson-Billings, G. (2014). Culturally relevant pedagogy 2.0: A.k.a. the remix. *Harvard Educational Review, 84*(1), 74–84.

Leafstedt, J., Richards, C., & Gerber, M. (2004). Effectiveness of explicit phonological awareness instruction for at-risk English learners. *Learning Disabilities Research and Practice, 19*(4), 252–261.

Lesaux, N., Rupp, A. A., & Siegel, L. S. (2007). Growth in reading skill of children from diverse linguistic backgrounds: Findings from a 5-year longitudinal study. *Journal of Educational Psychology, 99*, 821–834.

Lesh, J. L., Roberts, C., Cavitt, D., & Morales, D. L. (2021). Urban secondary school administrators and faculty perceptions of multitiered system of supports/response to intervention. *NASSP Bulletin, 105*(4), 225–249. https://doi.org/10.1177/01926365211060798

Leverson, M., Smith, K., McIntosh, K., Rose, J., & Pinkelman, S. (2021). *PBIS cultural responsiveness field guide: Resources for trainers and coaches*. Center on PBIS: Positive Behavioral Interventions & Supports. https://www.pbis.org/resource/pbis-cultural-responsiveness-field-guide-resources-for-trainers-and-coaches

Linan-Thompson, S., Ortiz, A. A., & Cavazos, L. (2022). An examination of MTSS assessment and decision-making practices for English learners. *School Psychology Review, 51*(4), 484–497. https://doi.org/10.1080/2372966X.2021.2001690

Marston, D., Mirkin, P., & Deno, S. (1984). Curriculum-based measurement: An alternative to traditional screening, referral, and identification. *The Journal of Special Education, 18*, 109–117. https://doi.org/10.1177/002246698401800204

Moll, L. C., & González, N. (1994). Critical issues: Lessons from research with language minority children. *JRB: A Journal of Literacy, 26*, 439–456.

National Association of Special Education Teachers (NASET). (2023). *Introduction to learning disabilities*. https://www.naset.org/publications/ld-report/introduction-to-learning-disabilities

National Center for Culturally Responsive Educational Systems. (2005). *Cultural considerations and challenges in response-to-intervention models: An NCCRESt position statement*. https://www.isbe.net/Documents/cultural-consid-rti.pdf

National Center for Education Statistics. (2024, May). English Learners in Public Schools. *Condition of Education*. U.S. Department of Education, Institute of Education Sciences. https://nces.ed.gov/programs/coe/indicator/cgf.

Nylén, K., Karlberg, M., Klang, N., & Ogden, T. (2021). Knowledge and will: An explorative study on the implementation of school-wide positive behavior support in Sweden. *Frontiers in Psychology, 12*, 1–20. https://doi.org/10.3389/fpsyg.2021.618099

O'Connor, R. E., Bocian, K. M., Beach, K. D., Sanchez, V., & Flynn, L. J. (2013). Special education in a 4-year response to intervention (RTI) environment: Characteristics of students with learning disabilities and grade of identification. *Learning Disabilities Research and Learning, 28*(3), 98–112. https://doi.org/10.1111/ldrp.12013

O'Connor, R. E., Fulmer, D., Harty, K., & Bell, K. (2005). Layers of reading intervention in kindergarten through third grade: Changes in teaching and child outcomes. *Journal of Learning Disabilities, 38*, 440–455.

Orosco, M. J., & Klingner, J. (2010). One school's implementation of RTI with English language learners: Referring into RTI. *Journal of Learning Disabilities*, 269–288.

Poed, S., & Whitefield, P. (2020). Developments in the implementation of positive behavioral interventions and supports in Australian schools. *Intervention in School & Clinic, 56*(1), 56–60. https://doi.org/10.1177/1053451220910742

Ronfeldt, M., Farmer, S. O., McQueen, K., & Grissom, J. A. (2015). Teacher collaboration in instructional teams and student achievement. *American Educational Research Journal, 52*(3), 475–514. https://doi.org/10.3102/0002831215585562

Rueda, R., & Windmuller, M. P. (2006). English language learners, LD, and overrepresentation: A multi-level analysis. *Journal of Learning Disabilities, 39*, 99–107.

Sabnis, S., Castillo, J. M., & Wolgemuth, J. R. (2020). RTI, equity, and the return to the status quo: Implications for consultants. *Journal of Educational and Psychological Consultation, 30*(3), 285–313. https://doi.org/10.1080/10474412.2019.1674152

Sailor, W., Skritc, T. M., Cohn, M., & Olmstead, C. (2021). Preparing teacher educators for statewide scale-up of multi-tiered system of support (MTSS). *Teacher Education and Special Education, 44*(1), 24–41. https://doi.org/10.1177/0888406420938035

Saunders, W., Foorman, B., & Carlson, C. (2006). Is a separate block of time for oral English language development in programs for English learners needed? *Elementary School Journal, 107*(2), 181–198.

Schiller, E., Chow, K., Thayer, S., Nakamura, J., Wilkerson, S. B., & Puma, M. (2020). *What tools have states developed or adapted to assess schools' implementation of a multi-tiered system of supports/response to intervention framework?* (REL 2020-017). U.S. Department of Education, Institute of Education Sciences, National Center for Education Evaluation and Regional Assistance, Regional Educational Laboratory Appalachia. https://ies.ed.gov/ncee/rel/regions/appalachia/pdf/REL_2020017.pdf

Shapiro, E. S. (2014). Tiered instruction and intervention in a response-to-intervention model. *RTI Action Network.* http://www.rtinetwork.org/essential/tieredinstruction/tiered-instruction-and-intervention-rti-model

Simmons, D. C., Coyne, M. D., Kwok, O., McDonagh, S., Harn, B. A., & Kame'enui, E. J. (2008). Indexing response to intervention: A longitudinal study of reading risk from kindergarten through third grade. *Journal of Learning Disabilities, 41*, 158–173.

Solano-Flores, G. (2008). Who is given tests in what language by whom, when, and where? The need for probabilistic views of language in the testing of English language learners. *Educational Researcher, 37*(4), 189–199. https://doi.org/10.3102/0013189X08319569

Sullivan, A. L. (2011). Disproportionality in special education identification and placement of English language learners. *Council for Exceptional Children, 77*(3), 317–334. https://doi.org/10.1177/001440291107700304

Sugai, G., & Horner, R. H. (2009). Responsiveness-to-intervention and school-wide positive behavior supports: Integration of multi-tiered system approaches. *Exceptionality, 17*, 223–237. https://doi.org/10.1080/09362830903235375

Sugai, G., & Horner, R. H. (2020). Sustaining and scaling positive behavioral interventions and supports: Implementation drivers, outcomes, and considerations. *Exceptional Children, 86*, 120–136. https://doi.org/10.1177/0014402919855331

Thorius, K. A. K., & Maxcy, B. D. (2015). Critical practice analysis of special education policy: An RTI example. *Remedial and Special Education, 36*(2), 116–124. https://doi.org/10.1177/0741932514550812

Thurlow, M. L., Ghere, G., Lazarus, S. S., & Liu, K. K. (2020). *MTSS for all: Including students with the most significant cognitive disabilities*. National Center on Educational Outcomes, TIES Center. https://nceo.umn.edu/docs/OnlinePubs/NCEOBriefMTSS.pdf

U.S. Census Bureau. (2020). *2020 U.S. population more racially and ethnically diverse than measured in 2010*. https://www.census.gov/library/stories/2021/08/2020-united-states-population-more-racially-ethnically-diverse-than-2010.html

Vaughn, S., Linan-Thompson, S., Mathes, P. G., Cirino, P. T., Carlson, C., Francis, D. G., Durodola, S. P., & Hagan, E. C. (2006). Effectiveness of Spanish intervention for first-grade English language learners at risk for reading difficulties. *Journal of Learning Disabilities, 39*, 56–73.

Vaughn, S., Mathes, P. G., Linan-Thompson, S., & Francis, D. (2005). Teaching English language learners at-risk for reading disabilities to read: Putting research into practice. *Learning Disabilities Research and Practice, 20*, 58–67.

Vellutino, F. R., Scanlon, D. M., Zhang, H., & Schatschneider, C. (2008). Using response to kindergarten and first grade to identify children at-risk for long-term reading difficulties. *Reading and Writing, 21*, 437–480.

Vincent, C. G., Randall, C., Cartledge, G., Tobin, T. J., & Swain-Bradway, J. (2011). Toward a conceptual integration of cultural responsiveness and schoolwide positive behavior. *Journal of Positive Behavior Interventions, 13*(4), 219–229. https://doi.org/10.1177/1098300711399765

Wanzek, J., & Vaughn, S. (2011). Is a three-tier reading intervention model associated with reduced placement in special education. *Remedial and Special Education, 32*, 167–175.

Warikoo, N., & Carter, P. (2009). Cultural Explanations for racial and ethnic stratification in academic achievement: A call for new and improved theory. *Review of Educational Research, 79*(1), 366–394. https://doi.org/10.3102/0034654308326162

Wiley, H. L., & Deno, S. L. (2005). Oral reading and maze measures as predictors of success for English learners on a state standards assessment. *Remedial and Special Education, 26*, 207–214.

Willis, A. I. (2019). Race, response to intervention, and reading research. *Journal of Literacy Research, 51*(4), 394–419.

Witzel, B., & Clarke, B. (2015). Benefits of using a multi-tiered system of supports to improve inclusive practices. *Focus on Inclusive Education, 91*(3), 215–219. https://doi.org/10.1080/00094056.2015.1047315

Young, C. Y., Wright, J. V., & Laster, J. (2005). Instructing African American students. *Education, 125*(3), 516–524.

Chapter 5
Engaging in Family–School Partnerships to Support Emergent Bilingual Youth Through Multitiered System of Supports

Rachel T. Santiago and Anisa N. Goforth

Families are foundational for youth development. They play a critical role in helping their youth learn and grow, and this role can look different across development, depending on the youth's age, strengths, and needs. Further, there are many ways to be a family (e.g., by relation, by marriage, or as chosen kin), with common themes of providing social support, shared time, and emotional intimacy (Jenicek & MacIntosh, 2023). Although there are commonalities, the conceptualization of family is shaped by culture. Parenting styles and disciplinary practices may differ based on underlying values of the youth's socialization (Domenech Rodríguez et al., 2009). For example, there may be cultural differences in parenting style, socialization goals, and parental practices; immigrant Chinese parents may emphasize more filial piety in their socialization goals for their children compared to white parents (Chao, 2000). Further, there may be differences within families, where differences in acculturation or language between families and their youth may impact their relationships. Differences in acculturation between Arab American adolescents and their parents, for example, were associated with more adolescent behavior problems (Goforth et al., 2015). Cultural differences across groups, as well as between parents and their children, reflect the importance of grounding supports within family context.

These cultural and contextual differences may pose particular challenges in the United States when youth enter formal schooling. Families' roles in their youth's

R. T. Santiago (✉)
Department of Educational, School, and Counseling Psychology and the Missouri Prevention Science Institute, University of Missouri, Columbia, MO, USA
e-mail: rsantiago@missouri.edu

A. N. Goforth
Department of Psychology, University of Montana, Missoula, MT, USA
e-mail: anisa.goforth@umontana.edu

D. Vega, J. N. Wolf (eds.), *Culturally and Linguistically Responsive Intervention and Assessment Practices with Emergent Bilingual Students*,
https://doi.org/10.1007/978-3-032-02084-0_5

development change as they encounter an educational system that may have different priorities and perspectives than their own. Given the role of schools in youth development (youth spend more time in school than any other non-home setting; Eccles & Roeser, 2010), it is essential for families and schools to collaborate with each other to best serve youth. These collaborations can occur within multi-tiered system of supports (MTSS), which is grounded in data-based decision-making, evidence-based practices, problem-solving, and team-based processes (Freeman et al., 2016). Intentional efforts to integrate families into the framework as active partners may enhance academic, behavioral, and social–emotional outcomes (Garbacz et al., 2017).

Although terms like family–school partnership, family educational involvement, and family engagement are often used interchangeably, they are distinct constructs (Sheridan et al., 2016). *Family–school partnerships* are youth-focused approaches in which families and schools work together with a shared goal of supporting youth development (Sheridan et al., 2012). *Family educational involvement* refers to the ways in which caregivers support youth development (Sheridan et al., 2012). These activities can take place at home, at school, and within communication between the two settings (Fantuzzo et al., 2000). *Family engagement* is generally unidirectional, moving from school to home, and can include things like invitations extended from schools to families to encourage participation (Sheridan et al., 2016). In short, family–school partnerships are about the relationship between families and schools, family educational involvement is about family behaviors, and family engagement is about information and invitations from school to home (Sheridan et al., 2012).

For specific groups of youth, such as emergent bilingual youth, the family–school partnership has unique considerations. Emergent bilingual youth and their families experience educational settings at the intersection of culture, language, and other dimensions of context. Thus, the purpose of this chapter is to highlight some of the unique considerations for family–school partnerships for emergent bilingual youth. First, we describe the theoretical underpinnings of family–school partnerships, emphasizing anti-oppressive frameworks that can be particularly relevant for working with emergent bilingual youth and their families who are often racially or ethnically minoritized. We then describe ways that family–school partnerships can be fostered within MTSS, providing recommendations that are useful for school personnel to consider. Finally, we highlight specific strategies that can be implemented across tiers that are grounded in strengths-based, culturally responsive approaches.

Relevant Developmental, Ecological, and Anti-oppressive Frameworks

When considering family–school partnerships for emergent bilingual youth, it is important to consider sociocultural contexts that shape those partnerships and the oppressive systems that may impact the youth, families, and schools. There are multiple theories that help guide our understanding of these contexts in fostering positive family–school partnerships. We have organized these theoretical underpinnings and frameworks into two categories: (a) developmental and ecological theories and (b) critical theories and anti-oppressive frameworks.

Developmental and Ecological Theories

To foster family–school partnerships, it is important to consider emergent bilingual youth's various sociocultural and ecological contexts. Ecological systems theory (Bronfenbrenner, 1979) provides a strong theoretical framework by highlighting the role of interconnected, nested contexts. Microsystems (the ecological contexts in individuals' immediate environments) include contexts like emergent bilingual youth's home, school, and community environments, while mesosystem (interactions among microsystems) reflects the family–school interactions and relationships. Thus, a youth's microsystem may include participating in their Catholic parish while their mesosystem includes family–parish interactions. Exosystems (more distal social and structural influences) include contexts like parents' work setting and local government policies. For example, state educational policies related to language immersion in schools may indirectly impact emergent bilingual youth. Finally, macrosystems (broader cultural and subcultural patterns in society) include the family's heritage, cultural norms, or perceptions of the educational system. All of these contexts are nested within chronosystems, which are historical events that occur within the course of one's lifetime (e.g., the COVID-19 pandemic).

These multiple systems influence youth's development, yet the foundational theories did not explicitly account for factors that affect the development of racially and ethnically minoritized youth. The Phenomenological Variant of Ecological Systems Theory (PVEST; Spencer et al., 1997), as well as García Coll et al.s' integrative model (1996), emphasize identity development, particularly for youth from minoritized communities, from a cultural ecological perspective (Hicklen House, 2020). PVEST posits that individuals continuously redefine their identities as they navigate environments. Importantly, there is an emphasis on how an individual experiences their environment within the broader context of cultural strengths and identities. Similarly, the integrative model emphasizes that development for minoritized youth must consider their environments (e.g., how specific contexts contribute to positive outcomes) while simultaneously acknowledging how racism, discrimination, oppression, and segregation uniquely affect minoritized youth. For example, a youth who is a first-generation immigrant from Guatemala may be navigating how to maintain their heritage culture and language (e.g., Spanish), integrating within the host culture (e.g., US culture) while simultaneously navigating the oppressive systems of the United States. Thus, these theories emphasize that for emergent bilinguals' development, there must be attention to cultural context.

These sociocultural factors must also incorporate the role of language in emergent bilingual youth development. Vygotsky's sociocultural theory posits that individual development originates in social sources—namely, that development occurs in a cultural context, is mediated by language, and is shaped by the historical context (John-Steiner & Mahn, 2003; Vygotsky, 1978). The role of language as a mediating factor in development is particularly important to understand for emergent bilingual youth, given the relevance of second (or third) language acquisition and how language shapes brain development. For example, in a fascinating study highlighting the connection between language and the conceptualization of time, Mandarin speakers tended to think about time vertically, even when thinking and communicating in English, which generally describes time horizontally (Boroditsky, 2001). Thus, language and brain development (particularly across different sociocultural contexts) may be particularly important contexts for supporting emergent bilingual youth.

In addition, the relationship between language and development is connected to broader macrosystemic influences. Linguicism (i.e., linguistic discrimination) contributes to English-centric practices and policies. For example, verbal English-language assessments may yield scores reflecting English proficiency or cultural knowledge rather than the construct of interest (Ortiz, 2019). This may influence disproportionalities in special education. Emergent bilingual youth are more likely than their white peers to be identified as having a learning disability or intellectual disability (Sullivan, 2011). These disproportionalities persist despite the decades-old legal requirement to attend to culture and language in assessment (Diana v. State Board of Education, 1970). Linguicism also shapes social discrimination based on language and accent (Liggett, 2014), which families teach their children to navigate. In short, language is both an important part of cultural identity and a target for discrimination (Murillo & Smith, 2011), which influences the social and developmental context of emergent bilingual youth.

Critical Theories and Anti-oppressive Frameworks

Emergent bilingual youth and their families have cultural strengths and assets that positively influence their development and education. These strengths can be supported within a liberation psychology perspective that centers empowerment, healing, and transformation (Comas-Díaz & Torres Rivera, 2020). This strengths-based, change-focused approach challenges existing paradigms of traditional theories because it involves approaches for understanding and addressing oppression in society. For emergent bilingual youth, this includes fostering their development of critical consciousness—which includes an awareness of systemic inequities and discrimination—as well as empowering them to advocate for their learning and well-being.

This development of critical consciousness and understanding of systems of privilege and oppression for emergent bilinguals are similarly promoted by critical theories. Much of this is grounded in critical race theory, which posits that racism is embedded into social structures and institutions (Crenshaw et al., 1995). By using critical race theory as an avenue for understanding the historical and contemporary context of education within the United States, we can begin to parse out the ways in which systems of privilege and oppression are embedded into educational systems, policies, and practices (Ladson-Billings, 2021). For example, official curricula implemented in educational systems are "culturally specific artifacts" that aim to maintain narratives of the dominant group as standard knowledge (Ladson-Billings, 1998, p. 18).

Although language is not synonymous with race, the ways in which US society approaches language are highly racialized; therefore, how we talk about language and multilingualism is influenced by systems of racial power, privilege, and oppression (Liggett, 2014). Other critical theories focus on cultural context. For example, in working with emergent bilingual youth and families from Latine communities, we can be informed by LatCrit, a complement to critical race theory that integrates considerations of language and Latinidad (Solórzano & Delgado Bernal, 2001). In integrating considerations of ableism and disability in supporting emergent bilingual youth receiving services within more intensive tiers of the MTSS continuum, we can be informed by DisCrit, which aims to clarify connections between racism and ableism (Annamma et al., 2013). Similarly, we can be informed by TribalCrit (Brayboy, 2005), which considers how colonization is endemic within the educational system and how honoring tribal sovereignty can be important in supporting Indigenous emergent bilingual youth. Overall, critical theories can play an important role in understanding the sociopolitical context that shapes how emergent bilingual youth and their families experience educational systems.

In translating these principles into action, it is essential to take strengths-based approaches which are inherently intertwined with youth and family cultural context. The community cultural wealth framework is derived from critical race theory and aims to shift away from deficit views to instead center cultural capital—the "cultural knowledge, skills, abilities, and contacts" that empower communities, foster survival, and provide avenues for resisting oppression (Yosso, 2005, p. 69). Yosso identifies six types of cultural capital: aspirational, linguistic, familial, social, navigational, and resistance. Emergent bilingual youth and their families have diverse forms of cultural capital at the intersection of language and cultural context. For example, families may prioritize multilingualism for their children as a path to reaching goals; this form of aspirational capital can be an important foundation for collaboration between families and schools (Project LEE et al., 2021) but is also a source of potential conflict when schools do not value, promote, or prioritize multilingualism.

In sum, across these theories and frameworks, a few key concepts regarding emergent bilingual youth and families become clear. First, emergent bilingual youth develop within interconnected social contexts that shape their identities and the mechanisms they develop for navigating educational settings. Second, these experiences are shaped by long-standing systems of oppression and discrimination, including on the basis of language and culture. Finally, challenging these systems and supporting the growth of emergent bilingual youth requires attention to youth and family cultural wealth. Overall, to foster positive family–school partnerships for emergent bilingual youth, we must consider all of these components and intentionally acknowledge emergent bilinguals' unique contexts and strengths.

Support for Family–School Partnerships Within MTSS

Family–school partnerships have been shown to be associated with positive youth outcomes through decades of research. Families' involvement in their children's education is associated with improved academic achievement (Castro et al., 2015), behavioral and social–emotional outcomes (Sheridan et al., 2019), and other educational outcomes (e.g., attendance, class preparation; Simon, 2001). Additionally, collaborative partnerships between families and schools have the potential to improve child outcomes. For example, a meta-analytic study found that interpersonal and relational factors in family–school relationships were associated with positive behavioral and social–emotional outcomes (Sheridan et al., 2019), suggesting that the relationship itself—beyond the contributions of one individual—has implications for youth.

Given the important role that families play in youth development and the clear positive outcomes for youth, family–school partnerships are well-aligned with MTSS structures (Garbacz et al., 2020). The overall aim of MTSS is to promote student outcomes using screening and evidence-based practices. Specifically, the objective of each tier of MTSS—Tier 1 (universal), Tier 2 (selected), and Tier 3 (intensive)—is to deliver appropriate student support based on their needs in an identified area (e.g., academics, behavior, mental health).

Families can be active partners throughout the MTSS continuum. For example, Weingarten et al. (2020) identified that at Tier 1, these partnerships could include forming positive relationships, maintaining ongoing bidirectional communication, and sharing information about the MTSS framework. At Tier 2, this partnership could include ongoing communication regarding interventions, goals, and progress updates, as well as sharing strategies that may be useful for supporting youth's learning and behavior outside of school. Finally, at Tier 3, this partnership could include problem-solving to ensure supports are contextually relevant and individualized to youth's strengths and needs, as well as actively collaborating to develop intervention plans and review data. These approaches to active partnership emphasize the positive relationships that build on emergent bilingual youth's strengths.

Families of emergent bilingual youth bring perspectives, values, and beliefs that can contribute to culturally responsive MTSS structures and practices. However, there is often a disconnect between these families and school personnel. Families are often not familiar with the dominant culture of school environments within the United States, and educators often do not know how family culture and language affect norms, expectations, and values (Zacarian, 2023). For example, in many Spanish-speaking families from Latine communities, the concept of *bien educado* dictates that a good education goes beyond academic learning to encompass moral development and respectful behavior (Perrigo et al., 2023); when school personnel are not familiar with that concept, their efforts to develop behavioral expectations may not align with families' values. Similarly, for Indigenous communities, the historical impacts of colonization and subsequent kidnapping of children to residential schools may influence the family's perspectives of contemporary public schools

(Evans-Campbell & Campbell, 2011). Thus, for Latine and Indigenous communities, families of emergent bilingual youth highly value their children's education (Vera et al., 2012), but their support may be less visible to school personnel (e.g., homework help, seeking resources outside of school; Vakil et al., 2023), resulting in school personnel erroneously believing that families are not involved or do not want to be involved.

Together, this suggests that developing effective MTSS for emergent bilingual youth requires fostering an understanding of both home and school contexts, as well as the use of both traditional and non-traditional strategies to foster collaborative partnerships between families and schools to support emergent bilingual youth (Tarasawa & Waggoner, 2015). To develop positive family–school relationships with emergent bilingual families, it is important for schools to work on bridging cultural divides, integrating family advocacy, connecting family involvement to learning, and working together in service of youth's best interests (Zacarian, 2023). These approaches can be embedded within MTSS frameworks to shape culturally responsive services across the continuum of supports.

Recommendations for Culturally Responsive Family–School Partnerships in MTSS

There are myriad ways that school personnel can engage in family–school partnerships within MTSS. In this section, we highlight a number of recommendations that educators, staff, and administrators may consider to effectively engage and partner with families and community members to support emergent bilingual youth. These recommendations (summarized in Fig. 5.1) include (a) building relationships and fostering equitable schools; (b) collaborative decision-making in assessment and intervention; and (c) establishing educator and staff professional development training and leadership in family engagement.

Building Relationships and Fostering Equitable Schools

Relationships between families and schools are essential for fostering equitable school environments. For families of emergent bilingual youth, this relationship is particularly important because of the unique ways linguistic and cultural context shape youth development and their school experiences. Consistent and multidirectional communication between schools and families is essential for fostering strong relationships. Indeed, authentic and equitable partnerships are an important aspect of culturally responsive practice (Goforth & Pham, 2023). Weingarten et al. (2020) emphasized that communication must be multidirectional between schools and families of emergent bilingual youth. For example, they suggested that all communication should focus on strengths and the sociocultural context. Multidirectional

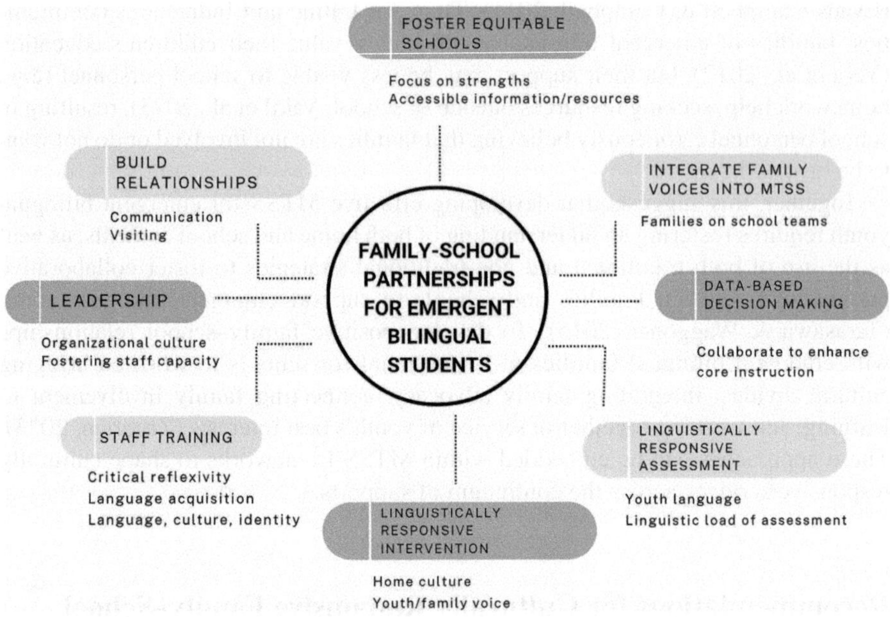

Fig. 5.1 Recommendations for family–school partnerships to support emergent bilingual youth

communication should also include diverse methods, such as home visits. Visiting, or being in relation across time and space, may be a particularly culturally responsive practice because it fosters respect and reciprocity (Tuck et al., 2023). Thus, when collaborating with a family of an emergent bilingual student, educators could visit their home and the initial conversations should focus on student strengths. Hospitality and visiting are often deeply cultural, and engaging with families in this way may enhance respect and trust and promote a positive relationship.

This focus on visiting and thus promoting authentic and equitable partnerships can be a foundation within an MTSS model with the goal of enhancing equity for emergent bilingual youth. Educators should also build awareness of MTSS and how special education fits within this model. Weingarten et al. (2020) suggested that schools provide a guide for families or post information on the school websites. For families of emergent bilingual youth, this also means ensuring that the information is not only appropriately translated but also culturally responsive. Educators could consider how to ensure that families' voices are part of the MTSS process (e.g., leadership teams). Bryan and Henry (2012) propose a School–Family–Community Partnership Process Model for building partnerships. The model has seven stages:

1. Preparing to partner (understanding attitudes and developing buy-in)
2. Assessing needs and strengths (gathering information from students, families, and community members to identify assets and priorities)
3. Coming together (meeting with potential team partners)
4. Creating a shared vision and plan (specifying a vision and goals for the partnership)

5. Taking action (collaboratively implement the plan)
6. Evaluating and celebrating progress (gathering information to identify what is going well and what needs changing) and
7. Maintaining momentum (revisiting and revising the plan for sustainability)

Empowerment, democratic collaboration, strengths-focused, and social justice are key elements across all stages (Bryan & Henry, 2012). These elements and stages highlight the importance of relationship-building and ongoing collaboration between families and schools.

Bryan and Henry also provide key questions to ask at each stage. For example, in Stage 1 (Preparing to Partner), relevant questions include "What are your beliefs, attitudes, and values about families?" and "Why should the administration give you the opportunity to build partnerships?" (Bryan & Henry, p. 412). In a more action-oriented stage (Stage 5, Taking Action), relevant questions to ask include "What is the timeline and implementation plan?" and "How will you overcome any barriers and challenges you expect in implementing your plan?" (Bryan & Henry, p. 412). We refer interested readers to Bryan and Henry's chapter (freely available) for an in-depth exploration of the stages, as well as a visual depiction of the model.

Collaborative Decision-Making in Assessment and Intervention

In addition to having positive relationships between school and families as the foundation for MTSS, there should also be collaborative data-based decision-making across all three tiers. This collaboration can foster use of culturally and linguistically responsive assessment and intervention to promote positive academic and social–emotional–behavioral outcomes.

Tiers 1 and 2

At Tier 1, families can be closely involved in enhancing core instruction and behavior expectations. Schools can also ensure the presence of culturally sustaining curricula for emergent bilingual youth (Garcia, 2019). For example, to support Indigenous youth, schools may need to consider how to effectively engage with families that acknowledge the colonization within the education system. Garcia (2019) provides a model of culturally sustaining Indigenous family engagement, where there is a "space for critical dialogues that empowers individuals, validates identities, and co-constructs spaces for collective agency for Indigenous education" (p. 84), thus acknowledging the harm of colonization and reclaiming Indigenous identity, history, and language. Given the close ties of language, identity, and culture, this model promotes family engagement in the school system where they are honored and supported.

At the Tier 1 and Tier 2, families also can be closely involved in the assessment and data-based decision-making process. Linan-Thompson et al. (2018) suggest that culturally responsive components in schools include providing explicit and systematic instruction as well as ongoing assessment. Schools could partner with families in making meaning from the assessment, and how the data gathered could inform intervention. That is, families could provide information about the youth's cultural background which provides context to the data. For example, in working with a Hmong second grader referred for Tier 2 reading intervention for decoding skills, educators should partner with the family to fully understand the Hmong cultural and language context. The family may provide information about the Hmong language structure and cultural norms that may be important in contextualizing student language and literacy development, which can guide the selection of appropriate reading intervention strategies, particularly if there are concerns that the student may have a reading disability.

It is important also for schools to consider how they make this collaborative decision-making accessible to families of emergent bilingual youth. Weingarten et al. (2020) recommended sharing screening data during conferences to ensure that there is consistent communication, and once the student is receiving Tier 2 or Tier 3 interventions, families should participate in intervention planning meetings. Importantly, they recommended that there be multiple formats for meetings that respect families' various work schedules, such as using video conference software. Across these activities, it is essential to use the services of a trained interpreter who is able to translate language as well as culture, to ensure mutual understanding between families and schools (Banerjee & Guiberson, 2012).

Tier 3 and Special Education

At Tier 3, family–school partnerships are essential for informing culturally responsive interventions. For example, in planning social and behavioral interventions or counseling, the cultural understandings of the family can shape how the family and student conceptualize mental health (Cauce et al., 2002). When an emergent bilingual youth is referred for Tier 3 interventions, it would be critical to consider how the family's conceptualization of the concerns may determine whether they allow the youth to obtain services, as well as how those services might be most effective. For example, some cultural groups, such as Chinese Americans, may perceive that somatic distress (e.g., stomach aches) would be more socially acceptable compared to other types of symptoms, such as feelings of depression (Kung & Lu, 2008). Given that language and culture are integrally tied, including families at this tier of support would help ensure that interventions are chosen that are culturally responsive.

Strong family–school partnerships can be helpful when navigating the special education process. When school psychologists are conducting testing as a component of the broader assessment, the family's perspectives and contributions would be critical. For example, the family could provide specific information about the student's language skills if the concerns were associated with a specific learning disability in reading. School psychologists or special educators should provide the family with information about the process, as well as ensure that families understand that they are valued members of the multidisciplinary team. Cultural brokers may also be useful within the special education process, as navigating the complex system can feel overwhelming for families. In one study, Latina mothers emphasized the importance of cultural brokers in the special education process, from understanding specific paperwork to discussing accommodations with educators (Mortier et al., 2021). Brokers and families provided specific recommendations for schools, highlighting that educators should be culturally humble, create a welcoming environment, and use strengths-based language.

Teachers may be concerned about referring emergent bilingual students for special education because of fears that the students would be overidentified (and given the data on overrepresentation in special education, this may indeed be justified; Sullivan, 2011). Yet, learning disabilities in reading occur across multiple languages (Peterson & Pennington, 2012), and it is important that emergent bilingual students have equitable access to accommodations and services if they indeed have a disability. For academic concerns, families can provide important information about their skills in their first language. In addition, given the linguistic demands of many assessments (Ortiz, 2002) and the lack of representation in many standardized assessments' normative samples (Vega & Wolf, 2023), families can provide perspective on considerations for choosing appropriate assessment tools and non-standardized approaches to yield a more accurate depiction of their child's skills. For example, schools and families could discuss how interviews, informal measures (e.g., language samples), observations, and permanent products (e.g., classroom work samples) could be used to gather comprehensive information on a student's strengths and needs (Vega & Wolf, 2023). We refer readers to Chap. 10 of this book for a more comprehensive overview of assessment with emergent bilingual students.

Staff Professional Training and Leadership to Support Family Engagement

Many educators do not receive specific training in developing family–school partnerships during their teacher preparation programs. Preservice training often focuses more on classroom teaching skills than on interpersonal skills for working with families (Hiatt-Michael, 2006); one study found that teacher educators and student teachers both reported concerns about preservice teachers' ability to work with families (D'Haem & Griswold, 2017). In addition, many teachers specifically feel unprepared to work with emergent bilingual youth and their families (Chen et al., 2008). Given the importance of developing positive, collaborative relationships with families of emergent bilingual youth across all tiers of MTSS, it is essential to support teachers in developing these skills. Thus, as a final recommendation, family–school partnerships can be fostered through professional development training and leadership.

Professional development could include engaging in critical reflexivity. Characterized as an intentional process of reflection and self-critique (Goforth &

Pham, 2023), critical reflexivity can be an important component of culturally responsive practices. Understanding one's own worldview and how one's lived experiences may shape these worldviews is important when engaging with families whose worldviews, cultures, and norms may be substantially different. Critical reflexive prompts or questions during professional development trainings may help foster more empathy and understanding within family–school partnerships. For example, prompts may include, "When interacting with a family of an emergent bilingual student, describe your immediate thoughts or feelings" or "When establishing partnerships, what aspects of your worldview overlap with the families? What might be different?" Administrators play a particularly important role in these efforts as part of their own culturally responsive leadership (Genao, 2021). This includes cultivating and sustaining an organizational climate that integrates critical reflexivity, as well as holding oneself accountable as a school leader.

In addition to critical reflexive prompts, educators and administrators may benefit from specific training on best practices related to second language acquisition and the connections among language, culture, and identity. The process of second language acquisition may not be incorporated in all pre-service training programs; thus, additional training can help educators not only understand the process of language acquisition for emergent bilinguals but also debunk any myths (e.g., learning an additional language "confuses" children). Further, there may be a lack of knowledge about the connection among language, culture, and identity. For example, for Indigenous youth, learning their Indigenous language is also about self-determination, sovereignty, identity, and their connection to place (McCarty et al., 2021).

Conclusion

Emergent bilingual youth develop within the sociocultural and ecological contexts of their communities and bring unique cultural strengths that shape their experiences. Families of emergent bilingual youth play a critical role in their development and are essential partners in their educational growth. As schools identify and develop MTSS structures to promote positive outcomes for all youth, it is important to emphasize approaches in structural (e.g., leadership and staff skills and capacity) and relational (e.g., communicating with families) domains, in order to ultimately foster equitable school environments and honor the cultural and linguistic assets of emergent bilingual youth and their families.

References

Annamma, S. A., Connor, D., & Ferri, B. (2013). Dis/ability critical race studies (DisCrit): Theorizing at the intersections of race and dis/ability. *Race Ethnicity and Education, 16*(1), 1–31. https://doi.org/10.1080/13613324.2012.730511

Banerjee, R., & Guiberson, M. (2012). Evaluating young children from culturally and linguistically diverse backgrounds for special education services. *Young Exceptional Children, 15*(1), 33–45. https://doi.org/10.1177/1096250611435368

Boroditsky, L. (2001). Does language shape thought?: Mandarin and English speakers' conceptions of time. *Cognitive Psychology, 43*(1), 1–22. https://doi.org/10.1006/cogp.2001.0748

Brayboy, B. M. K. J. (2005). Toward a tribal critical race theory in education. *Urban Review, 37*(5), 425–446. https://doi.org/10.1007/s11256-005-0018-y

Bronfenbrenner, U. (1979). *The ecology of human development: Experiments by nature and design*. Harvard University Press.

Bryan, J., & Henry, L. (2012). A model for building school–family–community partnerships: Principles and process. *Journal of Counseling & Development, 90*(4), 408–420. https://doi.org/10.1002/j.1556-6676.2012.00052.x

Castro, M., Expósito-Casas, E., López-Martín, E., Lizasoain, L., Navarro-Asencio, E., & Gaviria, J. L. (2015). Parental involvement on student academic achievement: A meta-analysis. *Educational Research Review, 14*, 33–46. https://doi.org/10.1016/j.edurev.2015.01.002

Cauce, A. M., Domenech-Rodríguez, M., Paradise, M., Cochran, B. N., Shea, J. M., Srebnik, D., & Baydar, N. (2002). Cultural and contextual influences in mental health help seeking: A focus on ethnic minority youth. *Journal of Consulting and Clinical Psychology, 70*(1), 44–55. https://doi.org/10.1037/0022-006X.70.1.44

Chao, R. K. (2000). The parenting of immigrant Chinese and European American mothers: Relations between parenting styles, socialization goals, and parental practices. *Journal of Applied Developmental Psychology, 21*(2), 233–248. https://doi.org/10.1016/S0193-3973(99)00037-4

Chen, C.-T., Kyle, D. W., & McIntyre, E. (2008). Helping teachers work effectively with English Language Learners and their families. *School Community Journal, 18*(1), 7–20.

Comas-Díaz, L., & Torres Rivera, E. (Eds.). (2020). *Liberation psychology: Theory, method, practice, and social justice*. American Psychological Association.

Crenshaw, K., Gotanda, N., Peller, G., & Thomas, K. (1995). *Critical race theory: The key writings that formed the movement*. The New Press.

D'Haem, J., & Griswold, P. (2017). Teacher educators' and student teachers' beliefs about preparation for working with families including those from diverse socioeconomic and cultural backgrounds. *Education and Urban Society, 49*(1), 81–109. https://doi.org/10.1177/0013124516630602

Diana v. State Board of Education. Civil Action No. C-70-37 (N. D. Cal. 1970).

Domenech Rodríguez, M. M., Donovick, M. R., & Crowley, S. L. (2009). Parenting styles in a cultural context: Observations of "protective parenting" in first-generation Latinos. *Family Process, 48*(2), 195–210. https://doi.org/10.1111/j.1545-5300.2009.01277.x

Eccles, J. S., & Roeser, R. W. (2010). An ecological view of schools and development. In *Handbook of research on schools, schooling and human development* (pp. 6–22). Taylor and Francis. https://doi.org/10.4324/9780203874844.ch2

Evans-Campbell, T., & Campbell, C. (2011). Historical trauma and native child development. In P. Farrell, P. Spicer, H. Fitzgerald, & M. Sarche (Eds.), *American Indian and Alaska Native children's mental health: Development and context*. Praegar.

Fantuzzo, J., Tighe, E., & Childs, S. (2000). Family Involvement Questionnaire: A multivariate assessment of family participation in early childhood education. *Journal of Educational Psychology, 92*(2), 367–376. https://doi.org/10.1037/0022-0663.92.2.367

Freeman, J., Simonsen, B., McCoach, D. B., Sugai, G., Lombardi, A., & Horner, R. (2016). Relationship between school-wide positive behavior interventions and supports and academic, attendance, and behavior outcomes in high schools. *Journal of Positive Behavior Interventions, 18*(1), 41–51. https://doi.org/10.1177/1098300715580992

Garbacz, S. A., Herman, K. C., Thompson, A. M., & Reinke, W. M. (2017). Family engagement in education and intervention: Implementation and evaluation to maximize family, school, and student outcomes. *Journal of School Psychology, 62*, 1–10. https://doi.org/10.1016/j.jsp.2017.04.002

Garbacz, S. A., Vatland, C. H., Kern, L., von der Embse, N. P., Novotnak, T., Minch, D. R., & Weist, M. D. (2020). Family–school partnerships within tiered systems of support to increase access, improve equity, and promote positive outcomes for all children and families. In C. S. Clauss-Ehlers, A. B. Sood, & M. D. Weist (Eds.), *Social justice for children and young people: International perspectives*. Cambridge University Press. https://doi.org/10.1017/9781108551830.013

García Coll, C., Lamberty, G., Jenkins, R., McAdoo, H. P., Crnic, K., Wasik, B. H., & Vázquez García, H. (1996). An integrative model for the study of developmental competencies in minority children. *Child Development, 67*(5), 1891–1914. https://doi.org/10.2307/1131600

Garcia, J. (2019). Critical and culturally sustaining Indigenous family and community engagement in education. In *The Wiley handbook of family, school, and community relationships in education* (pp. 71–90). Wiley. https://doi.org/10.1002/9781119083054.ch4

Genao, S. (2021). Doing it for culturally responsive school leadership: Utilizing reflexivity from preparation to practice. *Journal of Research on Leadership Education, 16*(2), 158–170. https://doi.org/10.1177/19427751211002226

Goforth, A. N., & Pham, A. V. (2023). *Culturally responsive school-based practices: Supporting mental health and learning of diverse students*. Oxford University Press. https://doi.org/10.1093/med-psych/9780197516928.001.0001

Goforth, A. N., Pham, A. V., & Oka, E. R. (2015). Parent–child conflict, acculturation gap, acculturative stress, and behavior problems in Arab American adolescents. *Journal of Cross-Cultural Psychology, 46*(6), 821–836. https://doi.org/10.1177/0022022115585140

Hiatt-Michael, D. B. (2006). Reflections and directions on research related to family-community involvement in schooling. *School Community Journal, 16*(1), 7–30.

Hicklen House, S. (2020). Implementing culturally responsive practices in family–school partnership programs. In S. A. Garbacz (Ed.), *Establishing family–school partnerships in school psychology: Critical skills* (pp. 135–151). Routledge.

Jenicek, A., & MacIntosh, H. (2023). What about our chosen kin? Determining who counts as family within family therapy. *Revue Intervention, Hors série, 2*, 81–89.

John-Steiner, V., & Mahn, H. (2003). Sociocultural contexts for teaching and learning. In I. B. Weiner (Ed.), *Handbook of psychology* (1st ed., pp. 123–151). Wiley. https://doi.org/10.1002/0471264385.wei0707

Kung, W. W., & Lu, P.-C. (2008). How symptom manifestations affect help seeking for mental health problems among Chinese Americans. *The Journal of Nervous and Mental Disease, 196*(1), 46. https://doi.org/10.1097/NMD.0b013e31815fa4f9

Ladson-Billings, G. (1998). Just what is critical race theory and what's it doing in a nice field like education? *International Journal of Qualitative Studies in Education, 11*(1), 7–24. https://doi.org/10.1080/095183998236863

Ladson-Billings, G. (2021). *Critical race theory in education: A scholar's journey*. Teachers College Press.

Liggett, T. (2014). The mapping of a framework: Critical race theory and TESOL. *The Urban Review, 46*(1), 112–124. https://doi.org/10.1007/s11256-013-0254-5

Linan-Thompson, S., Lara-Martinez, J. A., & Cavazos, L. O. (2018). Exploring the intersection of evidence-based practices and culturally and linguistically responsive practices. *Intervention in School and Clinic, 54*(1), 6–13. https://doi.org/10.1177/1053451218762574

McCarty, T. L., Noguera, J., Lee, T. S., & Nicholas, S. E. (2021). "A viable path for education"—Indigenous-language immersion and sustainable self-determination. *Journal of Language, Identity & Education, 20*(5), 340–354. https://doi.org/10.1080/15348458.2021.1957681

Mortier, K., Brown, I. C., & Aramburo, C. M. (2021). Cultural brokers in special education. *Research and Practice for Persons with Severe Disabilities, 46*(1), 3–17. https://doi.org/10.1177/1540796920975386

Murillo, L. A., & Smith, P. H. (2011). "I will never forget that": Lasting effects of language discrimination on language-minority children in Colombia and on the U.S.-Mexico border. *Childhood Education, 87*(3), 147–153. https://doi.org/10.1080/00094056.2011.10521714

Ortiz, S. O. (2002). Best practices in nondiscriminatory assessment. In *Best practices in school psychology IV* (Vol. 1–2, pp. 1321–1336). National Association of School Psychologists.

Ortiz, S. O. (2019). On the measurement of cognitive abilities in English Learners. *Contemporary School Psychology, 23*(1), 68–86. https://doi.org/10.1007/s40688-018-0208-8

Perrigo, J. L., Villamil Grest, C., Harris, T., & Samek, A. (2023). Spanish-speaking Hispanic/Latino families education-related parental involvement practices. *Journal of Latinos and Education*, 1–13. https://doi.org/10.1080/15348431.2023.2276781

Peterson, R. L., & Pennington, B. F. (2012). Developmental dyslexia. *The Lancet, 379*(9830), 1997–2007. https://doi.org/10.1016/S0140-6736(12)60198-6

Project LEE, Project ELLIPSES, & Project ELITE. (2021). *Meeting the needs of English learners with and without disabilities: Brief 4, Fostering collaborative partnerships with families of English learners within a multitiered system of supports*. U.S. Office of Special Education Programs. https://www.mtss4els.org/files/resource-files/Series2-Brief4.pdf

Sheridan, S. M., Holmes, S. R., Smith, T. E., & Moen, A. L. (2016). Complexities in field-based partnership research: Exemplars, challenges, and an agenda for the field. In S. M. Sheridan & E. Moorman Kim (Eds.), *Family-school partnerships in context* (pp. 1–23). Springer International. https://doi.org/10.1007/978-3-319-19228-4_1

Sheridan, S. M., Kim, E. M., Coutts, M. J., Sjuts, T. M., Holmes, S. R., Ransom, K. A., & Garbacz, S. A. (2012). Clarifying parent involvement and family-school partnership intervention research: A preliminary synthesis. CYFS working paper no. 2012-4. In *Nebraska Center for Research on Children, Youth, Families and Schools*. Nebraska Center for Research on Children, Youth, Families and Schools. https://eric.ed.gov/?id=ED537845

Sheridan, S. M., Smith, T. E., Kim, E. M., Beretvas, S. N., & Park, S. (2019). A meta-analysis of family-school interventions and children's social-emotional functioning: Moderators and components of efficacy. *Review of Educational Research, 89*(2), 296–332. https://doi.org/10.3102/0034654318825437

Simon, B. S. (2001). Family involvement in high school: Predictors and effects. *NASSP Bulletin, 85*(627), 8–19. https://doi.org/10.1177/019263650108562702

Solórzano, D. G., & Delgado Bernal, D. (2001). Examining transformational resistance through a critical race and LatCrit theory framework. *Urban Education, 36*(3), 308–342. https://doi.org/10.1177/0042085901363002

Spencer, M. B., Dupree, D., & Hartmann, T. (1997). A phenomenological variant of ecological systems theory (PVEST): A self-organization perspective in context. *Development and Psychopathology, 9*(4), 817–833. https://doi.org/10.1017/S0954579497001454

Sullivan, A. L. (2011). Disproportionality in special education identification and placement of English Language Learners. *Exceptional Children, 77*(3), 317–334. https://doi.org/10.1177/001440291107700304

Tarasawa, B., & Waggoner, J. (2015). Increasing parental involvement of English Language Learner families: What the research says. *Journal of Children and Poverty, 21*(2), 129–134. https://doi.org/10.1080/10796126.2015.1058243

Tuck, E., Stepetin, H., Beaulne-Stuebing, R., & Billows, J. (2023). Visiting as an indigenous feminist practice. *Gender and Education, 35*(2), 144–155. https://doi.org/10.1080/09540253.2022.2078796

Vakil, S., Byrd, D., & Smolen, L. (2023). Making connections with parents of English learners: Promoting culturally and linguistically diverse classrooms. *Journal of the International Society for Teacher Education, 27*, 5–14. https://doi.org/10.26522/jiste.v27i1.4231

Vega, D., & Wolf, J. N. (2023). Best practices in assessment of bilingual learners in schools. In P. L. Harrison, S. L. Proctor, & A. Thomas (Eds.), *Best practices in school psychology: Vol. 1. Data-based and collaborative decision-making* (7th ed., pp. 163–173). National Association of School Psychologists.

Vera, E. M., Israel, M. S., Coyle, L., Knight-Lynn, L., Moallem, I., Bartucci, G., & Goldberger, N. (2012). Exploring the educational involvement of parents of English learners. *School Community Journal, 22*(2), 183–202.

Vygotsky, L. S. (1978). *Socio-cultural theory: Mind in society*. Harvard University.

Weingarten, Z., Zumeta Edmonds, R., & Arden, S. (2020). Better together: Using MTSS as a structure for building school-family partnerships. *Teaching Exceptional Children, 53*(2), 122–130. https://doi.org/10.1177/0040059920937733

Yosso, T. J. (2005). Whose culture has capital? A critical race theory discussion of community cultural wealth. *Race Ethnicity and Education, 8*(1), 69–91. https://doi.org/10.1080/1361332052000341006

Zacarian, D. (2023). *Transforming schools for multilingual learners: A comprehensive guide for educators*. Corwin.

Chapter 6
Culturally Adapted Social-Emotional and Behavioral Interventions for Emergent Bilinguals

Sara Castro-Olivo, Wualú Altamira, and Natalie Vallarta

National data have documented that for decades, emergent bilinguals' (EB) scores on standardized state tests have been significantly lower than the scores obtained by monolingual English speakers (National Center for Education Statistics [NCES], 2023). Historically, this performance gap has mainly been attributed to EBs' limited English proficiency. Due to this perception, educators tend to focus their efforts on only providing EBs with additional English language development and support in academic content areas (Preciado et al., 2023); however, less focus is placed on their social–emotional and behavioral (SE/B) needs. Research has established a strong relationship between students' social–emotional and behavioral well-being and their academic performance (Durlak et al., 2022). Yet, EBs' social–emotional and behavioral needs tend to go unnoticed and unaddressed (Castro-Olivo et al., 2011).

Educators must increase their awareness of how unmet SE/B needs of EBs can be strong determinants of low academic performance, difficulties with learning English, making progress in other content areas, and establishing meaningful relationships in school and the broader US social networks (Castro-Olivo et al., 2011). Although more research is needed on the relationship between EBs' social–emotional well-being and EBs' academic performance, one way to illustrate how the SE/B needs of EBs go unnoticed is by looking at their disproportionate underrepresentation in special education under the Emotional Disturbance (ED) category (U.S. Department of Education, 2024). Recent national reports on the percentage of

S. Castro-Olivo (✉)
Counseling, Recreation and School Psychology, Florida International University, Miami, United States
e-mail: scastroo@fiu.edu

W. Altamira · N. Vallarta
Educational Psychology Department, Texas A&M University, College Station, TX, USA
e-mail: waltamira@tamu.edu; vallartan@tamu.edu

D. Vega, J. N. Wolf (eds.), *Culturally and Linguistically Responsive Intervention and Assessment Practices with Emergent Bilingual Students*,
https://doi.org/10.1007/978-3-032-02084-0_6

EBs who receive special education services indicate that only 1.9% of EBs received special education services under ED, compared to 5% of the overall public-school population (U.S. Department of Education, 2024). Although some could view the underrepresentation of EBs under the ED category as a strength in this community, indicating they are typically perceived by teachers as well-behaved and respectful (Harklau, 2000); others could argue that their quiet demeanor could easily be hiding symptoms of internalizing disorders such as depression and anxiety that usually go unnoticed by teachers (Gudiño et al., 2009). Further, the fact that EBs are overrepresented in other special education categories, such as Specific Learning Disabilities (EBs = 44.7%; non-EBs = 34.5%) and Speech Language Impairment (EBs = 18.9%; non-EBs = 17.6%; U.S. Department of Education, 2024), suggests that educators are more focused on EBs' academic and linguistic challenges, while inadvertently neglecting their broader social–emotional and/or developmental needs.

Not all EBs who are struggling socially, emotionally, and/or behaviorally will meet the criteria for special education, or even need to be considered for a formal evaluation; however, most could still benefit from targeted interventions that can support their transitions to their new language, culture, and social expectations. Educators must remember that children who qualify for English language development (ELD) services often come from families with a recent history of immigration to the United States (Toppelberg & Collins, 2010). Immigrant families often face many social, emotional, financial, and cultural challenges that make them more vulnerable to stress and other mental health issues. For example, EB youth are more likely to experience social–emotional problems due to the sociocultural factors associated with being immigrants or children of immigrants (Blanco-Vega et al., 2008). *Sociocultural factors* are the societal and cultural determinants of behavior and health outcomes among diverse groups.

The sociocultural factors that have been frequently associated with negative psychological outcomes of immigrant youth, which often go undiagnosed and untreated, are lower socioeconomic status, acculturation, acculturative stress, discrimination, immigration-related trauma, intergenerational trauma, etc. (Choy et al., 2021). It is important to note that in the rare occasions when evidence-based treatments (EBTs) are used to address the social–emotional and behavioral needs of EBs, the sociocultural factors that could be the root of their symptoms are likely not to be considered in treatment, leading to ineffective intervention outcomes (Martinez et al., 2011).

Although this chapter focuses on common social–emotional and behavioral needs of EBs, it is important to keep in mind that not all EBs will display social–emotional or behavioral issues in school. For decades, researchers have highlighted the *immigrant paradox* documented among different generations of immigrants in the United States. The immigrant paradox is a population phenomenon where newcomer immigrant children and adolescents show better developmental and academic outcomes than more acculturated (even US-born) youth despite their limited resources and English language dominance (Marks et al., 2014). Educators must always keep in mind that immigrant populations are often very resilient and highly motivated to do their very best in schools and the workplace (Cerna et al., 2021).

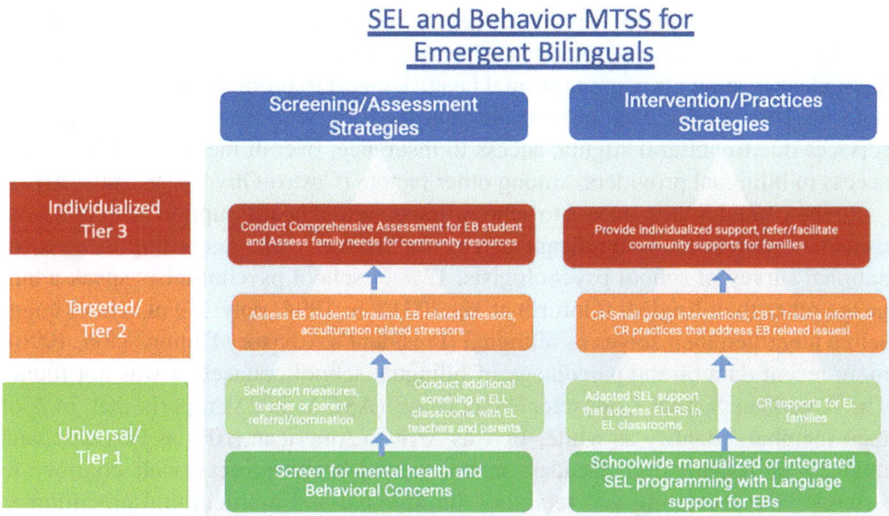

Fig. 6.1 SEL and behavior assessment and intervention/supports recommendations for EBs

While educators should expect the majority of emergent bilinguals (EBs) to thrive, this chapter focuses on recommending strategies for supporting those who may need additional supports adjusting to their new social networks. These strategies would also reinforce the ongoing success of students who are already meeting expectations by equipping them with coping and resilience-building skills that can further enhance their long-term outcomes. To that end, we propose a culturally responsive multi-tiered system of support that offers skill development beneficial to all EBs, while ensuring those with elevated needs are effectively identified and supported (see Fig. 6.1). The goal of this chapter is to raise awareness among school psychologists and educators about the unique social–emotional and behavioral needs of EBs. We also summarize current evidence-based practices and offer recommendations for implementing culturally sustaining social–emotional and behavioral supports in public schools.

The Role of Schools in EBs' Social–Emotional and Behavioral Health

Across the nation, mental health services are undersupported, particularly for youth. According to the Centers for Disease Control (CDC), only 20% of youth with mental health disorders receive specialized care (CDC, 2023). Further, Gudiño et al. (2009) found that children with internalizing problems (e.g., depression and anxiety) are less likely to receive services than students with externalizing behaviors (e.g., hyperactivity, defiance, etc). In that study, Gudiño et al. (2009) also found that youth who receive services are most likely to receive them in school settings. These findings illustrate the need for teachers to be well-versed in techniques that can help them identify students needing mental health support to promote their overall development. This need is even more prominent for EBs, who are less likely to receive services due to cultural stigma, access to insurance, overall mental health literacy, access to bilingual providers, among other factors (Castro-Olivo & Merrell, 2012).

In the United States, access to school-based mental health support with bilingual providers represents a significant barrier for EBs as well. According to a recent national survey of school psychologists, 12% of school psychologists speak a language other than English (Goforth et al., 2021). In 1994, only 2% of school counselors identified themselves as bilingual (President's Advisory Commission, 1996); more recent data on the percentage of bilingual school counselors was not found. The American School Counselor Association (ASCA, 2023) reports that 74% of their members identify as white, 11% as African American, 10% as Hispanic, and only 2% as Asian. After decades, school mental health professionals continue to struggle with recruiting and retaining multilingual and multicultural practitioners (ASCA, 2023; Goforth et al., 2021).

The limited number of multilingual and multicultural mental health professionals is not the only barrier EBs encounter to receiving culturally responsive mental health services in school settings. Research on developing and validating culturally responsive school-based interventions is also limited. For example, in 2020, Cuocci and Arndt reported finding only two social-emotional learning (SEL) programs that had been developed and validated with multilingual students' sociocultural reality (i.e., challenges related to being immigrants or children of immigrants who are navigating two different cultures and languages) in mind. Even informal social and academic mentoring programs are scarce for EBs. Castro-Olivo et al. (2023) found that only three evidence-based mentoring programs addressed social and emotional content specific to emergent bilinguals. See Table 6.1 for a list of studies that address the social–emotional and behavioral needs of EBs in a culturally responsive manner. Clearly, more research is needed to ensure the mental health services provided to EBs are effective at producing social-emotional and academic gains in a socially valid way (i.e., viewed as meaningful by members of the population the intervention is intended for) that is also perceived as culturally responsive/sustaining. See Paris (2012) for definitions of culturally responsive/sustaining practices.

Unique Social–Emotional and Behavioral Needs of Emergent Bilinguals

This section summarizes the different sociocultural factors contributing to EBs' unique social–emotional and behavioral needs. It is important to understand that universal or one-size-fits-all social–emotional and behavioral interventions will likely not address the root of many of EBs' social–emotional and behavioral

Table 6.1 Dimensions of culturally adapted social–emotional and behavioral interventions for EBs

Intervention (Authors)	Design	Focus	1	2	3	4	5	6	7	8
Castro-Olivo and Merrell (2012)	Pre-post	SEL	✓	✓	✓	✓	✓	✓	✓	✓
Castro-Olivo (2014)	Quasi RCT	SEL-resiliency building	✓	✓	✓	✓	✓	✓	✓	✓
Castro-Olivo et al. (2018)	Single Subject	Behavior	✓	✓	✓	✓	✓	✓	✓	✓
Cramer and Castro-Olivo (2016)	Pre-post	SEL/Internalizing	✓	✓	✓	✓	✓	✓	✓	✓
Kataoka et al. (2003)	RCT	PTSD	✓	✓				✓	✓	✓
Preciado et al. (2009)	Single Subject	Single Subject	✓	✓		✓			✓	✓
Pryce et al. (2019)	Qualitative	Sense of belonging	✓	✓				✓	✓	✓
Walker et al. (2009)	Single Subject	Behavior	✓	✓					✓	✓

Notes: 1: Language, 2: Persons, 3: metaphors, 4: content, 5: concepts, 6: context, 7: goals, 8: delivery problems. Given that the majority of EB families identify as immigrants or children of immigrants (NCES, 2022), educators must consider the factors described in this section when screening students in need of support, validating the need for support, selecting or developing interventions, and monitoring their effectiveness/impact on the students.

As previously stated, the sociocultural factors that are most cited in the extant literature as determinants of health and academic outcomes for EB youth include: acculturation, acculturative stress, familial acculturation gaps, perceived discrimination, low sense of belonging with their school and communities, low socioeconomic status (SES), higher risk of adultification (e.g., having to perform adult tasks such as taking care of a sibling), language and social brokering (e.g., having to serve as interpreters for parents), immigrant-related stress, limited access to multilingual culturally responsive mental health care providers, health insurance, and discrimination (Blanco-Vega et al., 2008). For children who have to cope with all these sociocultural challenges during key developmental stages in their lives, being exposed to SEL programs that cover skills such as self-awareness, social awareness, responsible decision-making, self-management, and relationship skills in a *one-size-fits-all* manner will likely feel superficial and not engaging (Castro-Olivo, 2010). Thus, there is a need for culturally responsive interventions that these youth can explicitly link to ways to help them cope with their cultural reality, or exposure to sociocultural factors (e.g., acculturation, perceived discrimination, language related stress), that make their life challenges different from the typical experiences of youth (Castro-Olivo & Merrell, 2012).

Most children rely on their caregivers to help them cope with most social–emotional and behavioral issues. Caregivers of EBs, who are likely to be immigrants to the United States, are also likely to be new to experiencing these sociocultural challenges or stressors, which highly limit their chances of having developed appropriate coping skills to pass down to their children (Lorenzo-Blanco et al., 2016). For a comprehensive review of sociocultural factors that EBs with an immigrant background experience, see Blanco-Vega et al. (2008). In the following section, we briefly summarize two of the most relevant sociocultural factors (according to extant literature) faced by EBs that must be addressed in any school-based social–emotional or behavioral intervention to be culturally responsive and ensure our interventions are socially valid. These factors are *acculturation* and *acculturative stress*.

Acculturation

The first sociocultural factor that must be addressed when discussing the needs of individuals new to a language and culture is acculturation, or the process of adopting a new culture's set of social norms, values, customs, and beliefs (Berry, 1997). Research from the last 30 decades demonstrates that for older populations, acculturation is associated with mental health problems (Choy et al., 2021). In youth, acculturation has been found to have equivocal findings. Some research has found that acculturation is associated with delinquent behavior, internalizing issues, and lower academic performance (Huq et al., 2016). Others have found that acculturation mediates English language proficiency (Jia et al., 2016; Yough et al., 2023).

School psychologists are encouraged to assess EB's acculturation to help determine language preference/use, which can guide decisions about when a child should be tested in English, home language, or both (Rhodes et al., 2005) and the language the intervention should be delivered in. The effects of acculturation on K-12 students' social–emotional and behavioral needs can be difficult to predict; however, acculturative stress, a common product of acculturation, has been found to be a more reliable predictor of negative outcomes for youth (Castro-Olivo et al., 2014). In the next section, we describe acculturative stress and the reasons to properly assess it and intervene with when working with EBs in school settings.

Acculturative Stress

Acculturative stress has been defined as the unique pressures individuals who are navigating two different cultures experience as they face conflicts between the two cultures' values, beliefs, and customs. Acculturating youth feel the pressure to conform to the host culture to avoid discrimination (Mena et al., 1987). Acculturative stress predicts internalizing issues (Albeg & Castro-Olivo, 2014), lower academic aspirations (Widales-Benitez et al., 2017), and a lower sense of belonging (Castro-Olivo et al., 2014; d'Abreu et al., 2021). EBs have also been found to report higher levels of acculturative stress than non-EB Latine populations (Castro-Olivo et al., 2014). Acculturative stress is often overlooked in school settings; however, given that school settings are the gates to the host society for acculturating children, they often become the main source of cultural conflicts for youth.

School mental health care providers would be the most ideal mental health providers to provide EBs with tools to cope with acculturative stress, which is moderated by perceived discrimination, or the feeling that others put you down based on your ethnic group membership (Garrison et al., 1999; Kataoka et al., 2003), and lower sense of belonging (Kayama & Yamakawa, 2020; Makarova, 2019). Both acculturation and acculturative stress can be influenced by school climate, federal, state, or local immigration policies, access to language supports, and culturally responsive practices by culturally competent teachers and mental health practitioners (Blanco-Vega et al., 2008). Schools prepared to support the EBs' social–emotional, behavioral, and cultural needs are better positioned to assess and understand the local climate and how it impacts the needs of EBs in their community. In the following section, we summarize social, emotional, and behavioral interventions validated and/or culturally adapted for work with emergent bilinguals in the United States or Canada.

Culturally Responsive Social–Emotional and Behavioral Interventions for EBs

To address the sociocultural factors listed in the previous section, some researchers have tested cultural adaptations of established evidence-based social, emotional, and behavioral interventions for use with EBs. The main aim of these adaptations is to ensure these interventions are more culturally responsive and explicitly address the unique sociocultural challenges EBs face within their school, home, and local communities. The most widely used model/framework for making cultural adaptations of evidence-based interventions is the Ecology Validity Model by Guillermo Bernal et al. (1995). The Ecology Validity Model requires practitioners and researchers working with populations different from those with which the manualized intervention program was originally validated to address eight different dimensions as they adapt the evidence-based interventions (Bernal et al., 1995; see Fig. 6.1).

Those dimensions are *language* (intervention provided in the native language of the participants/clients), *persons* (implemented by individuals who are bilingual and bicultural), *metaphors* (use metaphors or examples that are part of the participants' folk culture), *delivery methods* (deliver the intervention in ways that are aligned with delivery methods liked by the target population), *context* (social, political, and cultural context is taken into account from assessment to intervention), *content* (intervention includes content related to the unique sociocultural realities of target populations), *concepts* (intervention includes concepts that enhance the target's population connection of the intervention with their cultural reality), and *goals* (ensuring that researchers/implementers goals are aligned with the goals and values of the target population).

In the following section, brief summaries of the SEL and behavioral interventions that, to date, have been validated with EBs are provided. First, we summarize interventions that have endorsed the Ecological Validity Model to make the programs culturally responsive for EBs. We later summarize SE/B interventions validated with EBs but do not report endorsing a cultural adaptation model/framework. These summaries are included to increase awareness and illustrate how EBTs can be adapted to make interventions more culturally responsive and better address the sociocultural realities/needs of EBs. Table 6.1 summarizes how each of these dimensions was addressed in the SE/B interventions reviewed in this chapter.

Social–Emotional Interventions Validated for EBs

Jóvenes Fuertes

The first culturally adapted school-based SEL program for EBs documented in the school psychology literature was developed and validated by Sara Castro-Olivo et al. (2006). The first study was part of her dissertation at the University of Oregon under the supervision of Dr. Keneth Merrell, who, at that time, was finalizing the *Strong Teens* SEL program with members of the Oregon Resiliency Project (ORP; Merrell et al., 2007a, 2007b). As an immigrant and emergent bilingual herself, Dr. Castro-Olivo, who started learning English as a ninth grader in a newcomer English as a second language (ESL) program in Northern California, states that personal experiences influenced her view of the need to provide culturally responsive practices that focused on building social–emotional resilience in adolescent EBs.

From this experience, Dr. Castro-Olivo and Dr. Blanco-Vega (also a member of Dr. Merrell's ORP lab) adapted ORP's *Strong Teens* SEL program for use with Latine immigrant youth. *Strong Teens* is part of the *Strong Kids* SEL curricula (Merrell et al., 2007a, 2007b), a semi-scripted manualized program promoting resilience from a preventative framework. *Strong Teens* is a 12-lesson program that explicitly teaches the following core SEL skills: *self-awareness*, *social awareness* (including empathy training, emotion variation, and problem-solving), *self-managemen*t (including reframing and stress management), *relationship/social skills,* and *responsible decision-making* (including problem-solving and goal setting).

Strong Kids has a prevention focus that employs a cognitive–behavioral therapy (CBT) approach to manage emotions and make responsible decisions. The program has been shown to be effective at improving students' social–emotional knowledge and internalizing and externalizing issues with both EB and non-EB students (Merrell, 2010). *Strong Kids* and *Strong Teens* had not been tested with predominantly minoritized populations, particularly EBs. Thus, Castro-Olivo and Blanco-Vega endorsed the Bernal et al. (1995) Ecology Validity Model to make cultural adaptations to the *Strong Teens* program with the main goal of helping EB students cope with unique sociocultural factors (e.g., acculturation, acculturative stress, familial acculturation gap). The adapted program, called *Jóvenes Fuertes,* maintained the same number, order, and structure of all lessons in the *Strong Teens* program. The goal of promoting resilience was equally retained; however, the adaptations carefully addressed all eight dimensions of the Ecological Validity Model.

In Castro-Olivo and Merrell (2012), the authors explain that the intervention was translated into Spanish by native Spanish speakers (*language*). It was delivered by bilingual and bicultural interventionists (*persons*). Every lesson had new examples, or *metaphors,* added that connected the student's culture and *context* with the skills being taught, and the examples provided for modeling SEL skills were also adapted to match the student's cultural values, traditions, and realities (*content and context).* *Concepts* such as acculturative stress and ethnic pride were included to connect the student's cultural reality and context (considering the students' SEL outcomes based on their immigrant and EB status/treatment) to the skills being taught. The *delivery methods* and *goals* stayed the same but added culturally specific methods and goals that emphasized Latine values such as *respeto*/respect and *familismo*/familism. For a more comprehensive description of the cultural adaptation process, see Castro-Olivo and Merrell (2012).

Since its development and original validation, *Jóvenes Fuerte*s (Castro-Olivo et al., 2006) has been evaluated in multiple studies. In 2014, Castro-Olivo endorsed a quasi-experimental design to evaluate the effects of the culturally adapted intervention in 102 newcomer EB middle/high school students' social–emotional resiliency skills and knowledge. That study found that youth and teachers rated the program as highly socially valid. In addition, students in the intervention group reported statistically significant improvements in resiliency and SEL knowledge.

Two additional studies have been conducted on *Jóvenes Fuertes* since then. Castro-Olivo et al. (2016) evaluated the program with 86 Spanish-speaking high school students in four different classrooms. The main focus of this program was to evaluate the effects of the program following Tier 1 and Tier 2 intervention support. Castro-Olivo et al. (2016) endorsed a pre-post design with all 88 high school students in this study. Teachers from each classroom were asked to nominate three students (top 5%) of students they identified as high risk for social–emotional issues. Nominated students received three one-on-one booster sessions on problem-solving and cognitive restructuring.

The results of this study showed that the Tier 1 intervention was effective at improving SEL knowledge and resilience, as in previous studies. It was also rated as highly socially valid. Students who received Tier 2 interventions (three booster sessions) reported lower levels of acculturative stress and internalizing symptoms at post-booster assessment. In the third study, Cramer and Castro-Olivo (2016) reported the results of the adapted program with a diverse group of students, with the majority of the students identified as EBs. In this study, students also rated the program as socially valid and reported higher levels of resilience and lower levels of internalizing symptoms at post-intervention assessment.

Mental Health for Immigrants Program

The Mental Health for Immigrant Program (MHIP; Kataoka et al., 2003) is an eight-session CBT group for children. It is based on the cognitive-behavioral intervention for trauma in schools framework to target the mental health needs (e.g., PTSD, anxiety, depression) of Latine immigrant youth's traumatic experiences. Kataoka et al. (2003) piloted MHIP with Latine immigrant students exposed to community violence. Participants were recruited from nine public schools with high populations of immigrant youth. Eligibility criteria included: (1) being elementary-middle school aged (from third to eighth grade); (2) being from one of the nine schools that were participating; (3) being born outside of the United States; (4) being a recent immigrant (in the United States for less than 3 years); (5) and being a Spanish speaker. The quasi-experimental pilot study included 67 immigrant youth in the MHIP intervention group and 46 randomized youth in the waitlist control group (Kataoka et al., 2003). Results showed there was a decrease in PTSD and depression symptoms in the youth who received the intervention compared to those in the waitlist control group at the 3-month follow-up. Although the authors do not report employing a specific framework for making cultural adaptations of the EBT they adapted, the method section of their articles reports that they had bilingual and bicultural interventionists (*persons*), implemented the intervention in Spanish (*language*), provided *examples* that were unique to the target population, and made additions related to *content, context,* and *concepts.*

Conversation Club

Conversation Club (CC; Pryce et al., 2019) was created by the Canadian branch of the Big Brothers Big Sisters (BBBS) mentoring program as a group mentoring intervention for recent immigrant students to be delivered after school. Although this intervention was not an adaptation of an existing manualized EBT, it adapted mentoring practices for use with newcomer EBs. In this study, Pryce et al. (2019) evaluated the effects of a mentoring intervention on newcomer youth's experiences with connectedness, hopefulness, integration into Canadian society, and belonging. The study used a quasi-experimental design that included 67 newcomer youth in CC and 25 immigrant youth in the comparison group. Participants were recruited from public schools (i.e., high school, middle school), English Learner (EL) programs, libraries, and community centers in the Peel Region of Canada (Pryce et al., 2019). Results suggested that Conversation Club participation increased students' sense of belonging and connection with their community (Pryce et al., 2019).

Behavioral Interventions Validated with EBs

First Steps to Success

The First Steps to Success (FSS) program is an evidence-based behavioral program validated with EBs by Castro-Olivo et al. (2018) and Walker et al. (2009). FSS was originally developed for use with kindergarten through third-grade students who display significant behavioral challenges with the function of gaining adult and peer attention. The program includes a classroom management training/classroom component (for participating teachers), direct social skills training (for participating children), and a caregiver training/*HomeBase* component (for participating caregivers). FSS focuses on teaching students basic social skills such as keeping their hands and feet to themselves, following instructions, and raising their hand before speaking. These skills are taught through individualized instruction and behavior rehearsal, feedback, role-plays, and activity-based performance incentives in the classroom, individual, and *HomeBase* components. For more details on the FSS program, see Golly et al. (1998) and Walker et al. (1998).

Castro-Olivo et al. (2018) made cultural adaptations to this program, also endorsing the Ecology Validity Model by Bernal et al. (1995). Most of the cultural adaptations made to this intervention focused on the work with the adults. For example, to address *content*, *context*, and *concepts*, the authors started by adapting the teacher training by providing participating teachers additional training on risk factors for Latine EBs and best practices for working with Spanish-speaking students. To address the cultural reality of the students, the authors added lessons on English language vocabulary development interventions, allowing them to use English or Spanish interchangeably in the classroom and at home during the program as needed by the students.

The *HomeBase* interventions had more adaptations to better support immigrant caregivers' sociocultural needs. The program was adapted based on language delivery in Spanish; the program was delivered by a bicultural and bilingual interventionist, with examples/metaphors aligned with the caregivers' cultural reality. The adaptation added an entirely new lesson discussing the differences and similarities in the school systems in the United States and Latin American countries. This lesson also discussed the different expectations regarding caregiver involvement and positive reinforcement of expected/desired behaviors. A multiple-baseline across participants single-subject design was employed for this study. The findings showed that the intervention was effective at improving participating students' reading and behavioral outcomes. In addition, caregivers and teachers rated the intervention as socially valid.

In 2009, Dr. Walker and colleagues conducted a randomized trial of FSS where 200 students were randomly assigned to an intervention or control group. Although they did not conduct cultural adaptations or specifically recruit EBs, 58% of their sample identified as Latine and 22% as EBs. Teachers and caregivers rated students' behavior problems pre- and post-intervention. Students in the intervention group received statistically significant lower ratings of problem behavior at post-intervention, with effect sizes ranging from .62 to .73. Although it is hard to generalize to EBs, the results of this study show that FSS has resulted in positive outcomes for minoritized populations, including EBs.

Function-Based Behavioral and Reading Intervention for EBs

Another function-based intervention that supported EBs was published by Dr. Jorge Preciado et al. (2009). In this study, the authors combined reading and behavioral intervention. The intervention focused on supporting the needs of EBs who engaged in problem behavior to escape English reading instruction. To neutralize the effects of reading difficulties, participants received one-on-one reading instruction focused on pre-teaching reading skills and language/vocabulary-building intervention from bilingual graduate students. This study showed that function-based interventions with language and instructional support for EBs improved academic and behavioral outcomes for EBs. Teachers rated this intervention highly; ELD teachers reported endorsing the practice of these interventions at the district level so that more EBs can be supported by obtaining vocabulary-building support and additional direct reading instruction from bilingual interventionists in a one-on-one setting.

Although a systematic literature review was not conducted to identify the interventions listed in this section, Castro-Olivo and colleagues have regularly reviewed the literature on social–emotional learning and behavioral interventions for EB or immigrant populations in school settings. Most recently, Castro-Olivo et al. (2023) published a systematic literature review on mentoring interventions for EBs and found that only one of the five studies that met the criteria for inclusion in the systematic review (i.e., evaluation study of a mentoring program for EBs) had focused on social–emotional and behavioral outcomes (Pryce et al., 2019). The scarcity of social–emotional and behavioral interventions validated for use with EBs is alarming. Researchers are urged to focus on EBs' SE/B outcomes in addition to academic interventions (where there is more intervention research for EBs). Given the limited research in this area, in the following section, we provide suggestions for practitioners and educators to consider when working with EBs in the areas of social–emotional and behavioral supports. We urge practitioners to endorse a multitiered system of supports (MTSS) to ensure EBs with social–emotional and behavioral needs are given a chance to cope.

Recommendations for Culturally Responsive School-Wide MTSS of Social–Emotional Learning (SEL) and Positive Behavior Interventions and Supports (PBIS) for EBs

In Fig. 6.2, we illustrate a proposed MTSS model for assessing and supporting the social–emotional and behavioral needs of EBs within school settings. We recommend that schools interested in supporting the social–emotional and behavioral needs of EBs employ an adapted version of the Outcomes Driven Model (ODM) introduced by Good and colleagues in 2002. The ODM requires educators to (a) identify the need for support; (b) validate the need for support; (c) develop an intervention based on the skills needed; and (d) enter an intervention/progress monitoring loop where interventions can be constantly adapted until data demonstrates that students have made the desired progress/outcome (Good et al., 2002).

As explained below, an adapted ODM (see Fig. 6.3) for social–emotional and behavioral interventions of EBs would require schools to establish school-wide practices that would allow them to properly: (a) identify students' needs for support through the use of validated culturally relevant screening tools; (b) validate needs for support through semi-structured interviews with students, teachers, and caregivers to determine sociocultural factors to address in intervention; (c) provide culturally responsive interventions; () systematically assess students' progress/response to supports provided at each level in a multitiered system; and (e) promote cultural sustainability (i.e., ensuring intervention allows youth to sustain cultural views, values, and behaviors that promote resiliency) by evaluating social validity and potential need for further cultural adaptations of programs/practices provided to EBs.

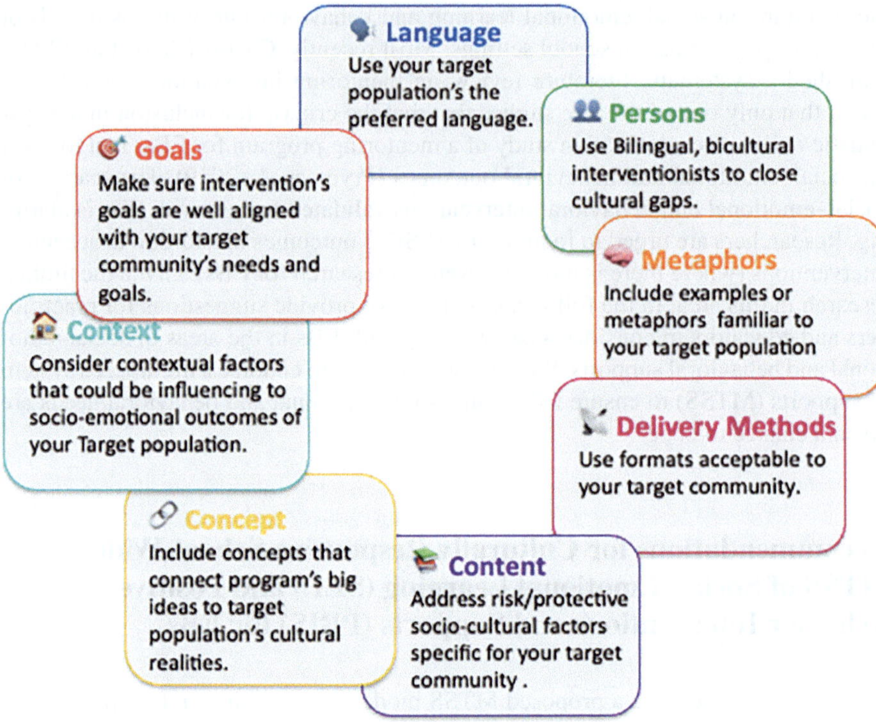

Fig. 6.2 Ecological validity model: dimensions to adapt

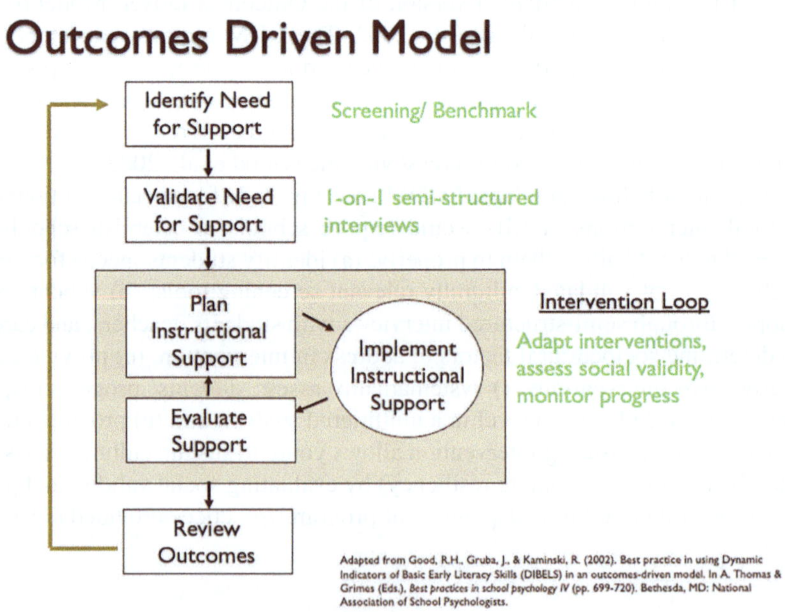

Fig. 6.3 Adapted version of outcomes-driven model

Identifying Need for Support

One of the first steps for any school team planning to endorse a school-wide MTSS system to address their students' social, emotional, and behavioral needs is to identify the type of support their students need and choose a strong universal intervention likely to meet most students' needs. We must emphasize that the social–emotional and behavioral needs of EBs must be considered in the context/climate of local communities and the sociocultural factors discussed in this article. Similarly to school-wide positive behavior interventions and supports (SWPBIS) programs, schools should be expected to develop their own implementation manual as the cultural adaptations needed will vary from school to school, and community to community. See Center on PBIS (2025) for recommendations on steps schools should consider when developing SWPBIS manuals.

Schools developing their own culturally responsive SEL/behavioral interventions must consider their students' contextual/sociocultural realities when identifying measures used to screen, monitor progress, and evaluate the need for special education services. These measures must be used to inform intervention decisions (i.e., how and what to adapt from evidence-based practices to make school-wide SEL and PBIS culturally responsive use with EB populations). For a list of validated measures commonly used to evaluate the sociocultural and social–emotional needs of EBs, see Table 6.2.

In 2014, Castro-Olivo and colleagues published the validation of the Coping with Acculturative Stress in American School (CASAS) scale for use as a screener to identify students struggling with high levels of acculturative stress and are likely to be at higher risk for mental health problems related to perceived discrimination, EB-related stress, familial acculturative gaps, and low sense of community/school

Table 6.2 Validated screening assessment tools for EBs

Author	Measure name	Focus	Language available
Castro-Olivo et al. (2014)	Coping with Acculturative Stress in American Schools (CASAS)	Acculturative stress—subscales: community belonging, EL-related stress, familial acculturation gaps, perceived discrimination	English, Spanish, Arabic
NCTSN (2025)	Refugee Services Core Stressor Assessment Tool	Trauma, acculturation, resettlement, isolation	English (web-based, culturally adaptable)
Ornelas et al. (2022)	Strengths and Difficulties Questionnaire (SDQ)	Emotional, behavioral, social difficulties	60+ languages
Scarpato et al. (2010)	Pediatric Symptom Checklist (PSC)	Emotional and behavioral symptoms	19+ languages
Steinberg et al. (2004)	UCLA PTSD Reaction Index (DSM-5)	PTSD symptoms	10+ (e.g., Spanish, Arabic, Korean)

belonging. Other measures of acculturation and a sense of school belonging could also be used as screeners that can help identify EBs in need of further assessment to determine the type of cultural adaptations the interventions provided to them must address.

Validate the Need for Culturally Adapted Support

School-based mental health providers or teachers of EBs would be excellent individuals to interview students identified as at-risk in the screening process. For example, students whose scores are within the top 75th percentile on the CASAS should have a one-on-one follow-up semi-structured interview with a trained professional to determine the need for culturally adapted SEL/PBIS support (Castro-Olivo et al., 2016). These interviews should ask questions that not only follow up on items endorsed in screening tools but also ask students about the specific coping skills they use to manage their cultural reality. For example, students could be asked: "Tell me about how connected you feel to this school and community?" "What do you do to help you feel connected?" "What could others do to help you feel more connected?" "What type of issues related to being made to be different by others, having caregivers telling you that you are becoming too Americanized, or struggles with feeling comfortable speaking English to native English speakers have you experienced, if any?" and "How do you cope with those issues?" (Castro-Olivo et al., 2016).

Developing Cultural Adaptations to Programs to be Delivered to EBs

As part of developing a culturally responsive MTSS for social–emotional and behavioral skills, all staff must be trained on the most common behavioral symptoms of internalizing disorders (e.g., socially withdrawn, low class participation, flat affect) and externalizing disorders (e.g., talking out of turn, defiance, aggression; Weisz et al., 2006). All staff should also learn about the most common sociocultural and contextual factors that influence EBs' social, emotional, behavioral, and academic difficulties (e.g., the community's stand on immigration legislation, familial acculturation gap, potential discrimination/bullying EB students could be experiencing due to their low English language proficiency).

Assuming *all* students in a school are exposed to universal (Tier 1) SEL or PBIS programming, a strong focus should be placed on ensuring EB students understand the language and can use the skills taught in the Tier 1 program in their cultural context/home and school. Data obtained in the screening and validating need for support stages should be used to select the program that would best address the social, emotional, and/or behavioral needs of most students. For EBs, the sociocultural factors that were identified as relevant for students in the local community and were mentioned by the students as concerns should be explicitly addressed in a culturally responsive/sustainable manner. The *Jóvenes Fuertes* program can be used as an example of a culturally adapted, evidence-based SEL program. Keep in mind that the examples will have to be changed to match the cultural reality of the students' local community.

Intervention Loop

Students identified as needing more support than what is provided in Tier 1 should be exposed to evidence-based/culturally adapted programming in Tier 2. These interventions would require a deeper discussion of sociocultural factors that students reported struggling to cope with during the validating need for support interview. Incorporating trauma-informed practices into SEL or PBIS programs should also be considered. Progress monitoring data should be collected regularly to determine if the students are making progress not only in learning SEL or behavioral skills taught in the program but also in their ability to adopt those new skills to their cultural reality (e.g., using the problem-solving model taught in class to manage cultural clashes with caregivers at home). In addition, students should be asked if they like the programs they are being exposed to and find the skills being taught to be useful for their lives and culture (i.e., social validity).

If progress monitoring data suggest that students are not making adequate gains with Tier 2 interventions, additional supports need to be developed. Students in need of Tier 3 interventions are likely to benefit from a multidisciplinary team that identifies additional supports and actively engages and provides services for both caregivers and students. These supports can vary from connecting them to community organizations that can provide financial support or just an opportunity to establish a social network in their new community, to referring them to counseling centers that can provide accessible family therapy. As mentioned previously, due to their immigration experiences, caregivers of EBs are likely to also need interventions that can help them cope with their own acculturation process, perceived discrimination, grief for leaving family, and stressors due to financial or language-related issues.

Districts with caregiver engagement centers have found that including caregiver groups in different languages and resources not only helps caregivers be more involved in school but also provides caregivers with an opportunity to form a social network with the other caregivers, validate their experiences, and gain valuable skills that will help them and their families for years to come (Barrueco et al., 2016). The cultural adaptation of the FSS program described in Castro-Olivo et al. (2018) can be used as an example of how to adapt a comprehensive intervention (i.e., multiple components that include students, caregivers, teachers, and community).

Conclusion

Emergent bilinguals are in great need of culturally responsive social, emotional, and behavioral interventions. In this chapter, we summarized the main programs that have been developed and validated with the specific social–emotional and/or behavioral needs of EBs in mind to date. Researchers and practitioners are urged to use a model similar to the Ecology Validity Model when making adaptations. Educators are also encouraged to follow an adapted Outcomes Driven Model approach to ensure school-based providers are constantly reminded of the need to evaluate progress, social validity, and adapt any part of the intervention that is not producing the desired outcomes.

The successful integration of EBs in the overall US society highly depends on what the support schools (which we view as the gates of US society) provide to these children during their most vulnerable developmental stages. Teachers and school-based mental health providers are in the best setting to make a difference for that "child." Your support makes a difference! I (SCO), dedicate this chapter to the many teachers and high school counselor who supported me when I was a newcomer EB in high school. Their support allowed my dream to become a reality. I owe who I am to those educators who believed in me and took the time to give me additional skills to shatter barriers. I am grateful to now be an educator who helps shatter barriers to new generations of EBs. I thank each person reading this book for your commitment to EBs.

References

Albeg, L. J., & Castro-Olivo, S. M. (2014). The relationship between mental health, acculturative stress, and academic performance in a Latino middle school sample. *Contemporary School Psychology, 18*, 178–186.

American School Counselor Association (ASCA). (2023). *Who are ASCA members?* Retrieved November 15, 2024, from https://www.schoolcounselor.org/Membership/Who-Are-ASCA-Members

Barrueco, S., Smith, S., & Stephens, S. A. (2016). Supporting parent engagement in linguistically diverse families to promote young children's life success. *Journal of Applied Research on Children: Informing Policy for Children at Risk, 7*(1), 13.

Bernal, G., Bonilla, J., & Bellido, C. (1995). Ecological validity and cultural sensitivity for outcome research: Issues for the cultural adaptation and development of psychosocial treatments with Hispanics. *Journal of Abnormal Child Psychology, 23*, 67–82.

Berry, J. W. (1997). Immigration, acculturation, and adaptation. *Applied Psychology, 46*(1), 5–34.

Blanco-Vega, C. O., Castro-Olivo, S. M., & Merrell, K. W. (2008). Social–emotional needs of Latino immigrant adolescents: A sociocultural model for development and implementation of culturally specific interventions. *Journal of Latinos and Education, 7*(1), 43–61. https://doi.org/10.1080/15348430701693390

Castro Olivo, S. (2010). One size does not fit all: Adapting SEL programs for use in our multicultural world. In K. W. Merrell & B. A. Gueldner (Eds.), *Social and emotional learning in the classroom: Promoting mental health and academic success*. Guildford Publications.

Castro-Olivo, S. M. (2014). Promoting social-emotional learning in adolescent Latino ELLs: A study of the culturally adapted Strong Teens program. *School Psychology Quarterly, 29*(4), 567–577. https://doi.org/10.1037/spq0000055

Castro-Olivo, S., Blanco-Vega, C., & Merrell. (2006). *Jóvenes Fuertes-Grades 6-12: A culturally adapted social and emotional learning curriculum* [Unpublished curriculum]. University of Oregon.

Castro-Olivo, S., Cramer, K., & Garcia, N. (2016). Manualized school-based intervention curricula for ethnic minority populations. In S. L. Graves & J. Blake (Eds.), *Psychoeducational assessment and intervention for ethnic minority children: Evidence based approaches*. APA Publications.

Castro-Olivo, S., Preciado, J., Le, L., Marciante, M., & Garcia, M. (2018). The effects of culturally adapted version of First Steps to Success for Latino English language learners: Preliminary pilot study. *Psychology in the Schools, 55*(1), 36–49. https://doi.org/10.1002/pits.22092

Castro-Olivo, S. M., Preciado, J. A., Sanford, A. K., & Perry, V. (2011). The academic and social-emotional needs of secondary Latino English learners: Implications for screening, identification, and instructional planning. *Exceptionality, 19*(3), 160–174. https://doi.org/10.1080/09362835.2011.579846

Castro-Olivo, S. M., & Merrell, K. W. (2012). Validating cultural adaptations of a school-based social-emotional learning program for use with Latino immigrant adolescents. *Advances in School Mental Health Promotion, 5*(2), 78–92.

Castro-Olivo, S. M., Palardy, G. J., Albeg, L., & Williamson, A. A. (2014). Development and validation of the Coping with Acculturative Stress in American Schools (CASAS-A) Scale on a Latino adolescent sample. *Assessment for Effective Intervention, 40*(1), 3–15. https://doi.org/10.1177/1534508413500983

Castro-Olivo, S., Witcher, K., Rivera, H., & Altamira, W. (2023). *A systematic review of the effects of mentoring programs in English Learners. Contemporary School Psychology*.

Center on PBIS. (2025). *Getting started with PBIS*. Retrieved March 30, 2025, from https://www.pbis.org/pbis/getting-started

Cerna, L., Brussino, O., & Mezzanotte, C. (2021). The resilience of students with an immigrant background: An update with PISA 2018. *OECD Education Working Papers, 261*, 0_1–69.

Centers for Disease Control and Prevention (CDC). (2023). *Improving access to children's mental health care*. U.S. Department of Health and Human Services. https://www.cdc.gov/childrensmentalhealth/access.html

Choy, B., Arunachalam, K., Gupta, S., Taylor, M., & Lee, A. (2021). Systematic review: Acculturation strategies and their impact on the mental health of migrant populations. *Public Health in Practice, 2*, 100069.

Cramer, K. M., & Castro-Olivo, S. (2016). Effects of a culturally adapted social-emotional learning intervention program on students' mental health. *Contemporary School Psychology, 20*, 118–129. https://doi.org/10.1007/s40688-015-0057-7

Cuocci, S., & Arndt, R. (2020). SEL for culturally and linguistically diverse students. *Journal of English Learner Education, 10*(1), 4.

D'Abreu, A., & Castro-Olivo, S., Ura, S. & Furrer, J. (2021). Hope for the future: A qualitative analysis of the resettlement experience of Syrian refugee adolescents and parents. *School Psychology International, 42*(2), 132–156. https://doi.org/10.1177/0143034320983595

Durlak, J. A., Mahoney, J. L., & Boyle, A. E. (2022). What we know, and what we need to find out about universal, school-based social and emotional learning programs for children and adolescents: A review of meta-analyses and directions for future research. *Psychological Bulletin, 148*(11-12), 765–782. https://doi.org/10.1037/bul0000383

Garrison, E. G., Roy, I. S., & Azar, V. (1999). Responding to the mental health needs of Latino children and families through school-based services. *Clinical Psychology Review, 19*(2), 199–219. https://doi.org/10.1016/s0272-7358(98)00070-1

Goforth, A. N., Farmer, R. L., Kim, S. Y., Naser, S. C., Lockwood, A. B., & Affrunti, N. W. (2021). Status of School Psychology in 2020: Part 1, Demographics of the NASP Membership Survey. *NASP Research Reports, 5*(2).

Golly, A. M., Stiller, B., & Walker, H. M. (1998). First step to success: Replication and social validation of an early intervention program. *Journal of Emotional and Behavioral Disorders, 6*(4), 243–250.

Good, R. H., Gruba, J., & Kaminski, R. A. (2002). *Best practices in using dynamic indicators of basic early literacy skills (DIBELS) in an outcomes-driven model.*

Gudiño, O. G., Lau, A. S., Yeh, M., McCabe, K. M., & Hough, R. L. (2009). Understanding racial/ethnic disparities in youth mental health services: Do disparities vary by problem type? *Journal of Emotional and Behavioral Disorders, 17*(1), 3–16. https://doi.org/10.1177/1063426608314160

Harklau, L. (2000). From the "good kids" to the "worst": Representations of English language learners across educational settings. *TESOL Quarterly, 34*(1), 35–67.

Huq, N., Stein, G. L., & Gonzalez, L. M. (2016). Acculturation conflict among Latino youth: Discrimination, ethnic identity, and depressive symptoms. *Cultural Diversity & Ethnic Minority Psychology, 22*(3), 377–385. https://doi.org/10.1037/cdp0000070

Jia, F., Gottardo, A., Chen, X., Koh, P., & Pasquarella, A. (2016). English proficiency and acculturation among Chinese immigrant youth in Canada: A reciprocal relationship. *Journal of Multilingual and Multicultural Development, 37*(8), 774–782. https://doi.org/10.1080/01434632.2015.1133630

Kataoka, S. H., Stein, B. D., Jaycox, L. H., Wong, M., Escudero, P., Tu, W., & Fink, A. (2003). A school-based mental health program for traumatized Latino immigrant children. *Journal of the American Academy of Child & Adolescent Psychiatry, 42*(3), 311–318. https://doi.org/10.1097/00004583-200303000-00011

Kayama, M., & Yamakawa, N. (2020). Acculturation and a sense of belonging of children in U.S. Schools and communities: The case of Japanese families. *Children and Youth Services Review, 119*, 105612. https://doi.org/10.1016/j.childyouth.2020.105612

Lorenzo-Blanco, E. I., Meca, A., Unger, J. B., Romero, A., Gonzales-Backen, M., Piña-Watson, B., et al. (2016). Latino parent acculturation stress: Longitudinal effects on family functioning and youth emotional and behavioral health. *Journal of Family Psychology, 30*(8), 966.

Makarova, E. (2019). Acculturation and school adjustment of minority students: School and family-related factors. *Intercultural Education, 30*(5), 445–447. https://doi.org/10.1080/14675986.2019.1643559

Marks, A. K., Ejesi, K., & García Coll, C. (2014). Understanding the US immigrant paradox in childhood and adolescence. *Child Development Perspectives, 8*(2), 59–64.

Martinez, C. R., McClure, H. H., Eddy, J. M., & Wilson, D. M. (2011). Time in U.S. residency and the social, behavioral, and emotional adjustment of Latino immigrant families. *Hispanic Journal of Behavioral Sciences, 33*(3), 323–349. https://doi.org/10.1177/073998631141281

Mena, F. J., Padilla, A. M., & Maldonado, M. (1987). Acculturative stress and specific coping strategies among immigrant and later generation college students. *Hispanic Journal of Behavioral Sciences, 9*(2), 207–225.

Merrell, K. W. (2010). Linking prevention science and social and emotional learning: The Oregon Resiliency Project. *Psychology in the Schools, 47*(1), 55–70.

Merrell, K., Carrizales-Engelmann, D., Feuerborn, L. L., Gueldner, B. A., & Tran, O. K. (2007a). *Strong Kids, Grades 6-8: A social and emotional learning curriculum* (Strong Kids Curricula). Brookes Publishing.

Merrell, K., Carrizales-Engelmann, D., Feuerborn, L. L., Gueldner, B. A., & Tran, O. K. (2007b). *Strong Teens, Grades 9-12: A social and emotional learning curriculum* (Strong Kids Curricula). Brookes Publishing.

National Center for Education Statistics. (2022). *English language learners in public schools.* U.S. Department of Education, Institute of Education Sciences. Retrieved April 28, 2025, from https://nces.ed.gov/programs/coe/indicator/cgf

National Center for Education Statistics. (2023). Reading performance. *Condition of Education.* U.S. Department of Education, Institute of Education Sciences. Retrieved December 12, 2023, from https://nces.ed.gov/programs/coe/indicator/cnb

National Child Traumatic Stress Network. (2025). *Refugee services core stressor assessment tool*. Retrieved March 30, 2025, from https://www.nctsn.org/resources/refugee-services-core-stressor-assessment-tool

Ornelas, J. H., Perreira, K. M., & Ayón, C. (2022). Validity of the Strengths and Difficulties Questionnaire among recently immigrated Latinx youth. *Psychiatry Research, 317*, 114860. https://doi.org/10.1016/j.psychres.2022.114860

Paris, D. (2012). Culturally sustaining pedagogy: A needed change in stance, terminology, and practice. *Educational Researcher, 41*(3), 93–97.

Preciado, J. A., Horner, R. H., & Baker, S. K. (2009). Using a function-based approach to decrease problem behaviors and increase academic engagement for Latino English language learners. *The Journal of Special Education, 42*(4), 227–240.

Preciado, J., Jalalian-Chursky, K., Norton, J., Rasikawati, I., & Eigenbrood, R. (2023). Achieving positive classroom experiences for Latino K-5 students. *Journal of Latinos and Education, 22*(3), 911–925. https://doi.org/10.1080/15348431.2021.1876696

President's Advisory Commission on Educational Excellence for Hispanic Americans. (1996). *Our nation on the fault line: Hispanic American Education.*

Pryce, J. M., Kelly, M. S., & Lawinger, M. (2019). Conversation club: A group mentoring model for immigrant youth. *Youth & Society, 51*(7), 879–899.

Rhodes, R. L., Ochoa, S. H., & Ortiz, S. O. (2005). *Assessing culturally and linguistically diverse students: A practical guide*. Guilford Press.

Scarpato, C., Verhulst, F. C., & Tiemeier, H. (2010). Cross-cultural application of the Pediatric Symptom Checklist. *European Child & Adolescent Psychiatry, 19*(6), 503–511. https://doi.org/10.1007/s00787-009-0078-y

Steinberg, A. M., Brymer, M. J., Decker, K. B., & Pynoos, R. S. (2004). The University of California at Los Angeles post-traumatic stress disorder reaction index. *Current Psychiatry Reports, 6*(2), 96–100. https://doi.org/10.1007/s11920-004-0048-2

Toppelberg, C. O., & Collins, B. A. (2010). Language, culture, and adaptation in immigrant children. *Child and Adolescent Psychiatric Clinics of North America, 19*(4), 697–717. https://doi.org/10.1016/j.chc.2010.07.003

U.S. Department of Education. (2024). *OSEP Fast Facts: Students with disabilities who are English Learners (ELs) served under IDEA Part B*. https://sites.ed.gov/idea/osep-fast-facts-students-with-disabilities-english-learners

Walker, H. M., Kavanagh, K., Stiller, B., Golly, A., Severson, H. H., & Feil, E. G. (1998). First step to success: An early intervention approach for preventing school antisocial behavior. *Journal of Emotional and Behavioral Disorders, 6*(2), 66–80.

Walker, H. M., Seeley, J. R., Small, J., Severson, H. H., Graham, B. A., Feil, E. G., Serna, L., Golly, A. M., & Forness, S. R. (2009). A randomized controlled trial of the first step to success early intervention: Demonstration of program efficacy outcomes in a diverse, urban school district. *Journal of Emotional and Behavioral Disorders, 17*(4), 197–212. https://doi.org/10.1177/1063426609341645

Weisz, J. R., McCarty, C. A., & Valeri, S. M. (2006). Effects of psychotherapy for depression in children and adolescents: A meta-analysis. *Psychological Bulletin, 132*(1), 132–149. https://doi.org/10.1037/0033-2909.132.1.132

Widales-Benitez, O., d'Abreu, A., & Castro-Olivo, S. (2017). The effects of acculturative stress on Latino ELL students' academic aspirations. In *Poster presented at the annual convention of the American Psychological Association: Washington, DC.*

Yough, M., Slaten, C. D., Sankofa, N., Li, J., & Anderman, E. M. (2023). English language learners perceptions of school climate and teacher–student relationships: Role of acculturation and implications for achievement. *Learning Environments Research*, 1–18.

Chapter 7
Culturally and Linguistically Responsive Interventions to Support Emergent Bilingual Students' Language and Literacy

Monica E. Romero and Linda O. Cavazos

Concerns are growing in the United States regarding the literacy achievements of emergent bilingual students (EBs), their language and reading instruction, and educators' effectiveness in understanding reading development and teaching strategies. Despite scientific advances that have deepened the field's understanding of language and reading acquisition, a significant gap remains in effectively supporting the language and literacy needs of EBs. A significant number of EBs continue to demonstrate low reading proficiency on state and national accountability assessments. In 2022, the National Assessment of Educational Progress found that only 10% and 4% of fourth- and eighth-grade EBs scored at or above proficient in reading (National Center for Educational Statistics [NCES], 2022). This persistent trend of underperformance has been documented for the past 30 years (NCES, 2022).

Achievement data indicate that teachers of EBs need to provide students with language and literacy support while delivering culturally and linguistically adapted interventions, which are defined here as high-quality interventions that address culture and language through culturally and linguistically responsive practices. Culturally and linguistically responsive practices involve changes to instructional practices and curricula to meet the linguistic and academic needs of EBs. They include providing linguistic accommodations and scaffolds, selecting materials that value language diversity and represent multicultural groups, assisting students in making connections between their experiences, cultural backgrounds, and academic content, and differentiating instruction for EBs at varying levels of language

M. E. Romero (✉)
Educational Psychology, The University of Texas at Austin, Austin, TX, USA
e-mail: mromero@austin.utexas.edu

L. O. Cavazos
English Learner Leadership Advocacy Support (ELLAS) Consulting, Austin, TX, USA
e-mail: linda@ellasconsulting.com

D. Vega, J. N. Wolf (eds.), *Culturally and Linguistically Responsive Intervention and Assessment Practices with Emergent Bilingual Students*,
https://doi.org/10.1007/978-3-032-02084-0_7

proficiency and abilities (Project ELLIPSES et al., 2021). Effective educators recognize the sociocultural influences on learning and implement practices that value and respect students' cultural differences. Educators must adopt an assets-based approach to instruction that values and affirms EBs' identities and cultural knowledge.

Teachers of EBs often lack an understanding of second language acquisition and the time required to become proficient in a second language (Project ELLIPSES et al., 2021). EBs typically need 4–6 years of language support to achieve the required levels of language proficiency to succeed in English instruction (Thomas & Collier, 2002). Even after attaining language proficiency, students may struggle to acquire the academic language needed to understand content (August & Shanahan, 2017). Learning to read in English can be challenging for EBs because the English pronunciation differs from other phonetic languages, which may introduce differences in learning literacy skills (Goldenberg, 2020). Moreover, EBs are expected to learn academic content while simultaneously acquiring English language proficiency (August & Shanahan, 2017). The challenge of learning academic language intensifies as EBs progress through grades and texts become increasingly complex. Hence, linguistic support for EBs should be commensurate with the language demands of texts and students' oral language proficiency levels.

Multi-tiered System of Supports

Multi-tiered System of Supports (MTSS) is a school-based prevention and early intervention framework that is, in part, based on accurately identifying appropriate support for students across three tiers (Project ELLIPSES et al., 2021). Tiered instruction within a culturally and linguistically responsive (CLR) MTSS framework includes targeted, intensive, differentiated instruction on specific learning and language objectives that proactively bridge learning gaps and accelerate learning for EBs. Figure 7.1 presents a CLR MTSS framework (Project ELLIPSES et al., 2021) that centers on EBs' oral language proficiency levels alongside reading achievement data for planning culturally and linguistically responsive instruction and intervention.

EBs' oral language proficiency levels set the foundation for literacy development in both the home language and English. English proficiency levels range from beginning (B) to advanced high (AH) proficiency. EBs at the beginning (B) language proficiency level need help understanding directions, use simplified language, rely heavily on context clues, visuals, and gestures, and provide yes or no, or one- to two-word responses. EBs at the intermediate (I) proficiency level have better comprehension skills and use simple sentences characterized by some pronunciation and grammatical errors. EBs at the advanced (A) proficiency level speak fluently, use more complex sentences, and make occasional errors, but they participate well in class discussions. Those at the advanced high (AH) proficiency level have near-native fluency and understand idiomatic expressions. Understanding EBs' language

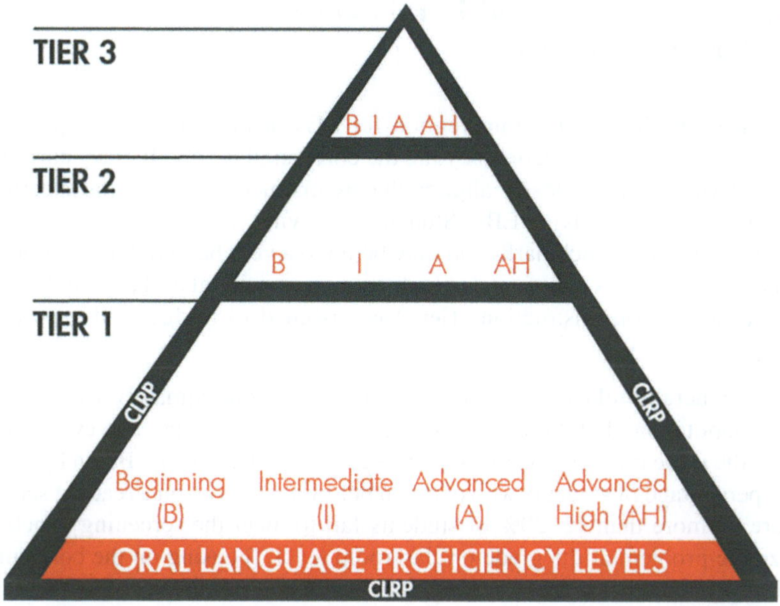

Fig. 7.1 Culturally and linguistically responsive MTSS framework (Source: Project ELLIPSES et al., 2021). *Note*: The MTSS framework addresses oral language proficiency levels and culturally and linguistically responsive (CLR) practices in every tier

proficiency levels is critical to planning tiered instruction and intervention lessons that meet students' language and literacy needs.

In Tier 1, differentiated core reading instruction is delivered within the general education classroom. *Differentiated instruction* involves focusing on individual student language and reading subskill needs during instruction. For example, within a differentiated small group in core instruction, teachers may support decoding for one student, fluency for another, and comprehension for others using the same text. School personnel are responsible for ensuring that quality core instruction, with differentiated class-wide support, is offered before considering Tier 2 and Tier 3 interventions within the MTSS framework. Tier 2 and Tier 3 interventions augment rather than supplant effective core instruction. Students who do not make adequate progress in Tier 1 receive targeted supplemental intervention, referred to as Tier 2, or intensive intervention, referred to as Tier 3. EBs benefit from small group intervention due to increased learning time, additional learning opportunities, more chances to participate, greater peer interaction, and opportunities to generalize skills (Project ELLIPSES et al., 2021). Language and literacy interventions are most effective in a safe environment where EBs can ask questions and receive instructional guidance, along with specific corrective and affirming feedback to promote skilled reading and deeper text comprehension (Cavazos, 2021). EBs may need language intervention separate from Tier 2 or 3 reading intervention in their language(s) of instruction if their language is not developing at a rate comparable to their peers.

Components of Tier 2 and Tier 3 Language and Literacy Intervention

Tier 2 Intervention Tier 2 intervention for EBs involves targeted supplemental language and literacy instruction beyond the core language and literacy curriculum. Tier 2 intervention must closely align with core instruction to meet the specific language and literacy needs of EBs. Students receiving Tier 2 intervention are not meeting grade-level benchmarks and may be up to a year behind. Furthermore, Tier 2 intervention employs a distinct curriculum or approach rather than simply extending the time for core instruction. Tier 2 is designed to bridge skill gaps in core instruction.

Tier 2 generally relies on a standard protocol for approximately 15–20% of the student population, but "standard protocol" does not mean that every student receives the same intervention (Truckenmiller & Brehmer, 2021). Begin by examining the percentage of students who perform below a cut score on a reading screening measure. If more than 15–20% of students fail to meet the screening benchmark, analyze the problem at the grade or classroom level, focusing on the core curriculum. It is possible that more than 20% of EBs will score below a cut score, or are at risk, on a screening measure. Low scores are not unusual as EBs progress through the second language acquisition process, particularly for those at lower language proficiency levels. If many EBs score below the cut score, analyze the linguistic support they receive in core and intensify oral language instruction. Additionally, the evidence base for the core curriculum, educators' implementation fidelity of the selected program, and student engagement and performance with the curricular materials must be reviewed to determine other necessary instructional adjustments.

Educational researchers have examined the effectiveness of Tier 2 intervention components and found positive outcomes when interventions are provided in small groups, delivered for 30–40 min 3–5 times a week, and designed to target specific skills (Truckenmiller & Brehmer, 2021). Effective interventions include explicit instruction, frequent opportunities to practice skills, and immediate teacher feedback (Gersten et al., 2020).

Tier 3 Intervention Tier 3 for EBs is more intensive support that addresses specific learning and language needs that have not been met with core instruction or Tier 2 intervention or for students with more intensive language and literacy needs (Linan-Thompson et al., 2022). Tier 3 intervention is intended for students who are significantly behind grade level (i.e., more than a year) and need additional materials and curricula to access grade-level content.

Schools and districts apply different criteria for identifying students for Tier 3 intervention. Typically, students who score in the bottom 5% on reading universal screeners or benchmark assessments are identified for Tier 3 intervention. Tier 3 intervention is designed to meet individual students' needs. Tier 3 intervention may require selecting materials at their ability levels but delivering them using

Table 7.1 Components of Tier 2 and Tier 3 interventions

Component	Tier 2	Tier 3
Eligible students	Bottom 15–20% of universal screeners or benchmark assessments	Bottom 5% of universal screeners or benchmark assessments
Grouping	4–6 students	1–3 students
Duration/ dosage	20–30 min, 2–5 days/week for 8–20 weeks	45–60 min, 4 or 5 days/week for 20+ weeks
Progress monitoring	Bimonthly	Biweekly or weekly
Interventionist	General education teacher, literacy specialist, or related service personnel	General education teacher, language or literacy specialist, English as a second language teacher, or special education teacher

Source: Project ELLIPSES et al. (2021). *Note*: Differences between Tier 2 and Tier 3 intervention

grade-level standards, for example, selecting simpler texts for a fifth-grade student reading at a third-grade level while helping them develop language and foundational reading skills to access grade-level text. This student would benefit from daily Tier 3 instruction.

Changes between Tier 2 and Tier 3 interventions include a decreased group size, increased frequency and duration, and the use of interventionists with deep expertise in second language acquisition who can address the language and literacy needs of EBs (Project ELLIPSES et al., 2021). To illustrate the difference between Tier 2 and Tier 3 interventions, see Table 7.1.

Evidence-Based Language and Literacy Practices for EBs

Evidence suggests that students can learn to read using a structured, code-based approach that is systematic, explicit, and sequential (Seidenberg, 2017). Effective literacy intervention emphasizes explicit and systematic instruction, prompt and targeted feedback, and data-based decision-making (Al Otaiba et al., 2023; Gersten et al., 2020). *Explicit* means that skills are taught directly, with modeling and clear explanations (i.e., concise, free of wordiness or extraneous information); children are not expected to learn foundational skills solely from exposure or introduction. *Systematic* refers to a planned sequence of instruction that gradually progresses from simple to complex skills.

Intervention practices and strategies must be validated for EBs and demonstrate effectiveness in improving their oral language and reading skills. Oral language development remains a priority and is an ongoing focus in interventions for EBs. Plan multimodal intervention lessons that activate the four language domains (listening, speaking, reading, and writing) to support language development. Ensure instruction is clear by delivering comprehensible input (e.g., adapting speech rate, enunciation, and simplification) aligned with EBs' language proficiency levels.

Provide clear task explanations, modeling, hands-on activities, demonstrations, and gestures (Echevarria et al., 2024). Incorporate ample discourse opportunities using strategies such as structured academic discussions with preplanned questions and set expectations for accountable talk (defined as understanding the norms of classroom discourse; Michaels et al., 2008). Understanding classroom norms, such as participating in discussions and answering in complete sentences using previously learned language structures, promotes educational equity and increased achievement for diverse learners (Michaels et al., 2008).

CLR teaching practices should include linguistic support in the students' home language, when possible, to ensure EBs understand the language and content of the lesson. Differentiate the language and literacy support based on EBs' oral language proficiency levels and abilities. Monitor students' responses to interventions and provide immediate corrective and affirming feedback to support their learning. Intervention materials must be culturally relevant and free of bias, stereotypes, or information that may be offensive to EBs from different cultures. Educators can begin by carefully reviewing materials and looking for representations of diverse individuals and cultures, with close attention to how they are portrayed. Ensure that curricular materials do not present any barriers to learning or cause anxiety for students.

Explicit and systematic oral language and literacy instruction for EBs should be provided daily, and skills should be taught to mastery. Allow EBs sufficient wait time to formulate appropriate responses after hearing a model response. Break intervention goals into smaller steps (e.g., chunking text) to reduce cognitive load on students. Explicitly draw attention to cross-linguistic transfer (i.e., use of the home language to understand English) and metalinguistic awareness (i.e., understanding the differences between languages) to help EBs identify and apply strategies independently. Build EBs' background knowledge by linking concepts to their lived experiences or prior learning and emphasizing key vocabulary (Echevarria et al., 2024). To activate or build background knowledge, present brief introductory information about the topic, question students to determine what they already know about it, share images or visuals, and display anchor videos (i.e., brief 1- to 3-min instructional videos). Building background knowledge helps EBs quickly learn information about a topic and stimulates interest in reading new text.

Target Reading Subskills for Intervention

Most EB teachers are familiar with the five components of reading identified by the National Reading Panel (2000) as essential for students to master to become proficient readers. These components are frequently referred to as the five components of reading: phonemic awareness, phonics, fluency, vocabulary, and comprehension. The components of reading apply to both home language and second language reading development. Mastering these components is dependent on EBs' oral language proficiency levels. For EBs, there are six components of reading, with oral language development driving the other five. Oral language development is the strongest predictor of EBs' reading comprehension and should be continuously developed alongside other reading subskills to achieve reading proficiency (Cavazos, 2021). Figure 7.2 illustrates the six components of reading that EBs need to become skilled readers in their home language and English.

Continue to develop EBs' oral language even after they achieve mastery of the components of reading, as increasing language and vocabulary will enhance comprehension of complex text as they progress through grade levels (Cavazos, 2021). EBs who have been reclassified or have exited language instructional programs need high levels of language and vocabulary for increased achievement.

Oral Language Development Oral language development is correlated with literacy development, and some EBs with reading difficulties may need language intervention in conjunction with reading intervention (Cavazos, 2021). Analyze current language data to determine if any difficulties in reading can be attributed to a lack of language proficiency. EBs need language to recognize words in a text, read them accurately and automatically, and comprehend their meaning as they read (Cavazos, 2021; Goldenberg, 2020).

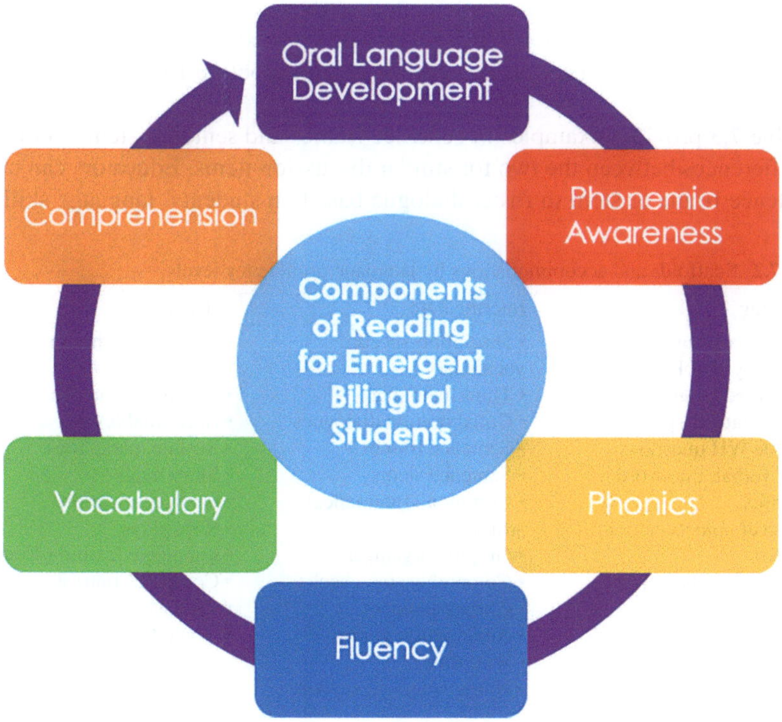

Fig. 7.2 Components of reading for emergent bilingual students. *Note*: Oral language development serves as the foundation for all reading components

Plan oral language goals for all language and reading intervention lessons with a specific focus on the target reading subskill goal based on student data. Oral language development provides EBs access to learning content and helps them navigate curricula. Strategically plan and incorporate explicit language goals into intervention to support the increased language demands of text (Cavazos, 2021; Goldenberg, 2020). Regularly assessing oral language development as part of an MTSS framework for EBs provides necessary language data to plan instruction and helps evaluate intervention effectiveness for students with oral language and literacy difficulties (Cavazos & Ortiz, 2020).

During language intervention, linguistic scaffolds and accommodations are essential for supporting students' comprehension of language and content. Table 7.2 presents examples of linguistic scaffolds and accommodations for EBs. The categories aid students at various language levels, though some may need scaffolds from all levels.

Some recommended language intervention strategies for EBs include structured academic discussions about the content being learned, extended accountable talk on instructional topics, daily dialogue with teachers and peers, and repeated exposure to new vocabulary (Cavazos, 2021; Dickinson & Porche, 2011). During language intervention, provide EBs with a model response and a sentence frame with blanks for students to fill in (e.g., *What I liked best about the story was _______ because of ______*). Sentence stems, or sentence starters, also help students generate responses (e.g., A connection I can make with the text is ____). These linguistic scaffolds allow EBs to hear an appropriate response before formulating their own responses.

Table 7.3 provides examples of sentence frames and sentence stems to illustrate the differences between the two for similar discussion items. Educators can choose a sentence frame or stem to foster dialogue based on students' language skills and

Table 7.2 Scaffolds and accommodations by language proficiency levels

Beginning	Intermediate	Advanced
• Functional language • Total Physical Response • Simplified language • Slower rate of speech • Simple WH questions • Non-verbal, one-word responses • Physical objects, actions, activities • Labels, visuals, objects • Think Alouds • Word banks; wall charts • Choral repetition • Read Alouds • Home language support	• Discipline-specific vocabulary • Think-pair-share • Collaboration dialogues • Sentence frames • Sentence stems • Common grammatical structures • Graphic organizers • Comprehension checks • Cloze passages • Anticipation guides • Wait time • Home language support	• Abstract, higher-order vocabulary • Complex sentence structure • Accountable talk • Restate, paraphrase • Story maps • Oral presentations • Role plays • Language learning strategies • Compare/contrast relationships • Home language support

(Adapted from Coelho, 2016; Levine et al., 2013). *Note*. Linguistic scaffolds to support EBs' oral language proficiency levels

Table 7.3 Sentence frames and sentence stems

Sentence frame	Sentence stem
My prediction is similar to ______, but I also think ___________.	One prediction I can make is ...
The main character can be described as ________ because of ________.	I would describe the character as ...
An experience I have had that relates to ______ in the story is _____.	The story made me think of ...

Note. Sentence frames and stems to generate dialog

ability to complete blanks or construct extended responses. It is recommended that both a sentence frame and a stem are used to ensure that students at different language proficiency levels can engage in the discussion.

Phonemic Awareness Phonemic awareness refers to the ability to hear and manipulate individual phonemes or sounds. It is a subskill of phonological awareness, a broader category that encompasses phonemes and groups of phonemes. EBs need to be able to discriminate individual phonemes to form words. Phonemic awareness is the foundational skill that precedes phonics, decoding, and encoding (National Reading Panel, 2000). Phonemic awareness is taught explicitly using phonemes (i.e., no graphemes or letters) during intervention. Phonemic awareness in an alphabetic and transparent language (i.e., predictable letter-sound correspondence), such as Spanish, may take less time to learn than in English (Cavazos, 2021). Learning to read in any language requires knowledge of phonemes and the ability to distinguish individual phonemes in spoken language.

During phonemic awareness intervention, provide ample opportunities for students to develop their skills. Phonemic awareness intervention is characterized by speech sound articulation and repetition, identifying phonemes in words through blending and segmenting phonemes and deleting or replacing sounds in words to form new ones. For example, after explicit instruction on phoneme segmentation with several modeled words and student practice, ask students to identify the phonemes in the word "duck" (/d/ /u/ /k/). Say the word slowly several times and let the students identify the phonemes. Conversely, after explicit instruction on phoneme blending, ask students to blend phonemes by listening to some sounds spoken slowly and identifying the word the sounds create (e.g., /d/ /u/ /k/ makes "duck"). Another example of phonemic awareness is to say the word *"can"* and ask students to change the phoneme /c/ to /m/ to make a new word ("man").

Phonics/Decoding Phonics instruction involves teaching the relationships between phonemes and graphemes (i.e., sounds and letters), also known as the alphabetic principle, which means that letters represent sounds in speech. Phonics includes letter recognition, matching letter sounds to letters, decoding, and learning to read. Decoding involves applying letter-sound knowledge to sound out and read words. EBs receiving intervention for reading may have difficulty mapping sounds to letters and translating written letters into words. If students come from language backgrounds with an opaque orthography (i.e., unpredictable letter-sound correspondence), it can be challenging for them to learn to decode. EBs must understand the alphabetic principle and its predictable relationships to decode and become fluent readers. They require explicit instruction on the six syllable types in English to learn to decode and encode words. In a language such as Spanish, where reading instruction is typically taught at the syllable level, students can learn to decode easily, while English phonics can be more challenging for EBs.

During phonics intervention, incorporate hands-on activities and manipulatives (e.g., plastic letters, letter cards, Elkonin boxes, etc.) to create words. Intervention teachers can assist students in decoding words, reading sentences, and navigating longer text passages with appropriate support. In the early decoding stages, EBs may require substantial linguistic support to comprehend unknown words. As they learn letter-sound patterns, they may struggle to tackle letter combinations that produce multiple sounds (e.g., /ou/ in out, pour, bought). Explicit instruction on the various sounds will aid them in understanding these patterns. As a fluent reader, the teacher should provide a daily model of 'good reading' while students learn to decode. Students who develop strong phonics skills in the early grades will gain a learning advantage as they advance through grades (Shanahan, 2020).

Fluency Reading fluency is the ability to read with speed, accuracy, and prosody (i.e., expression). Once EBs can decode, they can work on building fluency to become fluent readers. Fluency development is integral to skilled reading and highly correlates with text comprehension. EBs may need intervention for reading fluency if they exhibit slow, choppy, or labored reading with long pauses and lack of expression while reading aloud. During fluency intervention, explicitly teach and model fluency strategies such as reading aloud with students, letting students take turns reading aloud, using timed readings, and reading fluency phrases (i.e., short text sections; Cavazos, 2021).

Repeated text readings can help improve fluency and build students' confidence in reading familiar material. Reading smaller text sections aids EBs in developing fluency and reduces the cognitive load of lengthy passages. Listen for fluent reading at an appropriate rate (i.e., similar to speech rate or how students talk), with few hesitations, expression, and accuracy to identify any fluency issues. Address these issues as they arise, incorporating linguistic scaffolds to support skilled reading and oral language development. EBs may face fluency challenges due to a lack of word recognition, highlighting the importance of oral language development and broad vocabulary knowledge (Cavazos, 2021). Students require numerous daily opportunities to read to cultivate fluency. Researchers have found that reading fluency is a stronger predictor of reading comprehension in languages like Spanish, which have transparent orthographies, than accurate reading (Florit & Cain, 2011).

Vocabulary Vocabulary development is an essential skill for reading growth and is closely linked to oral language development and comprehension. EBs need exposure to extensive vocabulary in various contexts to recognize words in print and understand texts. Teach cross-curricular vocabulary and high-utility words, which appear more frequently in texts. EBs must practice using newly learned vocabulary and engage with content through meaningful language opportunities that activate the four language domains (i.e., listening, speaking, reading, and writing). As EBs learn to read and acquire language simultaneously, they will encounter many unfamiliar words. Therefore, they must learn an extensive academic vocabulary to access complex texts. Pre-teach vocabulary essential for comprehending the text and provide practice opportunities, including using vocabulary words in sentences.

Vocabulary intervention includes explicit instruction of a select set of academic words that are pre-taught before reading (Baker et al., 2014), teaching word learning strategies (e.g., syllable types, word analysis, multiple-meaning words, morphology), and providing embedded vocabulary instruction during reading (Hendrix & Griffin, 2017; Lesaux et al., 2010). Embedded vocabulary words are defined in the text and are easily understood in context. Explicit vocabulary instruction to support vocabulary development features student-friendly definitions, a visual or image, part of speech, cognate (shared word between the home language and English), and usage in sentences (Cavazos, 2021). Figure 7.3 depicts the information to include in vocabulary word cards for EBs.

Ensure that EBs repeat the words several times, create sentences with the words, and integrate them into writing (Baker et al., 2014; Lesaux & Harris, 2017). Provide home language support, if possible. Assist EBs in making cross-linguistic connections to vocabulary in their home language. Using the home language as a linguistic scaffold can help EBs learn new words in the second language. Using cognates supports language development and cross-linguistic transfer; if the student does not know the word in either language, knowing it is a cognate provides the word and definition in both languages.

Comprehension Understanding text eludes many EBs who may not grasp all the words they read because they are simultaneously learning to read in a language in which they are not yet proficient. To comprehend text, EBs need to be fluent readers who read automatically and accurately, have strong word recognition skills, and know the vocabulary they encounter. EBs may struggle with unknown words, both simple and complex. Text comprehension depends on the student's language development and vocabulary knowledge. These skills allow students to use cognitive energy to make sense of and comprehend text. If these skills are underdeveloped,

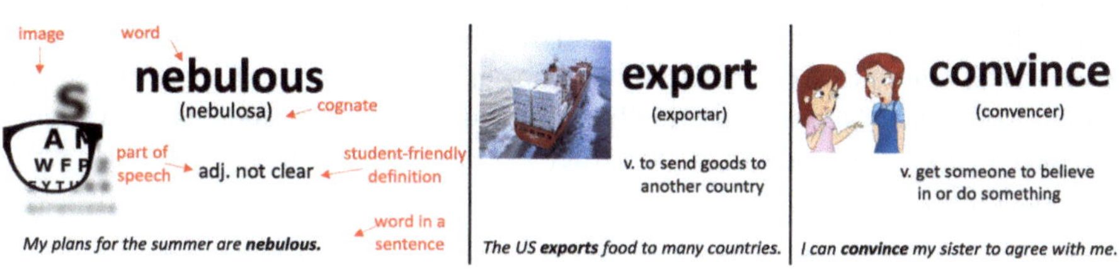

Fig. 7.3 Sample vocabulary word cards for EBs (Cavazos, 2024). *Note*: Vocabulary cards featuring images, student-friendly definitions, parts of speech, and example sentences

EBs expend most of their cognitive energy on decoding, fluency, and vocabulary, leaving less cognitive energy for text comprehension.

Interventions to improve comprehension include strategy instruction on analyzing text, drawing conclusions, making inferences, etc. Facilitate text comprehension for EBs by activating or building students' background knowledge about the text topic before reading. Chunk the text and ask comprehension questions for each section, engaging students in extensive dialogue before, during, and after reading. Utilize graphic organizers or semantic maps to organize text ideas. Every EB has a different language proficiency level in their home language (L1) and English (L2), so task differentiation is required to meet their individual needs. The level of linguistic and academic scaffolding provided to EBs will vary based on their language proficiency levels and academic performance data. Continuous comprehension checks should be conducted, and EBs should be allowed to demonstrate their text comprehension through both oral and written modalities.

Writing Writing is the fourth language domain and is often considered the most difficult to develop because of the heavy language and cognitive demands associated with it. EBs need knowledge of grammar, language, and sentence and paragraph structures to write effectively and communicate the ideas they are trying to convey (Cavazos & Cardenas-Hagan, 2020). They need well-developed oral language and vocabulary to draw from as they organize their ideas. It is critical for students with writing difficulties to determine whether these difficulties arise from low language proficiency levels or the challenge of organizing ideas around a topic to create a cohesive product. Begin by reviewing language proficiency data to make intervention decisions.

Students receiving intervention for writing need explicit instruction in writing strategies, including prewriting and educator support that encompasses modeling, guided practice, and both corrective and affirming feedback. Educators should model short and extended writing examples and discuss them (think aloud) to help students conceptualize the task and develop their respective writing assignments. Educators can assist students in organizing their ideas through group brainstorming, conceptual maps, and graphic organizers. Discuss vocabulary associated with the topic and create a word bank from which students can draw as they arrange their ideas into sentences, paragraphs, and longer writing products (Cavazos & Cardenas-Hagan, 2020). Plan daily writing opportunities and provide frequent feedback to students as they navigate the writing process of planning, brainstorming, organizing ideas, drafting, receiving feedback, and revising the draft for a final product (Cavazos & Cardenas-Hagan, 2020; Graham et al., 2012). For EBs at lower language proficiency levels, strategically pair them with other students with higher language proficiency levels to co-construct writing assignments until they can write independently.

Data-Based Decision-Making for EBs

A critical MTSS element is assessment and progress monitoring, which drives intervention decisions within and across tiers (e.g., matching students to intervention, increasing, decreasing, or maintaining support). Analyze assessment data to determine the skills students need. It is recommended that educators screen for all literacy skills to identify the specific skill in which the student needs additional support (Hoover et al., 2020). For example, if a student struggles with reading fluency, screen decoding skills to ensure that the root problem is not decoding—difficulty decoding will affect fluency. School personnel must match assessment data to specific interventions (Fuchs & Fuchs, 2006). When identifying intervention supports, consider these three essential decisions:

- Identifying individuals who require additional support (i.e., screening decision)
- Determining which interventions students might require (i.e., diagnostic decisions)
- Determining whether the intervention is effective (i.e., progress monitoring)

All instruction and intervention planning and decisions for EBs are guided by current language and reading assessment data. Data-based decision-making (DBDM) is driven by valid and reliable data and by implementing universal screeners and progress monitoring to inform instructional decisions (Linan-Thompson et al., 2022). For EBs, focusing on language skills is imperative for identifying instructional needs and planning interventions. Language and literacy development depend significantly on the amount of language input, opportunities for language production, and exposure to high-quality instruction in each language (Ortiz et al., 2018). When deciding if EBs need supplemental intervention, interpret assessment results while considering the amount and quality of literacy instruction students received in the target language(s).

Grade-level teams monitor trends in EBs' performance, identify needs, and determine group composition. An instructional change is necessary if an EB does not make adequate progress toward established language or literacy goals. For instance, possible changes may include different intervention materials, an increase or decrease in frequency or duration, a new intervention tier, or other instructional adjustments, such as the educator's pacing or amount of linguistic support. The same research-based reading intervention may not be effective for every EB. When selecting interventions, ensure they are effective for EBs, provide ample, differentiated linguistic support, and address culture and language (Linan-Thompson et al., 2022). Critical data-based decision-making components for EBs include:

- Establish a school team (e.g., principal, teacher, school psychologist, literacy specialist, and English language development specialist).
- Identify students by reviewing literacy and language assessments and consider their educational history, including instructional languages, grades, attendance, and vision or hearing.

- Select evidence-based interventions that address the language and literacy needs of EBs.
- Implement the intervention using language supports in the language(s) of instruction. Monitor and adjust intervention by examining progress monitoring and fidelity data

After collecting language and literacy screening or progress monitoring data, a decision rule is applied to analyze EBs' progress toward their language and literacy goals. Figure 7.4 highlights a data-based decision-making flowchart for EBs.

What Can Educators Do?

Educators of EBs must assume a proactive role in ensuring that current language and literacy data are used to inform instructional planning and decisions for EBs. Additional actions to take include:

- Apply assessment tools validated for EBs by reviewing the norming sample.
- Assess the four language domains: listening, speaking, writing, and reading.
- Triangulate data from various information sources, such as curriculum-based measurement and language and literacy state accountability assessments.
- Utilize assessment data to analyze growth rates.
- Implement language and literacy interventions.
- Regularly monitor student progress and EBs' responses to interventions.

If students are not progressing at expected rates, consider whether the reason may lie in the instruction or curricula used. Information gathered from student data is twofold: (1) how well the student responds to instruction/intervention; and (2) how effectively instruction was delivered. Both require immediate adjustments.

Considerations Before Special Education Referral for EBs

A prominent challenge facing educators is determining the extent to which an EB's reading difficulty can be attributed to the second language acquisition process or a learning difficulty or disability (Hoover et al., 2020; Ortiz et al., 2018). EBs are particularly vulnerable to misidentification in special education at higher rates than their monolingual English-speaking peers (Hoover et al., 2020). This pattern of misidentification occurs because educators may hesitate to refer students for eligibility determination when it is unclear whether slow reading skill acquisition arises from a difference in language ability and exposure or an underlying learning disability (Goodrich et al., 2023). Thus, educators must implement high-quality CLR instruction for EBs and carefully review oral language and reading data to identify the root cause of reading difficulties.

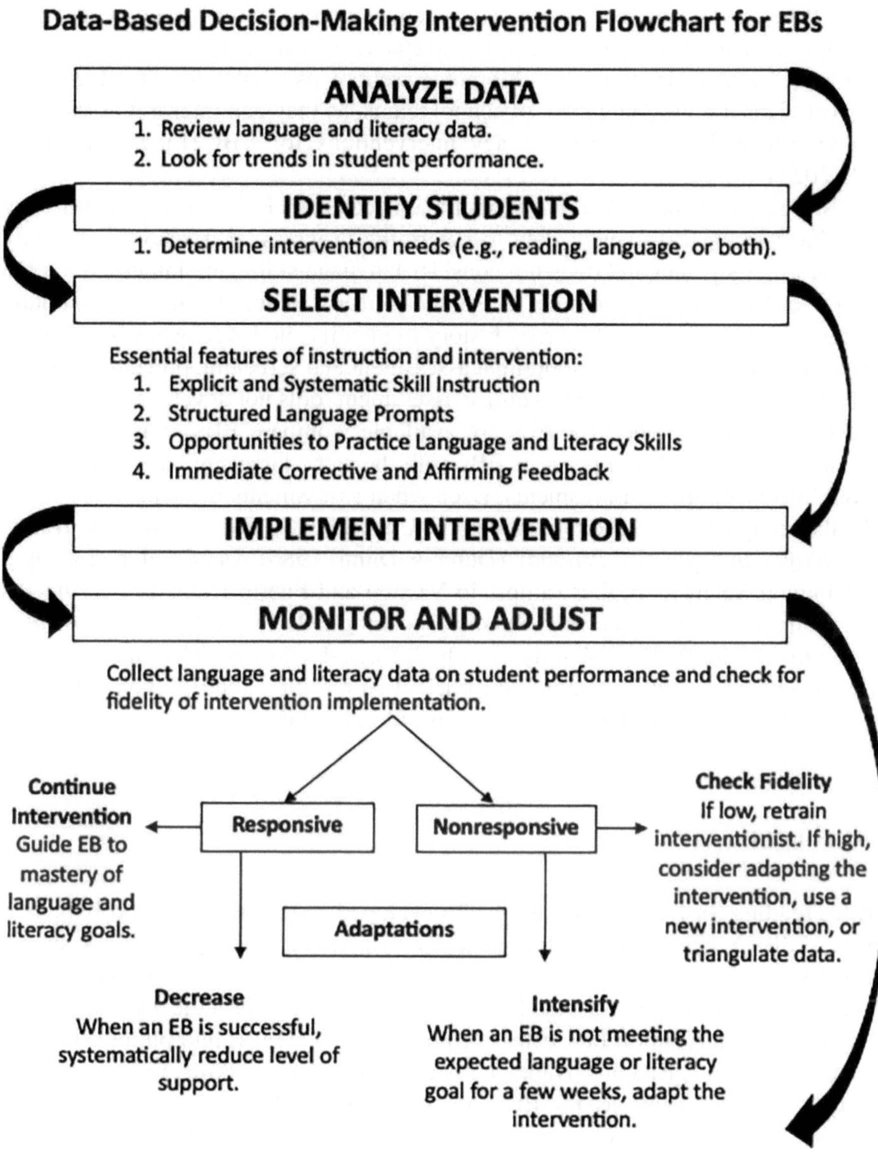

Fig. 7.4 Data-based decision-making intervention flowchart for EBs. *Note.* School-level data-based decision-making process

Besides literacy data, it is recommended that school teams collect and monitor oral language proficiency in L1 and L2 for EBs. Educators who understand L1 and L2 language acquisition and the relationship between language and literacy development will be better prepared to distinguish between EBs who need additional academic support and those who need intervention in language skills (Marrs et al.,

2022). When establishing a school team, include a member with deep expertise in language acquisition and multilingualism to ensure decisions consider language and its role in literacy development. Moreover, school psychologists or educational diagnosticians are vital members of school teams, as they can interpret assessment data to inform language and literacy interventions for EBs (Linan-Thompson et al., 2022).

It is highly recommended that school teams consider EBs' background history while interpreting assessment data to determine progress. If a school team only examines literacy data and does not consider language skills, the intervention plan may fail or be insufficient to meet the student's needs. School teams need to obtain a longitudinal language and literacy history to identify the languages EBs speak or have received instruction in for optimal assessment and screening procedures (Ortiz et al., 2018). It is inappropriate to utilize assessment tools not developed for EBs. If no assessments developed for EBs are available, compare EBs' performance on assessments to that of true peers or EBs with the same language backgrounds and school history on those assessments. Even when assessments in Spanish are available, they may not be normed for EBs in the United States. For example, the *Test de Vocabulario en Imágenes Peabody* (Dunn & Dunn, 1986) was developed using a monolingual Spanish speaker sample in Mexico and Puerto Rico. These students were instructed in Spanish only. Spanish-speaking EBs in the United States may receive instruction in English only or in both English and Spanish simultaneously. Select language assessments normed for EBs that resemble the EBs you instruct to inform intervention adaptations and improve literacy skills.

Conclusion

Skilled reading for EBs necessitates well-developed and continuously evolving language skills. A culturally and linguistically responsive MTSS framework should guide the provision of language and literacy instruction and intervention for EBs. Interventions should be informed by current oral language proficiency and reading data at every intervention tier. Effective phonemic awareness and phonics instruction to mastery give EBs an advantage in developing literacy skills. Evidence-based practices and interventions for EBs are those validated and demonstrated to be effective for them, characterized by extensive linguistic scaffolds and language opportunities. Continue linguistic support for EBs, including those who have been reclassified or are considered proficient in English, to ensure their ongoing language development and academic success. Key components of adapted interventions for EBs include the significance of oral language development in literacy intervention, evidence-based practices for EBs, and data-based decision-making for language and literacy intervention planning. This chapter emphasizes integrating CLR practices to support EBs' language and literacy needs. Guidance is provided on special education referral considerations for EBs and the importance of including specialists in second language acquisition who understand the role of language in literacy development in all data-based decisions for EBs.

Chapter Reflection Questions

- Is there a language proficiency progress monitoring system in place?
- Do EBs have a good language model for effective articulation and enunciation?
- Do EBs have sufficient oral language proficiency to understand literacy instruction?
- Are EBs receiving appropriate linguistic support to understand and access language and literacy instruction?
- Are differentiated language and literacy tasks and support provided regularly?
- Does the MTSS framework reflect a CLR model that supports the needs of EBs?
- Do school data teams include experts on language development in L1 and L2?
- Do school data teams review language and literacy data to inform literacy instruction and intervention?
- Are classroom conditions conducive to ample daily language opportunities for EBs?
- Does the classroom reflect a positive climate that values and encourages appreciation for language diversity?

References

Al Otaiba, S., McMaster, K., Wanzek, J., & Zaru, M. W. (2023). What we know and need to know about literacy interventions for elementary students with reading difficulties and disabilities, including dyslexia. *Reading Research Quarterly, 58*(2), 313–332. https://doi.org/10.1002/rrq.458

August, D., & Shanahan, T. (2017). *Developing literacy in second-language learners: Report of the National Literacy Panel on Language-Minority Children and Youth*. Routledge.

Baker, S., Lesaux, N., Jayanthi, M., Dimino, J., Proctor, C. P., Morris, J., ... & Newman-Gonchar, R. (2014). *Teaching academic content and literacy to english learners in elementary and middle school. IES Practice Guide*. NCEE 2014-4012. What Works Clearinghouse.

Cavazos, L. (2024). *Effective structured literacy for adolescent English Learners in Grades 6-12*. Canvas Course, New Mexico Public Education Department.

Cavazos, L. (2021). *The science of reading for emergent bilinguals in New Mexico*. https://webnew.ped.state.nm.us/wp-content/uploads/2022/01/The-Science-of-Reading-for-Emergent-Bilinguals-in-New-Mexico_Jan-2022-.pdf

Cavazos, L. O., & Cardenas-Hagan, E. (2020). Writing development among English Learners. In E. Cardenas-Hagan (Ed.), *Literacy foundations for English LE\arners: A comprehensive guide to evidence-based instruction* (pp. 189–206). Brookes Publishing.

Cavazos, L. O., & Ortiz, A. A. (2020). Incorporating oral language assessment into MTSS/RTI frameworks: The potential of personal narrative assessment. *Bilingual Research Journal, 43*(3), 323–344.

Coelho, E. (2016). *Adding English: A guide to teaching in multilingual classrooms* (2nd ed.). University of Toronto Press.

Dickinson, D. K., & Porche, M. V. (2011). Relation between language experiences in preschool classrooms and children's kindergarten and fourth-grade language and reading abilities. *Child Development, 82*(3), 870–886.

Dunn, L. M., & Dunn, L. M. (1986). *Test de vocabulario imágenes Peabody: adaptación española*. Mepsa.

Echevarria, J., Vogt, M., Short, D., & Toppel. (2024). *Making content comprehensible for Multilingual learners: The SIOP model* (6th ed.). Pearson.

Florit, E., & Cain, K. (2011). The simple view of reading: Is it valid for different types of alphabetic orthographies? *Educational Psychology Review, 23*, 553–576.

Fuchs, D., & Fuchs, L. S. (2006). Introduction to response to intervention: What, why, and how valid is it? *Reading Research Quarterly, 41*(1), 93–99.

Gersten, R., Haymond, K., Newman-Gonchar, R., Dimino, J., & Jayanthi, M. (2020). Meta-analysis of the impact of reading interventions for students in the primary grades. *Journal of Research on Educational Effectiveness, 13*(2), 401–427. https://doi.org/10.1080/19345747.2019.1689591

Goldenberg, C. (2020). Reading wars, reading science, and English learners. *Reading Research Quarterly, 55*, S131–S144.

Goodrich, J. M., Fitton, L., Chan, J., & Davis, C. J. (2023). Assessing oral language when screening multilingual children for learning disabilities in reading. *Intervention in School and Clinic, 58*(3), 164–172. https://doi.org/10.1177/10534512221081264

Graham, S., Bollinger, A., Olson, C. B., D'Aoust, C., MacArthur, C., McCutchen, D., & Olinghouse, N. (2012). *Teaching elementary school students to be effective writers: A practice guide*. NCEE 2012-4058. What Works Clearinghouse.

Hendrix, R. A., & Griffin, R. A. (2017). Developing enhanced morphological awareness in adolescent learners. *Journal of Adolescent & Adult Literacy, 61*(1), 55–63.

Hoover, J. J., Soltero-González, L., Wang, C., & Herron, S. (2020). Sustaining a multi-tiered system of supports for English learners in rural community elementary schools. *Rural Special Education Quarterly, 39*(1), 4–16. https://doi.org/10.1177/8756870519847466

Lesaux, N. K., Kieffer, M. J., Faller, S. E., & Kelley, J. G. (2010). The effectiveness and ease of implementation of an academic vocabulary intervention for linguistically diverse students in urban middle schools. *Reading Research Quarterly, 45*(2), 196–228.

Lesaux, N. K., & Harris, J. R. (2017). An investigation of comprehension processes among adolescent English learners with reading difficulties. *Topics in Language Disorders, 37*(2), 182–203.

Levine, L. N., Lukens, L., & Smallwood, B. A. (2013). *The GO TO strategies: Scaffolding options for teachers of English language learners, K-12*. For Project EXCELL, a partnership between the University of Missouri-Kansas City and North Kansas City Schools, funded by the U.S. Department of Education, PR (T195N070316).

Linan-Thompson, S., Ortiz, A., & Cavazos, L. (2022). An examination of MTSS assessment and decision making practices for English learners. *School Psychology Review, 51*(4), 484–497. https://doi.org/10.1080/2372966X.2021.2001690

Marrs, H., De Leon, M., & Lawless, T. (2022). Use of English language proficiency data to better assess reading growth for English language learners. *School Psychology Review, 51*(4), 427–440. https://doi.org/10.1080/2372966X.2021.1917971

Michaels, S., O'Connor, C., & Resnick, L. B. (2008). Deliberative discourse idealized and realized: Accountable talk in the classroom and in civic life. *Studies in Philosophy and Education, 27*, 283–297.

National Center for Education Statistics. (2022). *National Assessment of Educational Progress (NAEP) data*. National Center for Educational Statistics. https://www.nationsreportcard.gov/dashboards/achievement_gaps.aspx

National Reading Panel. (2000). *Report of the National Reading Panel—teaching children to read: An evidence-based assessment of the scientific research literature on reading and its implications for reading instruction*. National Institute of Child Health and Human Development.

Ortiz, A. A., Robertson, P. M., & Wilkinson, C. Y. (2018). Language and literacy assessment record for English Learners in bilingual education: A framework for instructional planning and decision-making. *Preventing School Failure: Alternative Education for Children and Youth, 62*(4), 250–265. https://doi.org/10.1080/1045988X.2018.1443423

Project ELLIPSES, Project ELITE, & Project LEE. (2021). *Meeting the needs of English learners with and without disabilities: Brief 3, English learners with significant learning difficulties or disabilities: Recommendations for practice*. U.S. Office of Special Education Programs.

Seidenberg, M. S. (2017). Dyslexia in a computational model of word recognition in reading. In *Reading acquisition* (pp. 243–273). Routledge.

Shanahan, T. (2020). What constitutes a science of reading instruction? *Reading Research Quarterly, 55*, S235–S247.

Thomas, W., & Collier, V. (2002). *A national study of school effectiveness for language minority students' long-term academic achievement*. Center for Research in Education, Diversity, & Excellence.

Truckenmiller, A. J., & Brehmer, J. S. (2021). Making the most of Tier 2 intervention: What decisions are made in successful studies? *Reading & Writing Quarterly, 37*(3), 240–259. https://doi.org/10.1080/10573569.2020.1768612

Chapter 8
Culturally Adapted Practices and Interventions to Support the Mathematics Needs of Emergent Bilingual Students

Genesis D. Arizmendi and Jennifer E. Kong

In today's increasingly diverse classrooms, it is imperative to recognize and respond to the unique needs of emergent bilingual students. The term "emergent bilingual" (EB) refers to those acquiring proficiency in a new language, often while maintaining their native language skills (García et al., 2008). In addition to building language proficiency in English, these students also engage with specialized academic content such as mathematics, requiring targeted instructional approaches to support their growth. For EB students, language-related factors can significantly impact their performance in specialized academic subjects like mathematics, creating disparities between their abilities in math calculation and math word problems. To bridge this gap and ensure equitable educational opportunities, practitioners must understand the unique needs of emergent bilingual students in their mathematical development and how to implement culturally adapted interventions tailored to their specific needs.

Throughout this chapter, we will explore the utility and necessity of culturally adapted interventions in the context of mathematics education for emergent bilingual students. We equip educators and practitioners with strategies to distinguish between features of second language development and mathematics-related

Competing interests: The author(s) declare none.

G. D. Arizmendi (✉)
Department of Speech, Language, and Hearing Sciences and Cognitive Science Program, College of Science, University of Arizona, Tucson, AZ, USA
e-mail: genesis@arizona.edu

J. E. Kong
Department of Special Education, Attallah College of Educational Studies, Chapman University, Orange, CA, USA
e-mail: jekong@chapman.edu

D. Vega, J. N. Wolf (eds.), *Culturally and Linguistically Responsive Intervention and Assessment Practices with Emergent Bilingual Students*,
https://doi.org/10.1007/978-3-032-02084-0_8

disabilities, while also examining practical methods for aligning instruction with students' cultural backgrounds and linguistic skills. The implementation of culturally adapted teaching methods and interventions is essential for ensuring that emergent bilingual students succeed in mathematics. This chapter serves as a guide, offering practical, evidence-based strategies for supporting the academic development and growth of emergent bilingual students in mathematics.

Understanding the Unique Needs of Emergent Bilingual Students in Mathematics

Children learning English as their second language are the most rapidly growing demographic in US public schools (National Center for Education Statistics [NCES], 2024). The US educational system categorizes students who are not proficient in English, with a heritage language other than English, as English learners (ELs). The term 'emergent bilingual' (EB) will be used from here on to highlight an EL's linguistic assets and unique potential for bilingualism rather than a label focusing on the acquisition of English alone (García et al., 2008). Children whose first language is Spanish and second language is English make up 76.4% of EBs in US public schools (NCES, 2024). A challenge that these children face is that they often display difficulties in school because of the additional cognitive load of learning a new language, all while learning the expectations, routines, and academic demands and subjects of a subtractive school environment (i.e., one that focuses on acquiring a second language at the expense of one's home language; Valenzuela, 2010).

A significant number of EB students consistently struggle to attain proficiency in mathematics, as evidenced by data from the National Assessment of Educational Progress (2011, 2013, 2017, 2019) and the National Center for Education Statistics (2020, 2023). Proficiency in mathematics is critical for academic success, providing a foundation for advancement in education, and has profound implications for future employment and socioeconomic opportunities. However, according to the National Center for Education Statistics and National Assessment of Educational Progress (2022), by fourth grade, 48% of emergent bilingual fourth-graders score below the basic level in mathematics. This figure escalates to approximately 76% scoring below the basic level by the time they reach eighth grade. These challenges often arise from the intersection of language barriers, cultural differences, and the intricacies of mathematical concepts (e.g., Arizmendi et al., 2021; Kong et al., 2022; Wolf & Leon, 2009), coupled with limited supports (e.g., Sugarman & Geary, 2018) and minimal teacher training related to EBs (e.g., Parkhouse et al., 2019), pointing to critical institutional failures in educational equity (e.g., De Brey et al., 2019). Understanding and addressing these challenges is crucial for providing equitable and effective mathematics education for this diverse group of students.

Emergent bilingual students are clearly a heterogeneous group; not all may experience math difficulties (MD) and/or a specific learning disability in mathematics. A specific learning disability in mathematics refers to students who are identified as having a specific learning disorder [IDEA Sec. 300.8(c)(10)] in one or more basic psychological processes, which significantly impact math calculation and problem-solving. However, many students may demonstrate low performance in mathematics without a formal diagnosis of a mathematics disability. For example, students may receive Tier 2 and Tier 3 interventions and supports within a multi-tiered system of supports (MTSS) model. Descriptions of example interventions, specifically for culturally and linguistically diverse students, are detailed below. For the purposes of this chapter, the term MD refers to students who experience difficulty in mathematics and are at risk for identification of a specific learning disability in mathematics (see Nelson & Powell, 2018, for more information).

The Role of Language

Emergent bilingual students encounter various challenges in mathematics education that are often rooted in access to the language of instruction, leading to vocabulary disparities and difficulties in reading and comprehension (Arizmendi et al., 2021). As language serves as the primary conduit for introducing, explaining, and practicing mathematical concepts, limited English proficiency becomes a significant obstacle for EBs in the United States enrolled in English-only programs (Wolf et al., 2023), who often have few supports (e.g., Sugarman & Geary, 2018) and minimal teacher training related to the unique considerations in instruction and assessment for EBs (e.g., Oh & Mancilla-Martinez, 2021; Parkhouse et al., 2019). Moreover, the specialized vocabulary and terminology prevalent in academic subjects such as mathematics present additional challenges. Mathematical terms such as "quadrilateral," "denominator," or "factor" can be particularly difficult, as they are both complex and often only heard and used in the classroom during instruction, leading to fewer opportunities to learn the mathematical language in English and potential misunderstandings that impede their grasp of essential math concepts (Ron, 1999).

Language skills can often pose a challenge to mathematical ability, particularly in the context of mathematical word problems (e.g., Barbu & Beal, 2010; Martiniello, 2008), which involve an element of text comprehension or receptive language (e.g., Swanson et al., 2021a). Word problems often feature complex syntactic structures, specialized mathematical vocabulary, and context-specific information (e.g., Moschkovitch, 2015), which require explicit instruction to comprehend the concepts. Emergent bilinguals can find word problems particularly challenging due to difficulties with comprehending complex language structures, along with the application of appropriate mathematical processes, which ultimately impacts their ability to accurately interpret and solve mathematical questions (e.g., Arizmendi et al., 2021; Driver & Powell, 2017; Powell et al., 2020; Swanson et al., 2021b). For students still developing their English language skills, comprehending the problem statement itself can be challenging. Without adequate instructional support, they may struggle to grasp the context, identify key information, and understand the connections between different elements of the presented information (i.e., ignoring distractors). Beyond language comprehension, EB students may also face challenges when converting verbal information into mathematical representations. This step involves not only changing words (e.g., "What is the sum of one and four?") into numbers (i.e., 1, 4) and symbols (i.e., +) but also understanding the mathematical concepts hidden within the problem (i.e., what is → perform the mathematical operation 1+4 = 5). Moreover, word problems often require higher-level thinking skills like problem-solving strategies, logical reasoning, and mathematical modeling. Emergent bilingual students might encounter difficulties applying these skills, not because they lack the ability, but because language-related barriers draw their cognitive resources away from solving the problem (e.g., Swanson et al., 2021b, 2022).

For example, Alt et al. (2013) administered the KeyMath-3, an English standardized mathematics test, to students classified by their schools as ELs. All EL students achieved notably lower scores than their monolingual English-speaking peers when the KeyMath was presented in English. However, when the researchers adjusted for language by administering a Spanish-language version of the test, the EL students' performance equaled that of their monolingual peers on the same assessment measures. These findings suggest that the EL students did not face challenges comprehending mathematical concepts (i.e., the fundamental constructs the test was designed to evaluate). Instead, their difficulties were rooted in the language specific to mathematical assessments. It is critical to emphasize that all EL students in this study demonstrated improved scores when they took the Spanish version, even those considered primarily proficient in English. Furthermore, research conducted by Alt et al. (2014) found that when math tasks were structured with reduced linguistic complexity, students classified as ELs performed just as well as their monolingual peers. These findings underscore: (1) the profound impact of language development in *both* languages on mathematical performance; (2) the intricate relationship between language and achievement in mathematics, and (3) the importance of developing evidence-based interventions in mathematics that focus on developing the language of mathematics (Arizmendi et al., 2021).

Theoretical Frameworks for Culturally Adapted Mathematics Interventions

One way to address the unique needs of EB students in mathematics instruction is through implementing culturally responsive pedagogy. A culturally responsive math education framework cultivates equitable learning environments by considering students' distinctive strengths, backgrounds, and needs from various cultures and languages (e.g., Kong et al., 2022). Culturally responsive pedagogy seeks to develop students' academic achievement and social and cultural competence (Gay, 2018). Students' unique cultural and social backgrounds are integrated and leveraged in a classroom setting to make learning relevant and engaging. That is, high levels of engaged learning are cultivated by bridging students' personal cultural experiences and curricular content, with literature supporting that integrating culturally responsive teaching in mathematics contributes to students' instructional engagement and success (Aronson & Laughter, 2016).

Culturally responsive pedagogy, which informs culturally responsive teaching practices, is rooted in sociocultural theory (Vygotsky, 1978). Sociocultural theory posits that social interactions and cultural contexts significantly influence individual development. Vygotsky proposed that a person's cognitive development is deeply intertwined with their social interactions and cultural experiences, highlighting the crucial role of social interactions, collaborative learning, and cultural influences in shaping how individuals learn and develop. According to this theory, learning is not solely an individual process; instead, it occurs within social contexts and is greatly impacted by the cultural tools, practices, and norms of one's environment. The norms of one's environment are often transmitted through language, and *language is culture* (Jiang, 2000; Lambert, 1973). Vygotsky emphasized the concept of the zone of proximal development, where learning occurs most effectively when individuals engage in tasks just beyond their current level of competence, with the guidance and support of others. This theory has profoundly impacted educational practices, emphasizing the importance of social interactions, scaffolding, and cultural context in facilitating learning and cognitive development. Therefore, mathematical cognition can be conceptualized as being shaped by language, everyday experiences, and social interaction with others.

Culturally Adapted Mathematics Curriculum and Instruction

A common misconception of mathematics is that it is considered a universal language (and culture) that can be understood regardless of one's own language and cultural background (e.g., Lee & Lee, 2017; Morita-Mullaney et al., 2021; Waller & Flood, 2016). However, learning math requires specific knowledge in the content area vocabulary, as well as complex language processing. Further, historical stereotypes of students of culturally and linguistically diverse backgrounds may negatively impact their own ability to do well in math and math identity (Miller-Cotto & Lewis, 2020; Nasir, 2002). Integrating student experiences and cultural experiences into math instruction supports positive self-perceptions and engagement in math (Abdulrahim & Orosco, 2020). Culturally adapted math curriculum and instruction represent an approach to teaching mathematics that recognizes and embraces students' diverse cultural backgrounds and identities. It is an educational framework designed to ensure that mathematics education is inclusive and relevant to all learners, regardless of their cultural background. In a culturally adapted mathematics curriculum, the content, materials, and instructional strategies are intentionally designed to incorporate elements that resonate with the cultural contexts and experiences of the students (e.g., Leonard, 2018). This approach acknowledges that culture plays a significant role in shaping students' perspectives and learning styles and leverages these cultural assets to enhance mathematical learning. These approaches acknowledge students' diverse cultural backgrounds and experiences, recognizing that one size does not fit all when it comes to learning. By adapting math curriculum and instructional strategies to reflect the cultural contexts and identities of the learners, educators can engage students more meaningfully and enhance their understanding of mathematical concepts (e.g., Abdulrahim & Orosco, 2020; Kong et al., 2021; Orosco & Abdulrahim, 2017; see Strutchens et al., 2023 for a review).

Culturally responsive education extends beyond emphasizing academic success. It seeks to initiate educational transformation by firmly anchoring pedagogy, curriculum, and assessment in local knowledge, culture, and language (e.g., Nicol et al., 2013). Culturally responsive mathematics instruction, particularly in the context of students with or at risk for MD, should not be viewed as a replacement for established effective instructional practices. Methods such as explicit instruction, the emphasis on conceptual comprehension, schema instruction, the utilization of visual aids and support, encouraging students to articulate mathematical concepts, and the systematic monitoring of progress (as evidenced in studies by Doabler et al., 2016; Fuchs et al., 2008; Kong et al., 2021; Woodward et al., 2012) remain essential in guiding quality mathematics education. Instead, culturally responsive mathematics instruction should be considered a complementary framework that enhances and sustains equitable and effective instruction for all students. It achieves this by integrating well-established principles of effective math instruction for students with MD with the principles of culturally responsive instruction.

One key aspect of a culturally adapted math curriculum as a part of Tier 1 instruction is incorporating real-world examples and problems that resonate with students' cultural backgrounds (e.g., Harding-DeKam, 2014; Ukpokodu, 2011). This makes mathematics more relatable and demonstrates its practical relevance for all learners. For example, incorporating culturally relevant word problems or mathematical challenges that draw from students' everyday experiences can inspire a deeper interest in mathematics (e.g., Costa et al., 2022). Furthermore, culturally adapted instruction can encourage diverse perspectives and approaches to problem-solving, with opportunities for students to relate to the content, engage in mathematics communication with peers, and promote student self-confidence (e.g., Hubert, 2014). When teachers tap into students' unique cultural lenses and experiences as assets instead of treating them as deficits, it empowers those students to draw from their full repertoire of strengths and assets (Bottoms et al., 2017). In essence, culturally adapted math curriculum and instruction are essential tools in promoting equitable and inclusive math education, bridging achievement gaps, and fostering greater opportunities for all students.

Another instructional practice that teachers may consider during Tier 1 instruction is the use of structured peer-assisted learning strategies (see Fuchs et al., 2011, *PALS Math Manuals* for review) while encouraging students to develop deep understandings in the students' native language. As mentioned above, culturally responsive math instruction does not replace typical evidence-based instructional practices but is a complementary framework for providing instructional strategies for all students, specifically emergent bilingual students. For example, previous literature has found that Tier 2 and Tier 3 interventions such as explicit instruction, teaching conceptual understanding, schema instruction, visual representations and supports, and ongoing progress monitoring are effective strategies for improving math outcomes for students with disabilities (Kong et al., 2021; Fuchs et al., 2008). Instructional strategies for EB students should also include these, with emphases on building and utilizing the rich background knowledge of students, teaching essential vocabulary, providing native language supports, including culturally engaging visual representations, and the use of linguistically and culturally appropriate assessments (Doabler et al., 2016; Kong et al., 2022; Foster et al., 2018; Orosco et al., 2013).

As an example, the National Center on Intensive Intervention (2016) provides a guide for designing interventions in math in specific skill areas. One strategy shown in the literature to improve students' math achievement by building conceptual understandings is using multiple representation models, the Concrete Representational Abstract (CRA) framework (Bouck et al., 2018; Gersten et al., 2009). Teachers can utilize this framework to provide Tier 2 and Tier 3 interventions for students struggling in math. In the Concrete phase, teachers can use physical manipulatives such as realia, base-10 blocks, clocks, or fraction tiles to introduce new concepts to students. Building upon students' background knowledge, teachers may incorporate familiar household objects and ask students to verbalize understandings with peers in their primary language. In the Representational phase, teachers may use drawings, diagrams, and pictorial representations to help solve problems. Visual diagrams are best used when explicitly connected to the conceptual understanding of the problem. Finally, numbers and symbols are used during the Abstract phase. Best practices for teaching EB students, such as teaching relevant vocabulary and the use of native language supports, can then be integrated with these careful instructional sequences.

Assessment and Monitoring of Student Progress

One essential element of culturally responsive instruction is using culturally and linguistically sensitive assessment practices. Emergent bilingual students face the challenge of simultaneously acquiring academic language in addition to content area knowledge in their second language. Thus, many EB students may struggle academically upon entering a class taught primarily in English (August et al., 2009). When EB students struggle academically, they may be referred for special education services and often inaccurately identified as needing academic services and support based on their performance on assessments administered only in English. Assessing EB students using English-based assessments is problematic because lower scores may reflect language proficiency rather than academic knowledge or skills. Conversely, the belief that students' academic difficulties result from low language proficiency may delay the referral of students who have an actual need for special education services. This leads to the paradoxical over- and under-representation of EB students receiving special education services (Morgan et al.,

2018; Morgan, 2021). This highlights the importance of correctly assessing students' skills in both their first and second language to determine if these difficulties result from language acquisition or learning disability. Further, clearly explaining tasks and directions in the native or comprehensible language is also vital in administering culturally appropriate assessments.

In addition to selecting the appropriate initial assessments for EB students, ongoing progress monitoring has been identified as a key instructional component for students with learning disabilities (Fuchs et al., 2008). Frequent progress monitoring allows educators to make informed data-based decisions to adjust instruction and understand the student's actual skill ability. Currently, curriculum-based measures are frequently used to monitor ongoing progress in math. While some assessment offerings are emerging in alternate languages (most commonly Spanish), most typical assessments may not accurately capture the skills of EB students because they do not have the appropriate psychometric properties, nor reflect EB students in the norming sample. As such, educators must be mindful of the assessments they select and determine their practical application to the EB students they serve. Educators may consider examining items to determine if language and/or cultural biases in assessments may impact a student's ability to demonstrate knowledge or skills. That is, educators might adjust assessment items that require specific contextual knowledge (particularly cultural and linguistic in nature) to answer correctly. For example, an item on an assessment may say, "How many buoys are by the dock?" For an EB child from a rural desert town in the southwest, there is likely no prior knowledge to draw upon about most of the vocabulary terms presented, regardless of the mathematics required, if there are no supports to understand the content. These considerations in selecting and adapting assessment items to be administered in a non-standardized way would allow for more accurate data to establish needs for targeted interventions.

Case Study and Best Practices

To apply these aforementioned concepts into practice, we offer a framework for implementing culturally sustaining practices in the classroom (as outlined in Kong et al., 2022). As mentioned previously, culturally responsive instruction for math does not replace current best practices for effective instruction; rather, it is a framework for integrating already established practices found effective in research with key features of culturally responsive instruction. This framework (see Table 8.1) includes the following four key features: (a) using culturally and linguistically appropriate assessment tools and approaches; (b) including anti-biased contextual supports within math instruction; (c) providing linguistic supports; and (d) sustaining home-school collaborations (Kong et al., 2022). A case study adapted from Kong et al. (2022) will be presented to provide examples of actual classroom implementations of these key features.

Table 8.1 Examples of culturally and linguistically responsive activities

Area	Specific skill	Sample activity
Culturally and linguistically appropriate assessment	Providing assessments that consider the child's language ability and cultural experiences	• Teacher provides directions and explanation of task in comprehensible language or with native language support. • Assessments are controlled for vocabulary and language ability, if appropriate. • Each assessment targets one skill to identify areas of need.
Antibiased contextual supports	Integrating students' experiences and cultural background into math instruction	• Teacher introduces the concept of part and whole by displaying pictures of food that can be cut into equal parts (e.g., apples, oranges). • Students provide examples and draw pictures of food that may be shared from their respective cultures. • Utilize student examples to cut foods into equal parts.
Linguistic supports	Providing language support in math instruction	• Teacher explicitly preteaches academic and mathematic specific vocabulary by: – Modeling pronunciation – Providing a student-friendly definition – Providing examples of appropriate usage – Providing native language translation, if appropriate. • Teacher models strategy usage in comprehensible language.
Home-school collaborations	Sustaining positive relationships between school and home	• Send home positive notes of successes (translated, if necessary). • Provide visual representations of progress in math (e.g., progress monitoring graphs). • Ask caregivers and students to identify ways math is used in the community. • Value home input on expectations and responsibilities.

Mr. Cruz is a new special education teacher in an urban school district in the southwest region of the U.S. His class is comprised of culturally and linguistically minoritized learners, many of whom are from marginalized and underserved communities. Additionally, many of his students are also in the process of acquiring English in addition to learning the content curriculum. Mr. Cruz would like to implement a culturally sustaining framework within his math teaching to support the diverse needs of his classroom.

Culturally and Linguistically Appropriate Assessments *Mr. Cruz knows that it is crucial to obtain accurate and valid data on his students. For this reason, he decides to administer assessments in math that are both culturally and linguistically*

appropriate. For example, he assesses all math skills in both the child's native language in addition to English to better understand the child's actual math skills. By assessing the student's native language, Mr. Cruz can determine if difficulties are arising due to a language issue or a difficulty related to the actual math skills. Additionally, Mr. Cruz might review the assessments he plans to use to investigate if any items require knowledge outside of a student's cultural experience to answer correctly. In line with this, Mr. Cruz could also adapt the assessment to control for general academic vocabulary and/or reading level. If difficulties in specific skills in math are evident across languages, Mr. Cruz can conclude that these areas may need to be addressed with intervention.

Anti-biased Contextual Supports *Given this new information that Mr. Cruz has acquired through appropriate assessments, Mr. Cruz can provide culturally responsive math instruction integrating the experiences of his students. For example, Mr. Cruz may utilize the students' collective knowledge of sharing and food to introduce the math concepts of part and whole. He could ask students to draw or find photos of different types of food they eat at home, which can be cut and shared equally. He could also ask about jobs and careers that require math, integrating past experiences of students and families. Mr. Cruz would be careful not to perpetuate negative and harmful stereotypes but to approach each student and their experiences with curiosity and openness.*

Linguistic Supports *Mr. Cruz knows that vocabulary and language are critical to engagement and learning in math. Before the start of any lesson, he would make sure to present the lesson objectives in student-friendly language, ensuring that he explains the directions of the task in a comprehensible manner and spends time teaching new vocabulary terms and their meaning. During instruction, Mr. Cruz could integrate native language supports by providing native language definitions, texts, and encouraging students to discuss with their peers in their native language, allowing for higher-level math processing while also validating the students' linguistic wealth.*

Home-School Collaborations *Mr. Cruz has the option to send home regular updates, whether weekly, biweekly, or monthly, about the classroom curriculum and their child's progress. The availability of free online translation tools like the TalkingPoints app or Google Translate enables consistent communication with families, even for teachers who do not speak multiple languages. This collaboration serves to involve parents in the curriculum and reinforce learning at home. For instance, if the current week's lesson focuses on multi-step word problems, Mr. Cruz could suggest a homework assignment where parents engage their child by creating structured activities. These activities might involve counting items of their choice around the house and then using sentence templates to form multistep word problems. For instance, "I have (number) shirts, (number) toys, and (number) pillows in one room. In another room, I have (number) shirts, (number) toys, and (number) pillows. Create a question asking how many items there are altogether and then solve it together." This approach extends math learning beyond the classroom, integrating it into everyday activities at home to further enhance mathematical development.*

Teacher Preparation and Professional Development

Throughout the developmental progression of mathematics, educators play a crucial role in providing guidance, scaffolding, and tailored interventions to support students' mathematical growth. Understanding the various stages of mathematical development and recognizing the diverse needs of EB students within this context is essential for designing effective and culturally adapted lesson plans that address their specific math needs while honoring their linguistic and cultural backgrounds (e.g., Kong et al., 2022). However, little is known about teachers' beliefs about language and mathematics. Much of the work done in this area has been focused on instructional practices that educators implement rather than teachers' perspectives and training, and those impacts on instruction (e.g., Li et al., 2022a, 2022b; McLeman et al., 2012).

With the rising demographic of EB students in the United States, educators must be equipped with an understanding of language development. Language is the vehicle for learning in the classroom, and for students who are simultaneously acquiring a new language while maintaining their native language, a nuanced understanding of language development is essential for understanding learning patterns and managing expectations in the classroom. As such, educators are encouraged to partner and consult with their school speech–language pathologist as a key resource for understanding the needs of EB students and how to best support them in the classroom based on the development of each of their languages. Ultimately, educators should be aware of the critical stages of language development, understand common challenges EB students face, and learn strategies to foster language development effectively.

By understanding the intricacies of language acquisition, educators can tailor their teaching methods to align with the specific needs of emergent bilingual students. They can provide targeted support to help these students bridge the gap between their home language and the language they are in the process of learning in school. Moreover, educators can implement differentiated instruction that acknowledges where each student is in developing their proficiency and provides support that can lead to a greater understanding of the content that is presented. When educational professionals understand how language develops, they can provide evidence-based recommendations regarding concerns in student learning and can dispel myths about second language acquisition, they foster a learning environment where EB students can build confidence in their language skills, excel academically, and feel valued as members of the learning community.

We recognize that a major challenge to providing bilingual instruction is largely a result of a shortage of bilingual practitioners, particularly highlighting the difficulty in providing bilingual instruction to an increasingly diverse student population. With this in mind, we emphasize the importance of culturally competent educators and a proficient understanding of language acquisition. By this, we mean that educators are responsible for setting the expectations and tone for the culture of their own classrooms. We encourage practitioners to examine their own biases and cultural expectations and how these perceptions may shape the classroom environment. Our hope is that these reflections could contribute to an environment in which diversity and inclusivity of all learners are celebrated. Finally, as it relates specifically to math instruction, educators are encouraged to investigate the extent to which culture is embedded within the math learning process. As discussed, while the common misconception is that math is universal and language-free, we know that language and culture are deeply steeped in the engagement and learning of math. The more educators can make the language and culture of math accessible to all students, the more students can engage with, feel success in, and build positive self-identities in math.

Challenges and Current Directions

Supporting EB students in mathematics faces ongoing challenges, notably stemming from a shortage of bilingual practitioners, which impacts the ability of an educator to readily provide tailored, effective instruction that bridges linguistic and mathematical concepts. The challenge extends beyond language proficiency to encompass cultural nuances and understand diverse learning needs. Addressing this scarcity requires concerted efforts in recruiting, training, and supporting educators with strong mathematical pedagogy, cultural knowledge, and linguistic proficiency.

Emerging trends across education spotlight a critical need for universities to develop specialized training opportunities that address the unique requirements of diverse student populations, particularly focusing on EB learners. Universities are now taking proactive measures by establishing targeted programs and courses dedicated to enhancing educators' capacity to support these students effectively. These training opportunities encompass diverse areas, including specialized courses in bilingual education, culturally responsive teaching methodologies, and language acquisition strategies. Additionally, universities are introducing programs emphasizing technology integration in language learning, adaptive curriculum development, and cross-disciplinary approaches that merge linguistic and mathematical concepts.

These initiatives are designed not only to equip educators with the necessary language instructional skills but also to cultivate a deeper understanding of culture and how to best address the learning needs of EB students. Collaborations with local communities and schools further enrich these training programs by providing hands-on experiences and practical exposure to diverse learning environments. Through these innovative solutions, universities have the opportunity to bridge the gap between theory and practice, preparing educators to navigate the complexities of teaching mathematics to EB students effectively. Ultimately, these initiatives seek to create a more inclusive and equitable educational experience by empowering educators with the tools and knowledge needed to support the diverse needs of EB learners.

Conclusion

Meeting the mathematical needs of emergent bilingual students is not just an educational imperative but a step toward a more inclusive and just academic system. We highlight the challenges EB learners face in English-dominant school systems, with disparities in math performance shaped by language barriers, cultural differences, the complexities of mathematical concepts, and limited change within the educational system to support learners of all backgrounds. This chapter serves as a guidepost, offering strategies and current best practices to empower educators in facilitating EB students' academic development and success in mathematics. In embracing this holistic approach, we strive toward a more inclusive and equitable educational system that supports the needs of all learners.

References

Abdulrahim, N. A., & Orosco, M. J. (2020). Culturally responsive mathematics teaching: A research synthesis. *The Urban Review, 52*(1), 1–25. https://doi.org/10.1007/s11256-019-00509-2

Alt, M., Arizmendi, G. D., Beal, C. R., & Hurtado, J. S. (2013). The effect of test translation on the performance of second grade English learners on the KeyMath-3. *Psychology in the Schools, 50*(1), 27–36. https://doi.org/10.1002/pits.21656

Alt, M., Arizmendi, G. D., & Beal, C. R. (2014). The relationship between mathematics and language: Academic implications for children with specific language impairment and English language learners. *Language, Speech, and Hearing Services in Schools, 45*(3), 220–233. https://doi.org/10.1044/2014_LSHSS-13-0003

Arizmendi, G. D., Li, J. T., Van Horn, M. L., Petcu, S. D., & Swanson, H. L. (2021). Language-focused interventions on math performance for English learners: A selective meta-analysis of the literature. *Learning Disabilities Research & Practice, 36*(1), 56–75. https://doi.org/10.1111/ldrp.12239

Aronson, B., & Laughter, J. (2016). The theory and practice of culturally relevant education: A synthesis of research across content areas. *Review of Educational Research, 86*, 163–206. https://doi.org/10.3102/0034654315582066

August, D., Shanahan, T., & Escamilla, K. (2009). English language learners: Developing literacy in second-language learners—Report of the National Literacy Panel on Language-Minority Children and Youth. *Journal of Literacy Research, 41*(4), 432–452. https://doi.org/10.1080/10862960903340165

Barbu, O. C., & Beal, C. R. (2010). Effects of linguistic complexity and math difficulty on word problem solving by English learners. *International Journal of Education, 2*(2), 1–19.

Bottoms, S. I., Ciechanowski, K., Jones, K., de la Hoz, J., & Fonseca, A. L. (2017). Leveraging the community context of Family Math and Science Nights to develop culturally responsive teaching practices. *Teaching and Teacher Education, 61*, 1–15. https://doi.org/10.1016/j.tate.2016.09.006

Bouck, E. C., Satsangi, R., Park, J., & Maggin, D. (2018). The concrete-representational-abstract approach for students with learning disabilities: An evidence-based practice synthesis. *The Remedial and Special Education, 39*(4), 211–228. https://doi.org/10.1177/0741932517721712

Costa, M. C., Domingos, A. M. D., Teodoro, V. D., & Vinhas, É. M. R. G. (2022). Teacher professional development in STEM education: An integrated approach with real-world scenarios in Portugal. *Mathematics, 10*(21), 3944. https://doi.org/10.3390/math10213944

De Brey, C., Musu, L., McFarland, J., Wilkinson-Flicker, S., Diliberti, M., Zhang, A., ... & Wang, X. (2019). *Status and trends in the education of racial and ethnic groups 2018.* NCES 2019-038. National Center for Education Statistics.

Doabler, C. T., Clarke, B., Kosty, D. B., Baker, S. K., Smolkowski, K., & Fien, H. (2016). Effects of a core kindergarten mathematics curriculum on the mathematics achievement of Spanish-speaking English learners. *School Psychology Review, 45*(3), 343–361. https://doi.org/10.17105/SPR45-3.343-361

Driver, M. K., & Powell, S. R. (2017). Culturally and linguistically responsive schema intervention: Improving word problem solving for English language learners with mathematics difficulty. *Learning Disability Quarterly, 40*(1), 41–53. https://doi.org/10.1177/0731948716646730

Foster, M. E., Anthony, J. L., Clements, D. H., Sarama, J., & Williams, J. J. (2018). Hispanic dual language learning kindergarten students' response to a numeracy intervention: A randomized control trial. *Early Childhood Research Quarterly, 43*, 83–95. https://doi.org/10.1016/j.ecresq.2018.01.009

Fuchs, L. S., Fuchs, D., Powell, S. R., Seethaler, P. M., Cirino, P. T., & Fletcher, J. M. (2008). Intensive intervention for students with mathematics disabilities: Seven principles of effective practice. *Learning Disability Quarterly, 31*(2), 79–92. https://doi.org/10.2307/20528819

Fuchs, L., Fuchs, D., Yazdian, L., Powell, S., & Karns, K. (2011). *PALS math manuals*. The Fuchs Research Group. https://frg.vkcsites.org/what-is-pals/pals_math_manuals/

García, O., Kleifgen, J. A., & Falchi, L. (2008). *From English language learners to emergent bilinguals*. Equity Matters: Research Review, No. 1.

Gay, G. (2018). *Culturally responsive teaching: Theory, research, and practice*. Teachers College Press.

Gersten, R., Chard, D. J., Jayanthi, M., Baker, S. K., Morphy, P., & Flojo, J. (2009). Mathematics instruction for students with learning disabilities: A meta-analysis of instructional components. *Review of Educational Research, 79*(3), 1202–1242.

Harding-DeKam, J. L. (2014). Defining culturally responsive teaching: The case of mathematics. *Cogent Education, 1*(1), 972676. https://doi.org/10.1080/2331186X.2014.972676

Hubert, T. L. (2014). Learners of mathematics: High school students' perspectives of culturally relevant mathematics pedagogy. *Journal of African American Studies, 18*, 324–336. https://doi.org/10.1007/s12111-013-9273-2

Jiang, W. (2000). The relationship between culture and language. *ELT Journal, 54*(4), 328–334. https://doi.org/10.1093/elt/54.4.328

Kong, J. E., Yan, C., Serceki, A., & Swanson, H. L. (2021). Word-problem-solving interventions for elementary students with learning disabilities: A selective meta-analysis of the literature. *Learning Disability Quarterly, 44*(4), 248–260. https://doi.org/10.1177/073194872199484

Kong, J. E., Arizmendi, G. D., & Doabler, C. T. (2022). Implementing the science of math in a culturally sustainable framework for students with and at risk for math learning disabilities. *Teaching Exceptional Children*, 00400599221127385. https://doi.org/10.1177/0040059922112738

Lambert, W. E. (1973). *Culture and language as factors in learning and education.*

Lee, W., & Lee, J. S. (2017). Math instruction is not universal: Language-specific pedagogical knowledge in Korean/English two-way immersion programs. *Bilingual Research Journal, 40*(4), 353–371. https://doi.org/10.1080/15235882.2017.1380729

Leonard, J. (2018). *Culturally specific pedagogy in the mathematics classroom: Strategies for teachers and students*. Routledge.

Li, J. T., Arizmendi, G. D., & Swanson, H. L. (2022a). The influence of teachers' math instructional practices on English learners' reading comprehension and math problem-solving performance in Spanish and English. *International Journal of Bilingual Education and Bilingualism, 25*(10), 3614–3630. https://doi.org/10.1080/13670050.2022.2068346

Li, J. T., Arizmendi, G. D., & Swanson, H. L. (2022b). The role of language comprehension skills and instructional practices in cross-language influence of Spanish-speaking dual language learners' calculation skills. *Early Childhood Research Quarterly, 61*, 90–105. https://doi.org/10.1016/j.ecresq.2022.05.004

Martiniello, M. (2008). Language and the performance of English-language learners in math word problems. *Harvard Educational Review, 78*(2), 333–368. https://doi.org/10.17763/haer.78.2.70783570r1111t32

McLeman, L., Fernandes, A., & McNulty, M. (2012). Regarding the mathematics education of English learners: Clustering the conceptions of preservice teachers. *Journal of Urban Mathematics Education, 5*(2), 112–132. https://doi.org/10.21423/jume-v5i2a170

Miller-Cotto, D., & Lewis Jr, N. (2020). *Am I a "math person"? How classroom cultures shape math identity among Black and Latinx students*.

Morgan, P. L. (2021). Unmeasured confounding and racial or ethnic disparities in disability identification. *Educational Evaluation and Policy Analysis, 43*(2), 351–361. https://doi.org/10.3102/0162373721991575

Morgan, P. L., Farkas, G., Cook, M., Strassfeld, N. M., Hillemeier, M. M., Pun, W. H., et al. (2018). Are Hispanic, Asian, Native American, or language-minority children overrepresented in special education? *Exceptional Children, 84*(3), 261–279. https://doi.org/10.1177/0014402917748303

Morita-Mullaney, T., Renn, J., & Chiu, M. M. (2021). Contesting math as the universal language: A longitudinal study of dual language bilingual education language allocation. *International Multilingual Research Journal, 15*(1), 43–60. https://doi.org/10.1080/19313152.2020.1753930

Moschkovich, J. N. (2015). Academic literacy in mathematics for English learners. *The Journal of Mathematical Behavior, 40*, 43–62. https://doi.org/10.1016/j.jmathb.2015.01.005

Nasir, N. I. S. (2002). Identity, goals, and learning: Mathematics in cultural practice. *Mathematical Thinking and Learning, 4*(2–3), 213–247.

National Assessment of Educational Progress. (2011). *Achievement gap: How Hispanics and White students in public schools perform in mathematics and reading on the National Assessment of Educational Progress*. U.S. Department of Education.

National Assessment of Educational Progress. (2013). *Math report card*. U.S. Department of Education.

National Assessment of Educational Progress. (2017). *The condition of education (update 2017)*. U.S. Department of Education.

National Assessment of Educational Progress. (2019). *NAEP mathematics and reading assessments: Highlighted results at Grades 4 and 8 for the nation, states, and districts*. U.S. Department of Education.

National Center for Education Statistics. (2020). *Local Education Agency Universe Survey (Common Core of Data series)*. U.S. Department of Education.

National Center for Education Statistics. (2023). Mathematics performance. *Condition of Education*. U.S. Department of Education, Institute of Education Sciences. Retrieved June 11, 2024, from https://nces.ed.gov/programs/coe/indicator/cnc

National Center on Intensive Intervention. (2016). *Principles for designing intervention in mathematics*. Office of Special Education, U.S. Department of Education.

National Center for Education Statistics. (2024). English learners in public schools. *Condition of Education*. U.S. Department of Education, Institute of Education Sciences. Retrieved June 11, 2024, from https://nces.ed.gov/programs/coe/indicator/cgf

Nelson, G., & Powell, S. R. (2018). A systematic review of longitudinal studies of mathematics difficulty. *Journal of Learning Disabilities, 51*(6), 523–539. https://doi.org/10.1177/0022219417714773

Nicol, C., Archibald, J. A., & Baker, J. (2013). Designing a model of culturally responsive mathematics education: Place, relationships and storywork. *Mathematics Education Research Journal, 25*, 73–89. https://doi.org/10.1007/s13394-012-0062-3

Orosco, M. J., Swanson, H. L., O'Connor, R., & Lussier, C. (2013). The effects of dynamic strategic math on English language learners' word problem solving. *The Journal of Special Education, 47*(2), 96–107. https://doi.org/10.1177/0022466911416248

Orosco, M. J., & Abdulrahim, N. A. (2017). Culturally responsive evidence-based practices with English language learners with learning disabilities: A qualitative case study. *Educational Borderlands: A Bilingual Journal, 1*, 27–45.

Oh, M. H., & Mancilla-Martinez, J. (2021). Elementary schoolteachers' bilingual development beliefs and English learners' English reading comprehension achievement. *The Elementary School Journal, 122*(2), 165–190. https://doi.org/10.1086/716899

Parkhouse, H., Lu, C. Y., & Massaro, V. R. (2019). Multicultural education professional development: A review of the literature. *Review of Educational Research, 89*(3), 416–458. https://doi.org/10.3102/0034654319840359

Powell, S. R., Berry, K. A., & Tran, L. M. (2020). Performance differences on a measure of mathematics vocabulary for English learners and non-English learners with and without mathematics difficulty. *Reading & Writing Quarterly, 36*(2), 124–141. https://doi.org/10.1080/10573569.2019.1677538

Ron, P. (1999). Spanish-English language issues in the mathematics classroom. In *Changing the faces of mathematics: Perspectives on Latinos* (pp. 23–34).

Strutchens, M., Krause, G., White, D., & Bay-Williams, J. (Eds.). (2023). *Antiracist mathematics education: Stories of acknowledgment, action and accountability*. Amazon Publishing Agency.

Sugarman, J., & Geary, C. (2018). *English learners in select states: Demographics, outcomes, and state accountability policies. Fact Sheet*. Migration Policy Institute.

Swanson, H. L., Arizmendi, G. D., & Li, J. T. (2021a). The stability of learning disabilities among emergent bilingual children: A latent transition analysis. *Journal of Educational Psychology, 113*(6), 1244. https://doi.org/10.1037/edu0000645

Swanson, H. L., Arizmendi, G. D., & Li, J. T. (2021b). Working memory growth predicts mathematical problem-solving growth among emergent bilingual children. *Journal of Experimental Child Psychology, 201*, 104988. https://doi.org/10.1016/j.jecp.2020.104988

Swanson, H. L., Arizmendi, G. D., & Li, J. T. (2022). What mediates the relationship between growth in math problem-solving and working memory in English language learners? *Journal of Educational Psychology, 114*(7), 1608. https://doi.org/10.1037/edu0000718

Ukpokodu, O. N. (2011). How do I teach mathematics in a culturally responsive way?: Identifying empowering teaching practices. *Multicultural Education, 19*(3), 47–56.

U.S. Department of Education, Institute of Education Sciences, National Center for Education Statistics, National Assessment of Educational Progress (NAEP), various years, 1990–2022 Mathematics Assessments.

Valenzuela, A. (2010). *Subtractive schooling: US-Mexican youth and the politics of caring*. State University of New York Press.

Vygotsky, L. S. (1978). *The role of play in development*.

Waller, P., & Flood, C. T. (2016). Mathematics as a universal language: Transcending cultural lines. *Journal for Multicultural Education, 10*(3), 294–306. https://doi.org/10.1108/JME-01-2016-0004

Wolf, M. K., & Leon, S. (2009). An investigation of the language demands in content assessments for English language learners. *Educational Assessment, 14*(3–4), 139–159.
Wolf, M. K., Bailey, A. L., Ballard, L., Wang, Y., & Pogossian, A. (2023). Unpacking the language demands in academic content and English language proficiency standards for English learners. *International Multilingual Research Journal, 17*(1), 68–85. https://doi.org/10.1080/19313152.2022.2116221
Woodward, J., Beckmann, S., Driscoll, M., Franke, M., Herzig, P., Jitendra, A., ... & Ogbuehi, P. (2012). *Improving mathematical problem solving in Grades 4 through 8*. IES Practice Guide. NCEE 2012-4055. What Works Clearinghouse.

Chapter 9
Working with Interpreters During Intervention Implementation

Emilia C. Lopez

Working with Interpreters During Intervention Implementation

U.S. demographic data clearly point to a significant number of students and families who communicate primarily in languages other than English (LOTEs). As of 2021, 10.6%, or 5.3 million students, were classified as English language learners, with Texas, California, and New Mexico reporting the highest numbers (National Center for Education Statistics [NCES], 2024). The languages most frequently spoken by those emergent bilinguals are Spanish, Arabic, Chinese, Vietnamese, Portuguese, Russian, Haitian Creole, Hmong, and Urdu (NCES, 2024). The U.S. Census (2023) indicates that approximately 68 million people speak LOTEs at home, with Spanish, Chinese, Tagalog, Vietnamese, and Arabic being the five most frequent languages. The Census data also indicate that 26 million of those who speak LOTEs at home reported speaking English "less than very well," suggesting that a significant number of families may need support communicating in English via interpreters in schools.

Given these demographic data, schools are faced with the need to engage with students and families from diverse language backgrounds. However, providing support in LOTEs is a significant challenge due to the shortage of school staff proficient in various languages. The National Association of School Psychologists (NASP) reports that the majority of its members are monolingual school psychologists (79.6%), with only 19% being able to communicate in other languages and 14.9% providing services in 24 LOTEs (Goforth et al., 2021).

E. C. Lopez (✉)
Queens College, City University of New York, New York, USA
e-mail: emilia.lopez@qc.cuny.edu

D. Vega, J. N. Wolf (eds.), *Culturally and Linguistically Responsive Intervention and Assessment Practices with Emergent Bilingual Students*,
https://doi.org/10.1007/978-3-032-02084-0_9

Family members who are not proficient in English are frequently not provided with opportunities to fully participate in special education meetings or decision-making for special education placement, with immigrant parents reporting that their input is not valued (Rossetti et al., 2018). These findings suggest that providing interpreters and translators is potentially a valuable service to students and families who are primarily proficient in LOTEs.

Working with Interpreters: Research on Scope and Impact

In this chapter, **translation** refers to the process of changing messages produced in one language to another language. The term "**interpreter**" refers to professionals who translate spoken language, while the term "**translator**" refers to professionals who translate written language (e.g., translating IEP documents; Tribe & Raval, 2003). The language from which one translates is referred to as **the source language**, whereas the language into which the translation is made is the **target language**.

Research specifically investigating how school psychologists work with interpreters is scant and primarily focused on assessment practices. O'Bryon and Rogers (2010) reported that school psychologists working with emergent bilinguals used interpreters for 14% of their assessment cases in 58 different languages. Interpreters assessed students' language proficiency skills, adaptive behavior, academic achievement, and behavioral functioning using standardized and informal tools; they were also used to communicate with parents. Most recently, Vega et al. (2016) found that 55% of the school psychologists who responded to a survey investigating practices for assessing culturally and linguistically minoritized students indicated using interpreters for assessment purposes.

Literature examining intervention practices with interpreters is virtually nonexistent in school psychology. Lopez (2000) used a case-study methodology to explore working with interpreters to deliver instructional consultation services in a high school setting. Six interpreters engaged in the instructional consultation process provided translations in Arabic, Amharic, Farsi, Polish, and Mandarin. Findings indicated that working with interpreters facilitated communication during all phases of the instructional consultation process with consultees (i.e., teachers, parents) and clients (i.e., students). The interpreters were also an asset as cultural brokers as they shared cultural knowledge with the consultants and school staff, which enhanced their understanding of the families (i.e., consultees) and clients' backgrounds and concerns. Consultees (i.e., teachers, other school staff, parents) and students shared that rapport was enhanced when interpreters facilitated communication.

Research is growing in the medical and mental health fields regarding the scope and impact of the work of interpreters with adults and regarding treatment processes and outcomes. Reviews of the research examining the effects of using professional interpreters in the medical field show positive outcomes that include patients expressing feeling better understood and perceiving improvements in the quality of their healthcare (Karliner et al., 2007). Fennig and Denov (2021) conducted a review of the literature on the outcomes of mental health services to refugees via the use of trained interpreters. Overall, interpreters were found to facilitate trust in the therapeutic relationship and alliance. Several studies also reported that access to a trained interpreter "was associated with increased reporting of physical and psychological symptoms by the patients, as well as higher quality of screening and significant improvement in the appropriate referral to further health care" (p. 56).

Challenges of Working with Interpreters

Although providing support via interpreters can be an asset, it presents time, communication, and interpersonal challenges. Several studies have noted that using interpreters is time-consuming because it requires more time for communicative interactions (Garcia et al., 2023; Lopez, 2000). Lopez (2000) noted other time-related barriers, such as difficulties finding trained interpreters, scheduling conflicts between the interpreters and the consultants, and needing to provide training to interpreters before consultation sessions. Strategies to overcome time barriers include allocating time to locate qualified interpreters via community resources (e.g., locating trained interpreters via local agencies) and scheduling additional time prior to and during assessment and intervention sessions to meet with interpreters for planning and executing translation sessions. Building time to advocate at the district level for interpreter training and to obtain resources, such as funding to compensate interpreters, is also time-consuming, as it may require addressing systemic issues, such as increasing the awareness of administrators of the need to provide translations.

Communication barriers can emerge related to translation errors made by interpreters. For example, errors may include omitting information, adding details not included in the original message, or changing a message's content or intent by substituting words or sentences (Cheatham, 2011). Other translation challenges may be due to interpreters' lack of technical vocabulary needed to translate specifically in school settings and related to special education issues. Verbatim or word-by-word translation is often not possible because the same word may not exist when translating from the source to the target language, and interpreters must be able to find the appropriate vocabulary in the source language to preserve communicative intent and content.

Interpersonal challenges are also part of the process of working with interpreters (Lopez, 2000). The interpersonal challenges may include clients: a) avoiding eye contact with clinicians or turning their bodies away from the clinicians and towards the interpreters, causing clinicians to feel left out of the communication; b) establishing stronger bonds with interpreters than with the clinicians, leading clinicians to feel excluded from the therapeutic bond; c) feeling uncomfortable about sharing personal information via interpreters or feeling that they are being judged by interpreters; d) worrying that interpreters may not keep information confidential, especially when the interpreters may come from the same community as the clients; and/or e) feeling left out when professionals hold side conversations in English with each other, leaving clients out of communicative interactions (Fennig & Denov, 2021; Maul, 2015). Cultural differences in identities and affiliations between interpreters and clients across ethnicity, race, clans, regional identity, religion, socioeconomic class, and education may result in biases and distrust between interpreters and clients (Fennig & Denov, 2021). Barriers may also surface in cultural aspects of communication, such as how to deliver messages within the client's expectations about personal interactions (e.g., verbal tone, nonverbal language, directness of message) or discussing topics that are considered taboo in certain cultures.

Communication barriers and interpersonal challenges are part of the complexity of working within cross-cultural contexts with interpreters. Communicative interactions can be facilitated by making time for rapport building (Lopez, 2000; Tribe & Raval, 2003). For example, it is important for the student and/or family to know that an interpreter will be used prior to the translation session and that all present are bound by confidentiality. Making time for the school psychologist and interpreter to establish rapport with the student and/or family prior to starting an assessment session or an intervention meeting also facilitates communication and interpersonal interactions.

Another key component is working with interpreters who are trained to work in schools, as well as training school personnel to work with interpreters. Working with trained interpreters facilitates processes and outcomes when providing services via interpreter (Fennig & Denov, 2021; Karliner et al., 2007). Access to a directory of trained interpreters in various languages is a useful tool that can be shared among various school districts. Training for school psychologists and other school personnel focused on how to improve communication and interpersonal interactions when communicating via interpreters is also recommended. The training can include the phases of working with interpreters and strategies such as discussing goals for meetings, identifying specific or technical vocabulary that will be needed so that the interpreter can prepare ahead of time, and using the communication guidelines provided in Appendix 1 in this chapter.

Intervention Implementation Using Equitable and Culturally Responsive Frameworks

Upah (2008) defined interventions "as a set of procedures and strategies designed to improve student performance with the intent of closing the gap between current performance and expectations…" (p. 209). The NASP Practice Model Domains (2020) emphasize the delivery of direct and indirect interventions within a multi-tiered system of supports that also includes intervening at systemic levels (e.g., classroom, school-wide, home-school collaboration) to promote learning.

Domain 8 in the NASP Professional Standards (2020) specifically calls for school psychologists to implement “evidence-based strategies to enhance services in both general and special education and address potential influences related to diversity,” while also emphasizing advocacy for social justice and ensuring that all students have access to the supports that they need (p. 8). Central to equitable and social justice practices is students gaining access to interventions that will enhance their learning, behavioral, social-emotional, and mental health functioning. School personnel collaborating with culturally minoritized families to plan and deliver interventions is also pivotal.

From a social justice perspective, language barriers that result in our inability to communicate effectively with students and families during any intervention implementation efforts marginalize immigrant populations and all those who are unable to communicate proficiently in English (Li et al., 2021). Language barriers are clearly social justice issues in the intervention delivery process that can translate into silencing students and caregivers and denying them access to a voice in intervention decision-making and outcomes. The ability to communicate via interpreters is a powerful resource that provides students and families with access to information and opportunities to ask questions and engage with school personnel to promote students’ success (Lopez, 2014, 2000;).

Culturally responsive intervention planning and delivery involve engaging in an intentional process that approaches every problem-solving stage of intervention delivery by using effective communication strategies, including the process of working with interpreters. Culturally responsive practitioners work towards understanding the populations that they work with in terms of their values, beliefs, and worldviews (Castro-Villareal & Rodriguez, 2023). Language then becomes a vehicle for understanding and communicating the cultural components involved in culturally responsive intervention planning and delivery. For example, interventionists need to explore how open students and their families are to recommended interventions and strategies, as these are important components for treatment acceptability and integrity (Roach & Graybill, 2023). They also must approach every intervention understanding the strengths and needs of emergent bilingual students and their families.

Working with Interpreters in the Process of Intervention Implementation

Engaging interpreters in the intervention planning and delivery process is conceptualized as: a) a comprehensive problem-solving process that integrates interpreters within every stage to maximize communication and rapport; b) a team effort that provides opportunities for students, families, and interpreters to collaborate in the intervention delivery process with school psychologists, teachers, and other school personnel; and c) a systematic way of involving students and families who primarily communicate in LOTEs in all the stages of intervention planning and implementation with interpreters becoming conduits to enhance equitable and culturally responsive practices.

Problem Identification and Interpreters

In the initial stages of problem identification, the interpreter can assist in seeking parental consent for student involvement in intervention delivery. Identifying the problem entails the interpreter supporting the school psychologist and others on the intervention team to understand how the problem is viewed by the student, family, and school professionals (Castro-Villareal & Rodriguez, 2023). The target problem may indeed be viewed differently by culturally minoritized students and family members than by teachers, school psychologists, and other interventionists. A culturally responsive lens in problem-solving entails understanding the instructional, behavioral, and social-emotional expectations of the school environment, as well as the context of the students' cultural backgrounds (Castro-Villareal & Rodriguez, 2023; Lopez, 2014). Strengths as well as gaps must be framed ecologically and with an understanding of how culture influences learning, behaviors, and social-emotional functioning. Interpreters with knowledge about the student's cultures can serve as cultural brokers in situations where they share the same background as the student and family, have experience with the particular cultural group, and/or have received training in cultural responsiveness (Lopez, 2000).

Interventionists can use a variety of problem identification tools, such as interviews, observations, behavioral logs, and curriculum-based assessment (CBA), to gather background information about the target problem (Castro-Villareal & Rodriguez, 2023; Lopez & Velasco, 2017). The school psychologist and other members of the intervention team must ensure that the tools used are culturally sensitive and valid for culturally and linguistically minoritized students. An interpreter may support these processes when a language difference is present.

The information obtained during problem identification must be processed and discussed among the members of the intervention team with a complex understanding of interacting dimensions related to cultural values, beliefs, and identities. Meeting to plan interventions with the student, family, and school professionals is facilitated through the interpreter to discuss implementation roles and tasks (e.g., "Who will do what?", "When?", and "How?"). The school psychologist and other members of the intervention team must plan and implement evidence-based interventions that are acceptable to culturally minoritized students and families (Roach & Graybill, 2023). Through the interpreter, interventionists can explore with students and families whether the suggested interventions are a good fit by asking questions such as: Is this an intervention that you agree with and that is compatible with your beliefs and values? In what ways does the intervention fit within your beliefs or values, or in what ways does it conflict with your beliefs or values? What barriers do you foresee in implementing this intervention? Interpreters in the role of cultural brokers can be helpful when they are able to share cultural beliefs or values that may conflict with the strategies and interventions being recommended, so that interventions can be designed to be more culturally responsive.

Intervention Processes, Outcomes, and Interpreters

Interpreters also have a role in supporting school psychologists in examining the processes and outcomes related to intervention delivery (Lopez, 2008). Process evaluation during intervention delivery focuses on examining factors such as whether interventionists are using culturally sensitive tools conducive to establishing treatment outcomes. Interventionists and interpreters can collaborate to design and adapt interview questions, such as exploring intervention outcomes with family members. Jointly with interpreters, interventionists can also examine if the collaborative practices used were culturally responsive, such as when using the families' dialect, social greeting practices, and non-verbal communication styles.

Roach and Graybill (2023) refer to the importance of examining treatment integrity, and part of that task involves the interpreter helping to explore the variables impacting treatment implementation and outcomes when working with culturally and linguistically minoritized students and families. For example, school psychologists can check for communication and understanding of intervention steps and scripts via the interpreter. Students and family members can also be interviewed with the aid of an interpreter to explore how to overcome barriers to treatment implementation. Working with interpreters during the problem-solving stages can directly impact outcomes if communication, trust, and rapport are not clearly established, as those factors may potentially interfere with intervention implementation.

Considerations for Translating Documents

As part of the process, school psychologists and other interventionists must determine if they need written translations and should explore with interpreters if they have the skills to translate pertinent documents. Interventionists must take care to inquire about interpreters' credentials and training backgrounds focused on translating documents. When interventionists establish that an interpreter does not have the qualifications or skills needed, they must advocate and take action to locate a different interpreter.

The translation of documents is a complex process in and of itself. Interpreters may have the skills to translate documents such as letters and informal tools developed by interventionists (e.g., behavioral logs and ABC charts). However, informal tools with technical terminology may be difficult for interpreters to translate. For example, descriptors to label each point in a rating scale (e.g., Unsatisfactory, Meets Expectations) may be challenging to translate to another language or may not have the same meaning when translated. Intervention scripts that may have vocabulary specific to certain behavioral or instructional practices may also be complex for interpreters to translate without familiarity with the terms. Those scenarios require discussions between the interventionist and interpreter to ensure the translation is meaningful in the LOTE.

Tools such as validated rating scales, formal questionnaires, and standardized tests used during problem identification should not be translated as the translation process invalidates the tool and its outcomes (Lopez, 2014). Translating such tools will likely result in altering content, as the translation will not have the same meaning in the LOTE. Interventionists using formal tools are advised to use translated tools that have been validated in the target language. This is a sound but challenging recommendation because of the scarcity of tools that are validated and/or normed in LOTEs. Research shows that, given the lack of translated instruments, school psychologists rely on asking interpreters to translate tools prior to assessment sessions, assuming that the process will result in a better translated version of the tool (O'Bryon & Rogers, 2010). Another practice used by school psychologists is to ask interpreters to translate test items on the spot (i.e., during the session). However, such planning and foresight will not result in good practices because translating items may mean that the developmental level of the question may change in a standardized test, or the equivalent term may not be available when translating an item on a validated rating scale (Lopez, 2014). Translations may also be difficult because even regional differences may impact how an interpreter translates a concept or a vocabulary word. We can add to this complexity that interpreters can make errors that can result in poor translations.

Interventionists are encouraged to seek out trained interpreters who have expertise in translating written documentation. The translation of any documents, and particularly any tools used for problem identification, must be done with preparation that includes the interventionist and the interpreter meeting prior to the translation session to discuss the instrument's goals, purposes, and content. Careful attention should be paid to the validity of the items, with the interventionist clearly engaging the interpreter in discussing what the item means when translated into the LOTE. It is not just a matter of maintaining meaning but also ensuring that the translation is meaningful and valid for what is being measured. All results of problem identification tools and instruments obtained via interpreters must be translated with caution and reported qualitatively without scores. Reports generated for intervention purposes must clearly state that an interpreter was used in the process, specifying how the interpreter was used, for what purposes, and in what stages of the intervention and problem-solving process.

Integrating Interpreters in the Intervention Implementation Process

Interventionists can locate interpreters by using a variety of strategies. Large urban districts often work with translation agencies that provide per diem or per case interpreters at a cost to the district. State education departments and local districts may also have directories of interpreters. Rossetti et al. (2017) recommend strategies such as consulting with nonprofit organizations and community stakeholders who use interpreters and collaborating with community agencies with bilingual staff who can serve as interpreters. One of the biggest challenges is locating interpreters who have received training, including interpreters with training to work in schools. Partnerships can be formed with interpreter training programs that are seeking to supervise their students in educational settings as part of their preparation (Rossetti et al., 2017).

There is consensus in the translation field that the best interpreters for any scenario are interpreters who understand the processes involved within the situations that they are translating (Tribe & Raval, 2003). When translating for intervention purposes, interpreters should: a) understand schools, school policies, and education systems; b) demonstrate excellent interpersonal skills to interact with students, families, and school professionals; and c) have knowledge of the intervention delivery process, including vocabulary and terminology related to interventions and special education (Lopez, 2000, 2008, 2014). Interpreters should also know processes such as intervention acceptability and integrity so that they are fully aware of how clarity in communication and cultural beliefs can directly influence how interventions are accepted, perceived, and implemented. Ideally, interpreters are not just well-versed in the process of translation but also able to facilitate cultural understandings and demonstrate an openness to examining how they contributed to the process. Together with school psychologists and other interventionists, this process should be continuously monitored for improvement in service provision.

Ethical and professional conduct is also important for interpreters in the intervention delivery process. The National Council on Interpreting in Health Care (2005) and the American Association of Interpreters and Translators in Education (2023) both provide ethical codes that apply to interpreters providing services in schools. Some of the critical ethical behaviors include maintaining confidentiality, seeking training and supervision, engaging in appropriate and respectful ways, respecting the rights of the students and families they support, translating regardless of their own beliefs and views, and adhering to school and district policies.

The National Association of Interpreters of Educational Translators and Interpreters of Spoken Languages (https://naetisl.org/) provides several helpful resources for practitioners, interpreters, and multilingual families. For example, handouts are available in multiple languages designed to introduce the interpreter to students and/or families. Both practitioners and interpreters can download bilingual glossaries of terms used in education settings. Families have access to resources in multiple languages, including a description of the knowledge and skills that interpreters and translators should demonstrate in educational settings. These resources are helpful in the practice of working with interpreters as well as when providing training opportunities to graduate students, practitioners, and interpreters.

Five Phases of Working with Interpreters for Intervention Delivery Purposes

The process of working with interpreters is complex and involves several phases. The five phases to work with interpreters during intervention delivery are: a) planning, b) briefing, c) translating during meetings, d) debriefing, and e) process evaluation. Since intervention implementation is conceptualized in this chapter as a process that involves problem identification, problem analysis, intervention planning and delivery, and intervention evaluation, the interactions required to support students and families who are primarily able to communicate in LOTEs may then occur over multiple meetings and sessions. As a result, the phases proposed are conceptualized as iterative. For example, the school psychologist may meet with the student's parents and teacher for problem identification in the first session. The school psychologist must plan for that session and then work with the interpreter, including engaging in briefing and debriefing. When the school psychologist meets with the teacher and parent again to problem analyze and plan for the intervention, the school psychologist plans for the next translation session and revisits the phases involving interpreters (e.g., briefing, translation during the session, debriefing) and reflects on that session to then prepare for the next stage of intervention delivery, and so on.

Since the process is conceptualized as iterative, the recommendation is to aim to use the same interpreter for all intervention meetings. Research in the provision of counseling and psychotherapeutic services indicates that using the same interpreter during the entire sequence of the treatment results in better communication, rapport, and trust (Fennig & Denov, 2021), and in working with interpreters familiar with the process. Appendix 1 provides an outline of the recommendations for each phase.

Planning: The planning phase focuses on the preparation that school psychologists need to engage in prior to working with interpreters and, if needed, with other school staff members of the intervention team (Lopez, 2000; Tribe & Raval, 2003). Interventionists should have a clear sense of the languages and dialects spoken by the students and families needing interpreters to create a clear match between the two sides. Regional differences may mean that a family and an interpreter from the same country may not speak the same languages or dialects and may not be able to communicate effectively. Interpreters with prior experience in translating during intervention-related activities and training in this area should be prioritized. The school psychologist should work with the school staff involved in planning the intervention delivery (e.g., teachers) to establish the goals for the meeting and what needs to be accomplished during the meeting with students, families, and interpreters. Interventionists should also locate any documentation that needs translation before briefing with the interpreters and/or meeting with the students and families. Preparing an agenda for the translation session is helpful to review with the interpreters and the members of the intervention team.

Briefing: Briefing occurs before the actual session in which interpreters are needed and provides interventionists and interpreters with opportunities to discuss the goals of the meeting, the agenda for the meeting, and any documentation that will need to be translated (Langdon & Saenz, 2016). The style of translation that will be used during the meeting with the students and family should also be established during briefing (Tribe & Raval, 2003). Speakers deliver their messages in the source language and stop to allow interpreters to translate in the target language when translating consecutively. In simultaneous translation, interpreters translate at the same time that the speakers are communicating. Simultaneous translations are challenging, and they can result in students and family members feeling overwhelmed by the overlapping style of communication as the interventionist and interpreter both speak at the same time (Tribe & Raval, 2003). There is no research on using these two modes of translation and their impact on working with students and families in schools. Interventionists are cautioned to think carefully about the students' and families' potential level of comfort with each translation mode and the interpreters' skills in using consecutive or simultaneous translation. Seating arrangements and communication guidelines should also be discussed. Briefing is also the time to discuss any cultural behaviors, values, beliefs, and attitudes that should be taken into consideration when interacting and communicating with the student and family members, and to discuss why those cultural issues are important and their implications (Lopez, 2000).

Translation During Meetings: The meeting with students and family members is the actual time when the interpreter translates for all. Everyone should be introduced, and time should be allowed for rapport building. The goals of the meeting should be discussed, and students and family members should be informed that they can engage with any and all team members in all discussions and ask questions via the interpreter (Lopez, 2000, 2014). This is an important message as some students and families may hesitate to communicate through interpreters, expecting that interpreters are mostly there for the school professionals. The message also establishes that time must be spent on asking for input and feedback from students and family members, and checking for their understanding of the intervention process and tasks. The school psychologist or another member of the intervention team should mediate aspects of the communication, such as slowing down members of the intervention team who are speaking too fast or are not stopping to allow for translation. Specifics related to intervention implementation, such as tasks and intervention implementation details (i.e., "Who will intervene?", "When?", and "How?"), and relevant documents also need to be discussed and translated during this phase.

Debriefing: Debriefing is the last phase during which interventionists meet with the interpreter to discuss questions related to translation, communication, interpersonal, and cultural issues (Langdon & Saenz, 2016; Lopez, 2000). This stage is a time for all interventionists and the interpreter to discuss how well they worked together. The interpreter can also be asked a number of questions related to translation, communication, and interpersonal interactions during the meeting (see Appendix 1).

Process Evaluation: The last phase, process evaluation, is part of the process of intervention delivery as the intervention team reflects on how they worked together and on the validity of the process and outcomes, given the need to communicate via an interpreter (Lopez, 2008). This is a time to reflect on how the process of working with interpreters contributed to intervention delivery. It is also a time to examine how the process can be changed and improved to benefit emergent bilinguals and their families. Evaluation efforts should consider how working with interpreters impacted outcomes for all, including students, their families, and interventionists.

Lopez (2008, 2014) recommends similar phases when working with interpreters during assessment sessions. O'Bryon and Rogers (2010) surveyed bilingual school psychologists and found that 53% reported briefing with interpreters, and only 26% engaged in debriefing with interpreters after assessment sessions. These findings suggest that school psychologists are not consistently engaging in recommended practices when working with interpreters. Time constraints, a lack of knowledge and skills in how to work with interpreters, as well as systemic challenges, may be some of the issues impacting school psychologists' practices when delivering services via interpreters.

Systemic Challenges and Needs

At a systemic level, the school district or school benefits from having data on the primary LOTEs in the community to plan for the need to provide interpreters for various language groups. Identifying language needs and priorities will aid in the creation of interpreter directories for various languages and areas of expertise (e.g., assessment, intervention, district meetings). Training workshops and sessions can also be planned for potential school interpreters and school staff involved in delivering intervention services via interpreters.

Funding is a crucial aspect of any systemic plan, and specific allocations for the provision of interpreters must be available to create those opportunities and services for students and families. The ideal scenario is to allocate funding according to the number of students and families in the district that speak LOTEs, and not to rely solely on the number of emergent bilinguals in special education. Local school districts can provide school psychologists with data as to the number and language backgrounds of students receiving English as a new language services, and community outreach at the district level can also be used to establish the LOTEs spoken by students and families. Estimated needs derived from students needing support in Tiers 2 and 3 who are emergent bilinguals are also helpful to identify funding needs. School districts can collect those data as part of the evaluation process for multiple tiers of support. Vega et al. (2016) refer to challenges in obtaining resources allocated for school interpreters. They point out that providing interpreters adds to the budget costs at a time when schools are experiencing cuts, and administration may not recognize the value of or the need for interpreters' services. Competing needs may also exist. For example, districts may decide to allocate funding for students referred to or placed in special education, as those needs may be considered primary because of federal and state special education policies.

School psychologists in the role of interventions must become familiar with the policies in the district for locating and hiring interpreters. For example, does the district provide funding to hire interpreters for intervention delivery purposes? Communication with administration is key to advocating for project funding resources on short- and long-term bases and about how much funding is available for assessment versus intervention purposes in the district. Since intervention delivery may require several meetings with students and families for problem identification and intervention planning and delivery, interventionists need to project how many sessions they will need to work with interpreters and advocate for additional funding for intervention delivery.

In districts with a wide range of languages spoken by school staff and community members, opportunities can be created to provide training to translate during specific intervention activities. For example, bilingual school staff and community members can work with school psychologists to jointly create informal tools for outcome evaluation (e.g., behavioral logs, frequency tables) or to translate formal tools to use informally and qualitatively. They can also collaborate on conducting online searches for such tools in multiple languages. Bilingual staff with high levels of proficiency in English and the LOTEs, such as teachers, can also be trained to translate during intervention meetings and sessions.

Recommendations for Future Practice, Training, and Research

Practice

The practice of working with interpreters during intervention implementation is a neglected topic in the school psychology literature and research, as the focus is more on assessment practices. School psychologists working with interpreters during intervention delivery must advocate for the provision of qualified interpreters to ensure equitable practices when working with emergent bilinguals and their families during intervention delivery. Enlisting other school staff who also work with school interpreters (e.g., teachers, school counselors, speech and language therapists) to join in advocating for funding resources to hire interpreters during intervention delivery and home and school collaboration efforts is a potential systemic strategy for increasing the voices of our communities and school professionals.

Policies are needed from professional organizations addressing the provision of school psychological services via interpreters during various roles and functions.

The NASP standards minimally address working with interpreters. The NASP Principles for Professional Ethics (NASP, 2020), Standard II.39, states, "When interpreters are used to facilitate the provision of assessment and intervention services, school psychologists request the assignment of interpreters who are qualified and are acceptable to clients" (p. 47). That standard is under guiding principle II.3: Responsible Assessment and Intervention Practices, which is cross-referenced under cultural and linguistic diversity (CLD), diversity, and interpretation of assessment results. However, interpreters are not cross-referenced nor addressed under interventions or parental involvement. In the NASP Practice Model (2020), there is no mention of the need for school psychologists to receive training and demonstrate skills to work with school interpreters. Given the national shortage of school psychologists able to provide supports in LOTEs, qualifications to work with school interpreters are crucial for all school psychologists.

Training

Federal and state education policies should clearly state that interpreters must be qualified and credentialed to work in school settings, as available research suggests that school psychologists rely on unqualified interpreters' services. In a survey investigating assessment practices, Vega et al. (2016) reported that school psychologists rated 15.8% of the interpreters they worked with as poorly or very poorly trained. The research that is available about school psychologists' skills also shows that they lack the training to work with school interpreters. O'Bryon and Rogers (2010) found that bilingual school psychologists engaged in poor practices when working with interpreters to provide assessments, such as using untrained interpreters and family members to translate, asking interpreters to translate standardized tests on the spot, and writing psychological reports that did not include information about conducting assessments via interpreters.

Hernandez et al. (2022) recently surveyed graduate school psychology students regarding their training experiences in working with interpreters. The findings showed that the majority of graduate students surveyed reported not receiving training or receiving minimal training, including fieldwork experiences or professional development related to working with interpreters. In addition, the findings also indicated that school psychology graduate students lacked knowledge about fundamental practices involved in working with interpreters during psychoeducational evaluations and meetings held at schools. These findings align with Vega et al. (2019) reporting that faculty in graduate school psychology programs lacked experience in working with bilingual students, and those gaps were reflected in school psychology programs' curricula.

Both interpreters and school professionals working with interpreters should receive training to deliver intervention support to students and families who speak LOTEs (Langdon & Saenz, 2016). Interpreters need to demonstrate high levels of proficiency in both the source and target languages and should have specific training on translating in various roles and functions in schools, including during intervention delivery services (Tribe & Raval, 2003). School psychologists should receive training in understanding the roles and functions of interpreters and the phases of working with interpreters, and in evaluating the process of working with interpreters during intervention delivery.

Both interpreters and school psychologists need to develop skills in collaborating to create opportunities for improved communication, rapport, and positive intervention outcomes. Joint training between interpreters and school psychologists is potentially beneficial to reach those goals. Research shows that training interpreters with the professionals with whom they work benefits both the acquisition of knowledge and the level of confidence (Zhang et al., 2021).

Research

The lack of research focused on working with interpreters is vast in school psychology, particularly in areas related to intervention provision. Research investigating the use of interpreters during such functions as meeting with students and parents to plan and deliver interventions would help to understand current practices as well as challenges to plan for training and improved policies. Practices based on available technologies are also in need of investigation. Translation services via phone and telecommunication platforms are now being used in schools, but the impact of such services on the provision of psychoeducational services is unknown. The available research on the use of remote phone translation in the healthcare field is mixed, with some findings showing improved access to communication and healthcare, and other studies showing limitations during communication exchanges involving multiple speakers or discussing complex or detailed medical instructions (Garcia et al., 2023). As artificial intelligence (AI) becomes more sophisticated and available, it is possible that schools may turn to those platforms for translation services. At this point, artificial intelligence is in the early stages of development and is in danger of deploying biases based on algorithms created by humans and transmitting their own biases to AI platforms (Mittermaier et al., 2023). Translation is a human endeavor, and viewing it simply as an automatic language transaction means potentially missing the mark on understanding the complexity of the process at the interpersonal level, especially when situated in the context of delivering culturally responsive psychoeducational and mental health services in school settings.

Conclusion

The practice of working with interpreters will continue, and it is surely an equity issue as students and family members who primarily communicate in LOTEs are often unable to communicate with school professionals or are being provided with support that is not based on sound policies and best practices. School psychologists must continue to advocate for systemic changes that facilitate their work with interpreters. Engaging in intervention delivery via interpreters must be situated within culturally responsive and social justice frameworks that include engaging in recommended practices. Future research focused on how to work with interpreters and train interpreters and school psychologists to collaborate during intervention planning and implementation will enhance practices to support families who primarily communicate in LOTEs and emergent bilinguals' education, social, behavioral, and mental health functioning.

Appendix 1: Phases of Working with Interpreters During Intervention Delivery

Planning

- Identify specific language and/or dialect of student and family to recruit interpreter with specific language skills
- Locate interpreter needed for intervention meeting(s)
- Do not use family members or students as interpreters
- Establish who will need to be present for intervention meetings
- Discuss goals of the meeting with team members to identify what needs to be accomplished when communicating via the interpreter
- Identify vocabulary (e.g., technical language) that the interpreter will need to translate to share with the interpreter during briefing
- Identify written documents that need to be translated and determine if the interpreter has skills as translator to translate written documents, or locate translator with required skills
- Prepare agenda for meeting with interpreter and intervention team members

Briefing

- Discuss goals for the meeting with interpreter and members of the intervention team
- Share the agenda with all to have a clear vision of the meeting
- Identify and review documents that need to be discussed during the meeting with the students and family members
- Establish seating arrangements for all present and aim for members of the intervention team to sit where they can have eye contact or speak directly to the student and/or family members

- Establish communication guidelines with interpreter and intervention team, such as:
  - Establish if consecutive or simultaneous interpretation will be used
  - The interpreter should interpret everything said by all present during the meeting with student and family members
  - Members of the intervention team should not have side conversations that leave out the students or family from any communication
  - Speak directly to the student and/or family member(s) when communicating (i.e., avoid looking at the interpreter when speaking to the student and family)
  - Interpret everything that is said by all present in the first person
  - If the interpreter has any clarifying questions for the members of the intervention team, student and/or family, inform everyone present so that no one is left out of the communication
- The interpreter and members of the intervention team should take notes during the meeting about any issues, challenges, and questions that they want to discuss during debriefing
- Inform the interpreter and intervention team members that there will be an opportunity to debrief after the meeting
- Discuss the need to maintain confidentiality about any topics or issues discussed in the meeting
- Discuss with interpreter and members of the intervention team any cultural issues that need to be taken into consideration regarding behaviors, values, beliefs, and attitudes when interacting and communicating with the student and/ or family. Discuss: Why is it important to consider those issues? What are the implications for interacting with the student and or family during intervention delivery?

Meeting with Students, Family, and Interpreter

- Introduce everyone at the meeting, including the interpreter
- Allow time for all to establish rapport, and allow time for the interpreter to establish rapport with the student or family individually, if needed
- Establish goals for the meeting and what needs to be accomplished with specifics as to the intervention stage (e.g., goals for problem identification vs. problem analysis and intervention planning vs. intervention implementation vs. outcome and process evaluations)
- Communicate to the student and family members that they can ask questions and engage in the discussions via the interpreter
- Let the student and family know that everything will be translated so that they are aware of all that is discussed
- Follow guidelines for consecutive or simultaneous translation modes

- Allow time to clearly communicate about intervention implementation details and processes (e.g., intervention goals, how to implement the intervention, tools needed for intervention integrity and to monitor outcomes)
- Mediate translation modes (i.e., consecutive, simultaneous) and communication patterns (e.g., speed, timing, how much is translated) with the student, family members, and members of the intervention team
- Allow time to discuss documents and tools such as rating scales, intervention scripts, and intervention integrity checklists with students and family members

Debriefing

- Aim to debrief with the intervention team
- Discuss questions with all items such as:
  - Were there any challenges in interpreting certain vocabulary words, concepts, and/or messages? What were they? How did the interpreter handle those challenges? What were the implications for clarity of communication and rapport?
  - What were the interpersonal challenges during the meeting? How did they impact interactions and communication? How can those challenges be overcome?
  - What were the cultural behaviors, attitudes, values, and beliefs that emerged during the meeting and that should be considered in working with this student and family? What are the implications for intervention delivery?
  - What were topics that were easy or difficult to discuss? Why? What were the implications?
  - What needs to be revisited in future intervention delivery meetings to clarify communication?
  - Any challenges in translating documents? Any need to revisit translations?
- Discuss specific observations of behaviors (e.g., body language, verbal tone) and their implications for intervention implementation
- What could the intervention team and the interpreter have done differently? How can the process of working together be improved?
- Thank interpreter for their services and support

Process Evaluation

- Was the interpreter a good match for the student/family? Why? Why not? Any issues that need to be addressed or discussed to improve future meetings held via the interpreter? Should the interpreter be changed for future meetings?
- What was the quality of the translation and how did it impact the intervention delivery process?

- What was the quality of the interpersonal interactions when working with the interpreter and how did it impact the intervention delivery process?
- Were the goals of the intervention meeting accomplished?
- Are there any team dynamics that need to be improved when working with interpreters?
- What culturally responsive strategies were used when working with the interpreter during intervention delivery?
- What could be changed or improved in the future to improve the process of intervention delivery when working with interpreters?
- What can be improved in the future to improve the process of intervention delivery when working with interpreters?
- How can I/we prepare the interpreter and other team members for the next stage of intervention delivery?
- Were best practices followed when working with interpreters for the purposes of intervention delivery?
- Evaluate processes in intervention delivery via interpreters by taking into consideration the quality of the interpretation and communication, interpersonal issues, cultural responsiveness, and professional interactions to explore the question: Were best practices followed when working with interpreters, and how did it impact intervention delivery outcomes for students, family, and interventionists?

References

American Association of Interpreters and Translators in Education. (2023). *National code of ethics and standards of practice for interpreters in education*. https://aaite.memberclicks.net/assets/docs/AAITE_%20CoE_Interpreters_v1.0.pdf.

Castro-Villareal, F., & Rodriguez, B. J. (2023). Best practices in teacher consultation for implementing culturally responsive practices in classrooms. In P. L. Harrison, S. L. Proctor, & A. Thomas (Eds.), *Best practices in school psychology 1: Data-based and collaborative decision making* (pp. 281–294). National Association of School Psychologists.

Cheatham, G. A. (2011). Language interpretation, parent participation, and young children with disabilities. *Topics in Early Childhood Special Education, 31*, 78–88. https://doi.org/10.1177/0271121410377120

Fennig, M., & Denov, M. (2021). Interpreters working in mental health settings with refugees: An interdisciplinary scoping review. *American Journal of Orthopsychiatry, 91*, 50–65. https://doi.org/10.1037/ort0000518

Garcia, M. E., Mutha, S., Napoles, A. M., Malevanchik, L., Williams, M., & Karliner, L. S. (2023). "Long overdue": Nurse and resident physician perspectives on implementation of dual-handset interpreter phones in the inpatient setting. *Health Equity, 7*, 100–108. https://doi.org/10.1089/heq.2022.0023

Goforth, A. N., Farmer, R. L., Kim, S. Y., Naser, S. C., Lockwood, A. B., & Affrunti, N. W. (2021). Status of school psychology in 2020: Part 1, demographics of the NASP membership survey. *NASP Research Reports, 5*(2).

Hernandez, J. A., Norwalk, K. E., & Kim, E. K. (2022). Training to work with interpreters in US school psychology graduate programs. *Contemporary School Psychology, 28*, 157–172. https://doi.org/10.1007/s40688-022-00426-4

Karliner, L. S., Jacobs, E. A., Chen, A. H., & Mutha, S. (2007). Do professional interpreters improve clinical care for patients with limited English proficiency? A systematic review of the literature. *Health Services Research, 42*, 727–754. https://doi.org/10.1111/j.1475-6773.2006.00629.x

Langdon, H. W., & Saenz, T. I. (2016). Working with interpreters to support students who are English language learners. *Perspectives of the ASHA Special Interest Groups, 1*, 15–27. https://doi.org/10.1044/persp1.SIG16.15

Li, C., Kruger, L., & Abdulkerim, N. (2021). Advancing social justice for English learners: Implications for school psychology training. *School Psychology Training and Pedagogy, 38*, 54–70.

Lopez, E. C. (2014). Best practices in conducting assessments via school interpreters. In P. L. Harrison & A. Thomas (Eds.), *Best practices in school psychology: Foundations* (pp. 113–128). National Association of School Psychologists.

Lopez, E. C. (2008). Best practices in working with school interpreters. In A. Thomas & J. Grimes (Eds.), *Best practices in school psychology V* (Vol. 5, pp. 1751–1770). National Association of School Psychologists.

Lopez, E. C. (2000). Conducting instructional consultation through interpreters. *School Psychology Review, 29*, 378–388. https://doi.org/10.1080/02796015.2000.12086022

Lopez, E. C., & Velasco, P. M. (2017). Supporting teachers of English language learners via instructional consultation. In E. C. Lopez, S. Nahari, & S. Proctor (Eds.), *Handbook of multicultural school psychology: An interdisciplinary perspective* (2nd ed., pp. 35–55). Routledge.

Maul, C. A. (2015). Working with culturally and linguistically diverse students and their families: Perceptions and practices of school speech–language therapists in the United States. *International Journal of Communication Disorders, 50*, 750–762. https://doi.org/10.1111/1460-6984.12176

Mittermaier, M., Raza, M. M., & Kvedar, J. C. (2023). Bias in AI-based models for medical applications: Challenges and mitigation strategies. *npj Digital Medicine, 6*, Article 113. https://doi.org/10.1038/s41746-023-00858-z

National Association of School Psychologists (2020). *The professional standards of the National Association of School Psychologists*. https://www.nasponline.org/standards-and-certification/nasp-2020-professional-standards-adopted.

National Center for Education Statistics. (2024). English learners in public schools. *Condition of education*. U.S. Department of Education, Institute of Education Sciences. https://nces.ed.gov/programs/coe/indicator/cgf.

National Council on Interpreting in Health Care. (2005). *National standards of practice for interpreters in health care*. https://www.ncihc.org/assets/z2021Images/NCIHC%20National%20Standards%20of%20Practice.pdf.

O'Bryon, E. C., & Rogers, M. R. (2010). Bilingual school psychologists' assessment practices with English language learners. *Psychology in the Schools, 47*, 1018–1034. https://doi.org/10.1002/pits.20521

Roach, A., & Graybill, E. (2023). Best practices in identifying, implementing, and evaluating quality school interventions. In P. L. Harrison, S. L. Proctor, & A. Thomas (Eds.), *Best practices in school psychology 1: Foundations* (pp. 221–233). National Association of School Psychologists.

Rossetti, Z., Redash, A., Sauer, J. S., Bui, O., Wen, Y., & Regensburger, D. (2018). Access, accountability, and advocacy: Culturally and linguistically diverse families' participation in IEP meetings. *Exceptionality*, 1–16. https://doi.org/10.1080/09362835.2018.1480948

Rossetti, Z., Sauer, J. S., Bui, O., & Ou, S. (2017). Developing collaborative partnerships with culturally and linguistically diverse families during the IEP process. *Teaching Exceptional Children, 49*, 328–338. https://doi.org/10.1177/0040059918758163

Tribe, R., & Raval, H. (Eds.). (2003). *Working with interpreters in mental health*. Routledge.

Upah, K. R. F. (2008). Best practices in designing, implementing, and evaluating quality interventions. In A. Thomas & J. Grimes (Eds.), *Best practices in school psychology V* (Vol. 2, pp. 209–223). National Association of School Psychologists.
Vega, D., Lasser, J., & Afifi, A. F. M. (2016). School psychologists and the assessment of culturally and linguistically diverse students. *Contemporary School Psychology, 20*, 218–229. https://doi.org/10.1007/s40688-015-0075-5
Vega, D., Wolf, J. N., Barton, D. O., Stathatos, M., Iurino, C., & Hammer, L. (2019). Identifying the training experiences and needs of bilingual school psychologists. *Psychology in the Schools, 56*, 1687–1699. https://doi.org/10.1002/pits.22288
Zhang, C. X., Crawford, E., Marshall, J., Bernard, A., & Walker-Smith, K. (2021). Developing interprofessional collaboration between clinicians, interpreters, and translators in healthcare settings: Outcomes from face-to-face training. *Journal of Interprofessional Care, 35*, 521–531. https://doi.org/10.1080/13561820.2020.1786360

Part III
Utilizing Culturally Responsive Assessment Practices

Chapter 10
Assessment of Emergent Bilingual Youth for Specific Learning Disabilities

Jaclyn N. Wolf and Desiree Vega

Assessment of Emergent Bilingual Youth for Specific Learning Disabilities

As of 2021, emergent bilingual (EB) learners represent 10.6% (5.3 million) of students enrolled in K-12 public schools in the U.S. (National Center for Education Statistics [NCES], 2024). Most recent estimates show that 15.8% of English language learners (ELL), or the designation given to youth identified as EBs formally in school, have one or more educationally related disabilities (U.S. Government Accountability Office [GAO], 2024). While this represents K-12 ELL youth in the U.S. overall, there is variability by state, ranging from 5.6% (Louisiana) to 23.8% (Wyoming; GAO, 2024).

For all youth, specific learning disabilities (SLD) represent the most common eligibility category for special education and related services (32%; NCES, 2024). Compared to youth not classified as ELLs, however, EB students are more likely to be found eligible for special education and related services due to an SLD. That is, 45% of students classified as ELLs have also been identified as having an SLD compared to 35% of non-ELL youth nationwide (World Class Instructional Design and Assessment [WIDA], 2023). This variability, at the local and national levels, contributes to the disproportionate enrollment of EB youth in special education and related services for SLDs (Sullivan & Artiles, 2011).

J. N. Wolf (✉)
Psychology Department, San Francisco State University, San Francisco, CA, USA
e-mail: jaclynwolf@sfsu.edu

D. Vega
Department of Disability & Psychoeducational Studies, University of Arizona, Tucson, AZ, USA
e-mail: dvega2@arizona.edu

D. Vega, J. N. Wolf (eds.), *Culturally and Linguistically Responsive Intervention and Assessment Practices with Emergent Bilingual Students*,
https://doi.org/10.1007/978-3-032-02084-0_10

Specific Learning Disabilities

Definitions for an SLD are offered by both the Individuals with Disabilities Education Act (IDEA; U.S. Department of Education, 2004) and the Diagnostic and Statistical Manual of Mental Disorders, Fifth Edition, Text Revision (DSM-5-TR; American Psychiatric Association, 2022). While school-based services are guided by IDEA, the lack of a universal definition can impact data-based decision-making and the understanding of eligibility requirements (particularly when children have been evaluated by outside providers and are then seeking services in the K-12 setting based on the results).

Regardless of where the diagnosis (DMS-5-TR) or label (IDEA) originated from, to qualify for special education and related services under SLD, a student must show:

> A disorder in one or more of the basic psychological processes involved in understanding or in using language, spoken or written, that may manifest itself in the **imperfect ability to listen, think, speak, read, write, spell, or to do mathematical calculations**, including conditions such as perceptual disabilities, brain injury, minimal brain dysfunction, dyslexia, and developmental aphasia. (U.S. Department of Education, 2004, Section 300.8)

A child can show the manifestations of a SLD in one or more of the three major academic areas (i.e., reading, writing, and math) at any one time. However, the IDEA (U.S. Department of Education, 2004) regulations present special considerations for EB youth.

"Understanding or Using Language"

As stated above, the IDEA guidelines define an SLD as a disorder in the "processes involved in *understanding* or in *using language*, spoken or written" (U.S. Department of Education, 2004, Section 300.8). For bilingual youth, this means it is essential to determine whether the presentation of difficulties in understanding or in using language is due to low English proficiency or a true learning difference. While it is entirely possible that a child can be both bilingual **and** have a learning disability, understanding the impact of learning a new language on emerging academic abilities is essential. The process of learning a second language can mimic features of an SLD; however, a **true** learning disability should be present in all languages of the child (Vega & Wolf, 2023).

This is a particularly important consideration given that language learning and the demonstration of academic difficulties (in the language being learned) can overlap. Though not exhaustive, this includes appearing not to follow or remember instructions (due to them being in an unfamiliar language), difficulty with phonological processing (potentially due to sounds that are not present in one's native language), challenges retelling or explaining elements of stories recently read because of expressive language demands (i.e., low reading comprehension), and/or low processing speed and difficulties with attention due to the mental load that accompanies learning and communicating in a new language (Klingner, n.d.).

Through the use of standardized and non-standardized (e.g., record review, curriculum-based measures [CBMs], interviews, observations) assessment practices, school-based evaluators can systematically collect data to better understand the role of language development on a child's ability to demonstrate their **true** academic skills. Before collecting data, academic assessment (formal and informal) must be contextualized within the language the child has predominantly been educated in. That is, if a child has only ever received educational programming in English, then administering academic assessments in their native language may not produce valid data (Vega & Wolf, 2023). Table 10.1, based on recommendations from Vega and Wolf (2023), outlines the data collection process.

Table 10.1 Guidance for determining the role of language on the demonstration of academic skills. Data considerations and sources

Question/concern	Sources of data
Are academic difficulties present in **all** languages? • **Ask**: Have they received educational programming in all languages? • **Ask**: Are they participating in any specialized language instruction (i.e., English language development courses, outside-of-school programs to further their academic skills in their native language, at-home tutoring, etc.)?	Historical report cards and educational records; interviews with caregivers, teachers, and other service providers; CBMs/work samples (in all languages); state/local testing data; response to previous intervention (if applicable); standardized academic assessments in the appropriate language(s)
Orthographic processing (e.g., low grammatical understanding, poor spelling) • **Ask**: What are the symbolic/character differences between the child's native language and the one they are learning (e.g., English alphabet versus Mandarin Pinyin characters)? • **Ask**: How much writing instruction have they received in each language?	Historical report cards and educational records; interviews with caregivers, teachers, and other service providers; CBMs/work samples (in all languages); state/local testing data; response to previous intervention (if applicable); standardized academic assessments in the appropriate language(s)
Phonological processing • **Ask**: What are the differences in the phonological (tonal) features of the child's native language and the one they are learning (e.g., English versus Arabic)? • **Ask**: How much exposure have they had to the sounds of each language and starting at what age?	Historical report cards and educational records; interviews with caregivers, teachers, and other service providers; CBMs/work samples (in all languages); language samples/observations (in all languages); state/local testing data; response to previous intervention (if applicable); standardized academic assessments in the appropriate language(s)

(continued)

Table 10.1 (continued)

Question/concern	Sources of data
Math • **Ask**: How do their math abilities change when language demands are reduced (e.g., word problems)? • **Ask**: Are visuals (e.g., graphs) or words culturally loaded?	Historical report cards and educational records; interviews with caregivers, teachers, and other service providers; CBMs/work samples (in all languages); state/local testing data; response to previous intervention (if applicable); standardized academic assessments in the appropriate language(s) that measure both math **calculation** and math **reasoning**
Memory • **Ask**: Are there differences between visual and auditory memory? Could this be explained by the cultural or linguistic loading of the test items? • **Ask**: Are there other plausible explanations for memory difficulties (e.g., attention-deficit/hyperactivity disorder, trauma)? • **Ask**: Are memory difficulties present in their preferred language, or do they appear to be a result of the mental fatigue associated with completing mental tasks in an unfamiliar language?	Historical report cards and educational records; interviews with caregivers, teachers, and other service providers; standardized memory assessment in the appropriate language(s) that include visual and auditory memory; list learning tasks (in both languages); observations
Reading fluency and accuracy • **Ask**: Are there qualitative differences between the structure (i.e., phonological and orthographic) of the text and the child's native language? • **Ask**: Is the child experiencing challenges with rapid naming abilities? If so, are they present in all languages? • **Ask**: Have there ever been concerns about the child's reading in their native language?	Historical report cards and educational records; interviews with caregivers, teachers, and other service providers; CBMs/work samples (in all languages); language samples/observations (in all languages); state/local testing data; response to previous intervention (if applicable); standardized academic assessments in the appropriate language(s), including measures of rapid naming and phonological processing
Reading comprehension • **Ask**: Are there separate memory or attention concerns that may explain low reading comprehension? • **Ask**: Is the child unable to comprehend what they are reading due to having to read material in a language they are unfamiliar with? Are similar difficulties present when asked to read in their native language? • **Ask**: Is the text commensurate with their reading level in any language? • **Ask**: Is the text culturally relevant? Does it assume a degree of acculturation for understanding?	Historical report cards and educational records; interviews with caregivers, teachers, and other service providers; CBMs/work samples (in all languages); language samples/observations (in all languages); state/local testing data; response to previous intervention (if applicable); standardized academic assessments in the appropriate language(s)

Exclusionary Criteria

IDEA also provides guidance about what an SLD **does not** include, such as learning problems due to “environmental, cultural, or economic disadvantage” (U.S. Department of Education, 2004, Section 300.8). Similarly, this provision mandates that school-based evaluators take a holistic approach to evaluating EB youth for an SLD, which includes assessing factors beyond language use and education history (e.g., unique risk factors faced by culturally and linguistically minoritized families, socioeconomic status, immigration-related stressors, acculturation challenges, etc.). This should also include considerations for the ways bilingual youth and their families were impacted by the coronavirus (COVID-19) pandemic.

While the percentage enrollment of EBs in K-12 public schools has steadily increased in the U.S., enrollment fell during the first school year of the COVID-19 pandemic (NCES, 2024). Some of the nation’s school systems with the greatest number of youth classified as ELLs estimated that less than half were logging in to online instruction (an important consideration for exclusionary criteria; Sugarman & Lazarín, 2020). For EB youth, the COVID-19 pandemic and associated school closures only further highlighted the educational inequities that exist between them and their non-EB peers (Sugarman & Lazarín, 2020). As Sugarman and Lazarín (2020) state, “Among the most significant barriers to ELs’ participation were: a lack of access to digital devices and broadband, parents’ limited capacity to support home learning, inadequate remote learning resources and training for teachers, and school-family language barriers” (p. 1).

As outlined by Sugarman and Lazarín (2020), EB youth and their families face a variety of unique risk factors compared to their monolingual peers that were exacerbated by the pandemic. This includes a lack of school-offered translation and interpretation services to support caregivers’ ability to help their child with homework in English. While not a monolith, many EB youth have immigrant caregivers. During the pandemic, immigrants were disproportionately represented in occupations considered “essential,” meaning they often had to choose between working and supporting their child’s academic skill development during distance learning. Moreover, with caregivers expected to work outside of the home, many EB youth were also tasked with providing childcare or taking on other responsibilities around the home, all while also juggling their schoolwork. Finally, the pandemic itself could have activated trauma from similar experiences in their home country, and immigrants in the U.S. also faced an onslaught of racist and anti-immigrant rhetoric from the Trump administration.

Thus, it is important to consider these factors’ unique and lingering impact on the academic development of EB students during the pre-referral process to prevent unnecessary evaluations. While research is still emerging, disruptions in schooling appear to have affected monolingual and bilingual learners differently. For example, Sun et al. (2022) found that school disruptions were related to lower progress in reading comprehension for bilingual learners compared to their monolingual peers. The authors also found that prolonged school disruptions during the COVID-19 pandemic appeared most impactful on literacy skills when children had a home language different from their language of schooling.

SLD Assessment Practices

The three widely recognized methods for identifying learning disabilities are the discrepancy model (e.g., APA, 2022), processing strengths and weaknesses (PSW; e.g., Ventura County SELPA, n.d.), and multitiered system of supports (e.g., Pennsylvania Training and Technical Assistance Network, 2020). The method guides data collection, but which method should be used is typically guided by district requirements. For a more detailed overview of each method and its appropriateness for EB youth, see Vega and Wolf (2023).

Language(s) of Testing

A crucial element at the start of the assessment process for EB youth is determining which language(s) are appropriate for testing. This complex process involves understanding a child's dominant language **and** the language in which they have primarily been educated (which may differ). Multiple sources of data should be used to make determinations about one's dominant language and proficiency in other languages, as attempts to quantify language via standardized tests do not demonstrate the full scope of a student's linguistic ability. This can include qualitative data gathered through language samples and observations (Elizalde-Utnick & Romero, 2017) as well as norm-referenced measures such as the Woodcock-Muñoz Language Survey III (Vega & Wolf, 2023) or other formal language assessments, like those given when a child is classified as an ELL student at school.

Though a child may be dominant in a language separate from the one they have primarily been educated in, the latter is particularly important when assessing for the presence of an SLD. As outlined by Vega and Wolf (2023), academic testing should be conducted in English when it is determined that English is both the child's dominant language **and** the predominant language in which they have been educated. Conversely, testing should be done in the child's native language when it is determined to be their dominant language **and** the predominant language of their education. One may also consider administering academic tests in both English and the child's native language concurrently to determine if difficulties are present in both languages.

Decisions about which language(s) to test can be complicated by factors such as the assessor not being fluent in a child's dominant language or not having a test available in that language. In these cases, consultation with appropriately trained bilingual colleagues who have an understanding of language development (e.g., speech-language pathologists, school psychologists, English as a second language teachers) is highly recommended. Similar considerations apply to cognitive testing. However, an additional factor to consider when deciding whether to use standardized nonverbal tests is that they should be considered last, as they are not completely free of language or culture and should not be assumed to be inherently valid for EB learners (National Association of School Psychologists, 2023). Nonverbal tests are generally a good option when cognitive tests are not available in the child's native language. For more discussion on the use of nonverbal cognitive measures, see Chap. 12.

Standardized Assessment Tools

The use of standardized assessments to make eligibility decisions is the likely reality for most school-based evaluators (especially those in districts that mandate the discrepancy or PSW models for the identification of SLDs). It is well documented that norm-referenced standardized tests are biased against culturally and linguistically minoritized students for a variety of reasons. Though not exhaustive, this includes test items that are culturally loaded (Rhodes et al., 2005), the necessity of English proficiency to engage in testing (Durán, 2008), and the lack of representation of bilingual youth in the norming sample (Calderón-Tena et al., 2022).

There is also a paucity of standardized academic assessments available in a language other than English, and administering them requires the availability of appropriately trained bilingual assessors. See Appendix 1 for a list of measures available in languages other than English for assessing academic skills (and related processes, like attention). In addition to the norming sample, assessors should be mindful of the publication year when selecting tests for use with EB students. While there is no rule for when a test must be updated or revised (Psychological Assessment Resources [PAR], 2024) it is advised that the assessor ensure its appropriateness based on "psychometrics and diagnostic accuracy, appropriateness of the normative sample, appropriate measurement of constructs of interest, clinical and cultural relevance of stimuli, and clinical utility" (Alberta College of Speech-Language Pathologists and Audiologists, 2022, p. 2).

Evaluators may also consider utilizing standardized tests more holistically. For example, both formally and informally, most measures allow for an error analysis. When assessing EB youth, reporting these data may be more helpful and equitable than uncontextualized standard scores (Lenski & Verbruggen, 2010). In many cases, the pattern of errors can be used to inform decisions about difficulties as being related to language learning, while also providing more specific areas to target in intervention (e.g., Parker & Riley, 2010). In a measure of phonological processing, for example, error types can be analyzed to see if they center around phonological differences between one's native and second language (e.g., trilled "r" in Spanish, a falling tone in Mandarin, etc.). Analyzing error types in reading assessments can be helpful as well. For example, is the youth inserting or omitting words consistent with differences in each language (i.e., adjective-noun order, challenges with pronouns, conjugation requirements, etc.)? In addition to thoughtful decisions about how to analyze and report scores, assessors can also increase the equity and appropriateness of standardized assessments by reducing unnecessary language demands (e.g., unfamiliar words, complex instructions) that do not impact the concepts the test is designed to measure (Vega & Wolf, 2023).

Local Norms

To address the flaws associated with norm-referenced standardized assessments, some scholars have called for the use of **local norms**, or a sample of a local population, which allows for comparison of their true peers (e.g., all the EB youth in one grade, school, district, etc.; Stewart & Silberglitt, 2008). As federal legislation focused on prevention has expanded, so has the collection of local norm data; most schools collect these data at multiple points throughout the school year and use them for universal screening, instructional planning, resource allocation, and program evaluation (Steward & Silberglitt, 2008). For school-based assessors, and germane to assessment for SLDs, it is also possible to utilize these data to establish more equitable and appropriate academic norms for comparing EB youth to other EB youth. As schools integrate a whole-school, problem-solving approach (i.e., MTSS), local norms can also be helpful for providing current and relevant information for the academic skills of EB youth and their response to intervention (Steward & Silberglitt, 2008). For a comprehensive guide to developing and using local norms, see Steward and Silberglitt's *Best Practices in Developing Academic Local Norms* (2008).

Non-Standardized Assessment Tools

Ultimately, to ensure a holistic and equitable evaluation for EB learners, assessors **must** incorporate both standardized and non-standardized approaches into their practice. Non-standardized assessment practices and sources of data can include interviews, a thorough review of educational records, language samples, observations, CBMs, and work samples (Vega & Wolf, 2023). These types of data allow for important triangulation when paired with standardized assessment data, particularly as it relates to understanding where a child's **true** ability lies when not conflated with language learning (Elizalde-Utnick & Romero, 2017; Vega & Wolf, 2023). To this end, it is advisable to collect and compare non-standardized data (e.g., work samples, CBMs) in each language wherever possible to see if similar patterns exist. To collect and integrate these data, school-based evaluators may need to collaborate with their school's bilingual education teacher, English as a second language teacher, speech-language pathologist, and/or a trained interpreter (Vega & Wolf, 2023). CBMs for use with EB students are listed in Appendix 1.

Interpretation and Decision-Making

Determining whether an SLD is present in EB learners is a complex task, as discussed throughout this chapter. School psychologists must utilize holistic and strengths-based practices when evaluating EB students, which may also require collaboration with appropriately trained bilingual colleagues (e.g., SLP, interpreter). Data should incorporate both standardized and non-standardized (e.g., CBMs, observations, interviews, etc.) sources, nested within an understanding of the child's dominant language **and** predominant language of education. The assessment process also demands that evaluators understand the impact of language learning on the demonstration of academic skills, and data collected should support similar learning challenges in **all** languages before a SLD determination is made.

School psychologists will need to examine the multiple sources of data collected for consistency and validity, and determine whether it aligns with what they know about the child. For example, an EB student may receive a test score in the below average range, but error analysis and/or examination of other sources of data may indicate that the student has average skills in that area. Thus, school psychologists must also keep in mind that assessment results are estimates of functioning and represent a snapshot of that particular day and time, so the EB student's abilities may not be fully captured by a single score. Non-standardized data from records reviews, CBMs, interviews, observations, and/or language samples are valuable in establishing patterns and understanding EB students' strengths and weaknesses. Moreover, while examining the data collected, the influence of EB students' cultural, linguistic, and acculturative information must also be considered (Elizalde-Utnick & Romero, 2017). The unique academic impact of the COVID-19 pandemic on EB students needs to be factored into decision-making and case conceptualization as well.

Conclusion

The assessment of EB students for SLDs requires special consideration. Due to systemic barriers (i.e., a lack of bilingual school personnel, inappropriate assessment practices, etc.), these youth are at risk of both over- and underrepresentation in special education and related services. Practically speaking, this means that EB students with true learning differences are less likely to get the academic support they need, while those demonstrating expected behaviors associated with learning a new language are more likely to be placed in educational environments that miscategorize them and reduce their access and opportunity.

This chapter offers a variety of strategies for increasing efficiency within this determination, such as examining error patterns, creating and using local norms, and comparing academic performance across languages. By utilizing a multi-method, multi-informant assessment approach that is culturally and linguistically informed, school-based evaluators can foster more appropriate intervention and educational practices for emergent bilingual youth.

Appendix 1: Assessment Measures Available in Languages Other Than English

Name	Published	Language	What it measures	Norms	Where to access/ purchase
aimswebPlus	2018	Some components in Spanish	Spanish CBMs in reading and math for grades PreK to 12	Evidence-based benchmarks; grade-specific norms	https://www.pearsonassessments.com
Aprenda 3	2005	Spanish	A standardized measures of academic achievement across content areas K to 12 students	U.S. national norms	https://www.pearsonassessments.com
Bracken School Readiness Assessment, Third Edition (BSRA-3)	2007	Some components in Spanish	A standardized measure of basic school readiness concepts (i.e., colors, letters, numbers/counting, size/comparison, and shapes) for children aged 3:0 to 6:11.	U.S. national norms; has been shown to be valid for Spanish speakers in Puerto Rico (Ortiz et al., 2014)	https://www.pearsonassessments.com
Batería IV Woodcock-Muñoz	2019	Spanish	A standardized measure of academic achievement for ages 2 to 90. When used with the English version, it allows for direct comparison of skills in Spanish and English	U.S. national norms	https://riversideinsights.com
Batería Neuropsicológica Para Preescolares (BANPE)	2015	Spanish	A standardized measure of attention, memory, language, motor skills, and executive functions in children aged 3:0 to 5:0	Spain national norms	https://www.pearsonassessments.com

Name	Published	Language	What it measures	Norms	Where to access/ purchase
Boehm test of basic concepts (Boehm-3)	2001	Spanish	A standardized assessment that evaluates 50 foundational classroom concepts in grades K to 2	U.S. national norms	https://www.pearsonassessments.com
Brown executive function/attention scales (Brown EF/A)	2020; 2025	Spanish, French	A rating scale that screens executive functioning skills in ages 5 to 18	Spain national norms; French national norms	https://www.pearsonassessments.com
easyCBM Spanish (free edition)	n/a	Spanish	A CBM that measures oral reading fluency in Spanish for grades 1 to 5	Evidence-based benchmarks; grade-specific norms	https://www.easycbm.com
easyCBM (deluxe edition)	n/a	Spanish (all reading and math items; Spanish audio read-aloud for math)	Suite of reading and math CBMs in Spanish for grades K to 8	Evidence-based benchmarks; grade-specific norms	https://www.easycbm.com
Evaluación del Desarrollo de la Lectura 2 (EDL2+)	2010	Spanish	A standardized measure of oral reading fluency and reading comprehension in grades K to 8	Norms are based on words read per minute	https://www.pearsonassessments.com
FastBridge Spanish CBMs	n/a	Spanish	Various literacy CBMs available for grades K to 5	Evidence-based benchmarks; grade-specific norms	https://www.fastbridge.org
Intervention central CBM tools	n/a	Spanish (directions only)	Provides CBMs with Spanish *directions* for letter reading fluency, passage reading, math computation, and written expression	Varies by CBM	https://www.interventioncentral.org
Logramos Tercera Edición	2014	Spanish	A standardized measure of academic achievement for grades K to 8.	U.S. national norms	https://riversideinsights.com

Name	Published	Language	What it measures	Norms	Where to access/ purchase
NEPSY-II Spain	2011	Spanish (Spain)	A standardized measure of executive functions and other cognitive processes for children aged 3:0 to 16:11	Spain national norms	https://www.pearsonassessments.com
NEUROPSI third edition	2015	Spanish (Mexico)	A standardized measure of attention, memory, and learning for ages 6:0 to 85:0	Mexico norms	https://www.pearsonassessments.com
Prueba de Habilidades Academicas Iniciales (PHAI)	2006	Spanish	A standardized measure of academic achievement for children aged 4 to 7:11; Spanish adaptation of the young children's achievement test (YCAT)	Standardized in Mexico (10 states) that represent its five geographic regions	https://www.wpspublish.com
Star CBM Lectura	n/a	Spanish	CBMs that measures Spanish literacy (i.e., phonics, fluency, etc.) for grades K to 6	U.S. national norms for Spanish speakers	https://www.renaissance.com
Tests of Dyslexia (TOD)	2024	Spanish (parent/ caregiver rating form only)	A questionnaire that identifies dyslexia/SLD in reading for ages 6 to 18	U.S. national norms	https://www.wpspublish.com
Test of phonological processing in Spanish (TOPPS)	2003	Spanish	A standardized measure of phonological processing for kindergarten through adulthood; Spanish adaptation of the comprehensive test of phonological processing (CTOPP)	Unknown	https://www.cal.org

Name	Published	Language	What it measures	Norms	Where to access/ purchase
Woodcock-Muñoz language survey III	2017	Spanish	A standardized assessment of academic language proficiency in listening, speaking, reading, and writing for ages 3 to 22:11	U.S. national norms	https://www.wpspublish.com
Work sampling system (WSS)	2014	Some components in Spanish	A curriculum-based observational assessment aligned to grade-level guidelines for children aged 3 to 9	U.S. national norms	https://www.pearsonassessments.com

References

Alberta College of Speech-Language Pathologists and Audiologists. (2022, October). Professional predicaments: Using outdated versions of standardized tests. *Alberta College of Speech-Language Pathologists and Audiologists*. https://www.acslpa.ca/wp-content/uploads/2022/10/2022-10_Using-Outdated-Versions-of-Standardized-Tests_Final.pdf.

American Psychiatric Association. (2022). *Diagnostic and statistical manual of mental disorders* (5th ed.). American Psychiatric Publishing.

Calderón-Tena, C. O., Styck, K. M., Vega, D., & Kranzler, J. H. (2022). Evaluating cultural and linguistic load of IQ scores for English language learners. *International Journal of School & Educational Psychology, 10*(1), 46–62. https://doi.org/10.1080/21683603.2020.1803164

Durán, R. P. (2008). Assessing English-language learners' achievement. *Review of Research in Education, 32*(1), 292–327. https://doi.org/10.3102/0091732x07309372

Elizalde-Utnick, G., & Romero, P. A. (2017). Assessment of English language learners. In E. C. Lopez, S. G. Nahari, & G. B. Esquivel (Eds.), *Handbook of multicultural school psychology: An interdisciplinary perspective* (2nd ed., pp. 193–217). Routledge.

Klingner, J. (n.d.). *Distinguishing language acquisition from learning disabilities*. NYC Department of Education Division of English Language Learners and Student Support.

Lenski, S. D., & Verbruggen, F. (2010). *Writing instruction and assessment for English language learners K-8*. Guilford Press.

National Association of School Psychologists. (2023). *The provision of school psychological services to multilingual students*. [Position Statement].

National Center for Education Statistics. (2024). *Report on the condition of education 2024 (NCES 2024-144)*. U.S. Department of Education. https://nces.ed.gov/pubs2024/2024144.pdf.

Ortiz, A., Clinton, A., & Schaefer, B. A. (2014). Construct validity evidence for Bracken school readiness assessment, third edition, Spanish form scores. *Psychology in the Schools, 52*(2), 208–221. https://doi.org/10.1002/pits.21816

Parker, F., & Riley, K. L. (2010). *Linguistics for non-linguists: A primer with exercises* (5th ed.). Allyn & Bacon.

Pennsylvania Training and Technical Assistance Network. (2020). MTSS, RTI, and SLD determination in Pennsylvania. https://www.pattan.net/CMSPages/GetAmazonFile.aspx?path=~%5Cpattan%5Cmedia%5Cpublications%5Cmtss-rti-sld-faqs_2-20_9-20-wba.pdf&hash=ea8783ac14a98f3920d34b25728cea04b0eead134649b06de82384298ad66b3a&ext=.pdf.

Psychological Assessment Resources. (2024, July 18). When should a test be updated or revised? PAR, Inc. https://www.parinc.com/learning-center/par-blog/detail/blog/2021/09/14/when-should-a-test-be-updated-or-revised.

Rhodes, R. L., Ochoa, S. H., & Ortiz, S. O. (2005). *Assessing culturally and linguistically diverse students: A practical guide*. Guilford Press.

Stewart, L. H., & Silberglitt, B. (2008). Best practices in developing academic local norms. In A. Thomas & J. Grimes (Eds.), *Best practices in school psychology* (5th ed., pp. 225–242). National Association of School Psychologists.

Sugarman, J., & Lazarín, M. (2020). *Educating English learners during the COVID-19 pandemic*. Migration Policy Institute. https://www.migrationpolicy.org/sites/default/files/publications/mpi-english-learners-covid-19-final.pdf.

Sullivan, A. L., & Artiles, A. J. (2011). Theorizing racial inequity in special education. *Urban Education, 46*(6), 1526–1552. https://doi.org/10.1177/0042085911416014

Sun, X., Marks, R. A., Eggleston, R. L., Zhang, K., Lau, C., Yu, C., Nickerson, N., & Kovelman, I. (2022). Impacts of the COVID-19 disruption on the language and literacy development of monolingual and heritage bilingual children in the United States. *Reading and Writing, 36*(2), 347–375. https://doi.org/10.1007/s11145-022-10388-x

U.S. Department of Education. (2004). *Individuals with disabilities education act* (H.R.1350). https://www.congress.gov/bill/108th-congress/house-bill/1350/text.

U.S. Government Accountability Office. (2024). *K-12 education: How states identify English learners, including those with disabilities (GAO-24-107376)*. https://www.gao.gov/assets/gao-24-107376.pdf.

Vega, D., & Wolf, J. N. (2023). Best practices in assessment of bilingual learners in schools. In P. Harrison, S. Proctor, & A. Thomas (Eds.), *Best practices in school psychology* (7th ed., pp. 163–173). National Association of School Psychologists.

Ventura County SELPA. (n.d.). *Pattern of strengths and weaknesses model for specific learning disability eligibility procedural manual*. https://www.vcselpa.org/Portals/0/For%20Educators/Pattern%20of%20Strengths%20and%20Weaknesses/PSW%20Manual%202019%20r9-6-19.pdf?ver=fRaj5GmYgYVlVsUz5obxnQ%3d%3d.

World Class Instructional Design and Access. (2023). *Identifying multilingual learners with specific learning disabilities: Data, advice, and resources for school teams* (Focus Bulletin). https://wida.wisc.edu/sites/default/files/resource/FocusBulletin-Identifying-Multilingual-Learners-Specific-Learning-Disabilities.pdf.

Chapter 11
Assessing Social, Emotional, and Behavioral Functioning in Emergent Bilingual Youth

Juanita Torres, Kelsey Kuperman, and Jaclyn N. Wolf

Assessing Social, Emotional, and Behavioral Functioning in Emergent Bilingual Youth

Learning within school settings inherently involves social, emotional, and behavioral (SEB) components that can facilitate and/or interrupt children's learning (Zins et al., 2007). For instance, social and emotional factors have been shown to affect students' academic engagement, utilization of coping skills for behavior regulation, ability to sustain focus on learning content and classroom tasks, and level of dedication to coursework (Durlak et al., 2011). Given that SEB skills are malleable and have been linked to positive outcomes across important life domains (Durlak et al., 2011; Nagaoka et al., 2015), SEB functioning represents an important target for early intervention. This highlights the essential need for quality SEB assessment to effectively identify children's mental health needs and connect youth with appropriate resources and supports for fostering healthy adjustment and positive outcomes. Further, researchers have viewed SEB assessment, particularly when accounting for strengths and resilience, as a more comprehensive form of evaluation and

J. Torres (✉)
Reaching HOPE, Thornton, CO, USA
e-mail: juanita.torres@reachinghope.org

K. Kuperman
Department of Psychiatry, Denver Health Hospital Authorities, Denver, CO, USA

Department of Psychiatry, Anschutz Medical Campus, University of Colorado, Aurora, CO, USA
e-mail: Kelsey.kuperman@dhha.org

J. N. Wolf
Psychology Department, San Francisco State University, San Francisco, CA, USA
e-mail: jaclynwolf@sfsu.edu

D. Vega, J. N. Wolf (eds.), *Culturally and Linguistically Responsive Intervention and Assessment Practices with Emergent Bilingual Students*,
https://doi.org/10.1007/978-3-032-02084-0_11

conceptualization of mental health in youth as compared to strictly assessing psychopathology (Hass & Kennedy, 2014).

Cultural factors, such as languages spoken, acculturation level, and access to social supports, have been shown to play important roles in shaping the SEB functioning of culturally and linguistically minoritized (CLM) youth (Elizalde-Utnick & Romero, 2017; Trent et al., 2018). This calls for attention to the growing group of emergent bilingual learners, who comprise 10.6% of the U.S. public school student population (National Center for Education Statistics, 2024). Research indicates that differences in SEB functioning exist both **within** this CLM group of students and **in comparison to** English-speaking children in the U.S. (Hass & Kennedy, 2014), highlighting that CLM students are not monolithic. Beyond the inherent difficulties of learning a second language in and of itself, emergent bilingual students often face unique challenges associated with the experience of navigating social circles and academic coursework in a second language (Geva & Weiner, 2015). Continuous exposure to these challenges might intensify feelings of frustration, lower self-efficacy, and potentially disrupt the ability to access and utilize SEB skills (Soland & Sandilos, 2021).

Further, emergent bilingual learners may hold intersecting identities that, due to systemic barriers and social inequities, may be associated with psychosocial stressors and limited access to resources and supports, which can also influence SEB functioning in youth (Hass & Kennedy, 2014; Nagaoka et al., 2015). For instance, the experience of living in poverty (Mclaughlin et al., 2012) and facing barriers to accessing quality health care (Hass & Kennedy, 2014) are two of many contextual factors associated with disruptions in SEB functioning. Beyond SEB concerns, evaluators must also incorporate an understanding of strengths, resources, and resilience factors to gain a more comprehensive, contextualized understanding of each student as a whole person (Hass & Kennedy, 2014).

Schools represent an important setting and, in some cases, the only feasible environment for providing, at minimum, the first line of accessible assessment services to students (Richter et al., 2022). School-based mental health professionals are often particularly familiar with students, as well as their families and academic teams, which can create more accessible, inclusive, and consistent services. Further, the provision of comprehensive and culturally informed, school-based assessment services can ultimately help address social inequities while also working to reduce stigma associated with receiving mental health services by integrating such services into the fabric of the school system (Farmer et al., 2021; McClain et al., 2022). In this way, school-based mental health evaluators can play a critical role in not only contextualizing SEB functioning for CLM students, but also utilizing culturally informed assessment to help tease apart SEB functioning from mental health symptoms associated with the challenging language learning process for CLM students. The complex interplay between sociocultural factors and academic learning highlights the need for culturally informed frameworks for understanding and assessing SEB functioning among emergent bilingual students.

Culturally Informed Approaches

As the unique needs and challenges faced by emergent bilingual students continue to be identified in the literature, the need for psychologists to be culturally and linguistically informed has become a priority (Fouad & Arredondo, 2007). This priority was emphasized by the American Psychological Association (APA) in 2002 when the organization published their first set of multicultural guidelines, titled *Guidelines on Multicultural Education, Training, Research, Practice, and Organizational Change for Psychologists*. The publication of said guidelines solidified cultural competence as a pillar of training for psychologists and identified goals to address multiculturalism and diversity factors across the field of psychology (APA, 2002). Subsequently, the field saw exponential growth in culturally informed theory and research, which led to the APA publishing revised multicultural guidelines in 2017 (Clauss-Ehlers et al., 2019). The National Association of School Psychologists (NASP) also has various position statements about the provision of school psychological services that are culturally and linguistically informed (e.g., *The Provision of School Psychological Services to Multilingual Students*; NASP, 2023).

Despite the steady increase in discussions about multiculturalism and applied resources for enhancing cultural competence, evaluators frequently struggle with integrating culturally informed practices into the assessment process. For example, evaluators continue to prioritize the use of standardized measures when evaluating emergent bilingual youth, despite having literature detailing why said measures may not be valid for bilingual youth populations (Raines & Crumpton, 2017). Ultimately, the training and resources that prepare school-based evaluators to become culturally informed are limited (Vega et al., 2019), and the gaps between theory and practice remain quite large. Given these discrepancies, a conceptual framework is of vital importance when assessing the SEB functioning of emergent bilingual students.

Culturally Informed Conceptual Framework

Geva and Weiner (2015) adapted Mash and Hunsley's (2007) developmental systems approach (DSA) to identify three basic principles that are recommended for the assessment of SEB functioning in children and adolescents:

1. Develop trust with youth and families in order to obtain valid assessment information.
2. Focus assessments on the specific thoughts, feelings, and behaviors of youth and families, along with more general personality characteristics and dispositions.
3. Evaluate youth and families from a systemic lens, within the context of how social, emotional, and behavioral information is expressed.

Geva and Weiner's (2015) framework emphasizes culture as a primary social system that impacts schools, families, and peer groups. Similarly to Mash and Hunsley's (2007) DSA, Geva and Weiner (2015) share the perspective that the thoughts, feelings, and behaviors of emergent bilingual students should not be viewed as underlying causes of pathology, rather, should be seen as insight to various domains of interest. Further, Geva and Weiner's framework was adapted to maintain a developmental approach with CLM youth in mind. CLM students may be referred for a psychological evaluation for various reasons, such as concerns about internalizing, externalizing, or social behaviors. Some behaviors that might be labeled as concerning in the U.S. may be normative in a student's country of origin, or vice versa. It is also possible that parents of CLM students may consent to a psychological evaluation without understanding the evaluation process, to please the student's academic team (Geva & Weiner, 2015). These various considerations make it particularly important to follow Geva and Weiner's principles for the assessment of SEB functioning with emergent bilingual youth.

Developing Trust

Unfortunately, the vast majority of CLM students and families exist within systems that were not designed for them, which can impact the development of trust. Thus, it is particularly important to invest time in establishing a collaborative, trusting relationship with the youth and their families. Rapport can be enhanced by communicating genuine curiosity about the student and making an effort to learn and understand the norms, beliefs, and lived experiences of the family (Geva & Weiner, 2015). Additional techniques include physically getting on the same level as the student, engaging in play, following their lead, informing youth of the structure of the evaluation process, and providing praise and encouragement throughout. Including parents in evaluation sessions may also have added benefits related to increasing trust and engagement (Sattler, 2018). Evaluators are encouraged to keep in mind that CLM families may be unfamiliar with school-based evaluations; therefore, it is particularly important to explain the assessment process in a client's primary language while using understandable terms throughout.

Thoughts, Feelings, and Behaviors

The employment of multiple methods and informants is necessary to sufficiently and more holistically evaluate the thoughts, feelings, and behaviors of emergent bilingual students (Mash & Hunsley, 2007). Many externalizing and some internalizing behaviors can be assessed by observing students across a range of settings (e.g., classroom, playground, home). Rating scales and interviews can and should be used in conjunction with behavioral observations. Unlike behaviors, thoughts are rarely observable unless the student expresses them verbally. Therefore, culturally informed interviews are critical for gaining insight into individuals' thought processes. While feelings may be observable at times, emotions can be expressed differently across distinct cultures. By directly asking students and families how they feel, evaluators can supplement observational data with self-report information (Geva & Weiner, 2015). Various cultural variables, such as protective factors, membership, and access to social support, can affect assessment results and the interpretation of those results; thus, it is important to understand the cultural variables that contribute to the thoughts, feelings, and behaviors of the students being assessed (Dana, 2000; Geva & Weiner, 2015; Kohn et al., 2007).

Systemic Context

Emergent bilingual students exist across a range of social contexts, including within their families and schools and amongst peers. Thus, evaluators must examine students through a contextually informed lens by assessing the multi-directional impacts of students' thoughts, feelings, and behaviors across distinct social contexts. For instance, assessing for membership (e.g., acculturation, enculturation, acculturative stress; see Chap. 3) can provide important perspectives about SEB presentations that may be culturally bound or specific to salient aspects of students' identities. Inquiring about the youth's level of social support, activity involvement, protective factors, and community belongingness may be particularly beneficial for understanding the families' strengths and unique needs (Bernard, 2004). Ultimately, focusing an evaluation on individual characteristics is not sufficient, especially when considering the variety of social transitions and cultural contexts that emergent bilingual students navigate daily in school.

Conducting Social-Emotional Assessment with Bilingual Youth

In building upon the framework of the aforementioned culturally responsive approaches to evaluating SEB functioning, practitioners are encouraged to apply an integrated approach to assessment that incorporates a multiculturally informed lens throughout the entire evaluation process. Of critical importance is attending to potential language barriers that can significantly affect interpersonal interactions and assessment procedures. Thus, as discussed in multiple previous chapters, a fundamental building block for culturally informed assessment includes the evaluation of language use and proficiency. By using such findings to inform assessment procedures, conceptualization, and interpretation of results, evaluators can more accurately assess symptoms and tease apart clinical presentations, which can yield more accurate results (Elizalde-Utnick & Romero, 2017; Hoover et al., 2016). Specifically, language-based data can provide insight into the extent to which SEB functioning might stem from stress, frustrations, or other behavioral/mental health concerns associated with the significant challenges of learning an additional language.

Consultation and collaboration also represent core methods for enhancing cultural responsiveness in evaluation procedures. First, direct collaboration with professional interpreters helps to reduce identified language barriers (see Chap. 9). Research indicates that the use of trained interpreters has been shown to significantly improve clients' experience across several domains (Karliner et al., 2007). Additionally, evaluators are encouraged to engage in frequent and ongoing consultation with other key personnel, including but not limited to caregivers, teachers, medical providers, occupational therapists, and social workers who work closely with students and their families. Furthermore, collaboration with school counselors, psychotherapists, and speech-language pathologists who are bilingual in the child's first language could be particularly helpful for obtaining language samples and insight into psychosocial and behavioral functioning (Vega & Wolf, 2023).

Assessment Framework: RIOT

The implementation of a holistic and culturally informed approach also requires clinicians to gather information from multiple sources across various contexts. The multi-method approach allows evaluators to more fully capture a range of internal and external factors that might be influencing CLM students' academic learning and SEB functioning (Elizalde-Utnick & Romero, 2017). Hass and Kennedy (2014) outlined the RIOT approach, a comprehensive assessment framework that pulls data from record review, interviews, observations, and tests. The following sections will apply the RIOT framework to discuss culturally informed SEB assessment for emergent bilingual youth.

Record Review

Thorough record reviews can help to contextualize data and create a more holistic understanding of each student. For instance, evaluators can gather critical information on a student's educational history both within the U.S. and in one's country of origin, as well as family education and socioeconomic backgrounds (Elizalde-Utnick & Romero, 2017). School-based records can also help to establish timelines for changes in SEB functioning and highlight potential correlations between observed or reported SEB concerns and disruptions in academic performance. Further, medical and health records can provide important information about a child's developmental history, changes in mood and behavior, health conditions, and/or medication use that might also affect the development and presentation of SEB functioning.

Interviews

Clinical interviews with students, caregivers, and teachers represent another integral part of culturally informed assessments (Elizalde-Utnick & Romero, 2017). Interviews provide firsthand insight into a student's lived experience, language use, and levels of functioning across different settings. Geva and Weiner's (2015) proposed framework for culturally informed assessment directly applies to clinical interviews. At its core, this framework integrates collaboration, transparency, genuine curiosity, interactive engagement, and a contextualized, strengths-based approach to engaging students and their families in the assessment interview. These factors can help to build strong rapport and foster trust with students and families, which is a top priority given the sensitive nature of questions that may be asked during assessment interviews. Further, interviewers must remain grounded in cultural humility, which includes an interpersonal stance that is other oriented, curious, and invites aspects of identities that are most salient to clients (Hook et al., 2013). Further, evaluators are encouraged to maintain awareness of their own language use while tuning into client preferences regarding personal or culturally embedded word choices and identity descriptors throughout the interview process.

Semi-structured and structured diagnostic interviews are commonly employed in SEB assessment to help identify and assess the frequency and severity of behavioral challenges, onset and duration of functioning, and degree of impairment across life domains (Geva & Weiner, 2015; Sattler, 2018). One example of a widely used diagnostic interview is the Kiddie-Sads-Present and Lifetime Version (K-SADS-PL), which involves interviewing primary caregivers and children. The K-SADS-PL incorporates the use of an initial unstructured Introductory Interview, a structured Diagnostic Screening Interview, supplemental diagnostic tools, and a global assessment of functioning (Geva & Weiner, 2015).

Observations

From an ecological perspective, direct observation of students across a range of natural and controlled settings is another critical form of data collection (Elizalde-Utnick & Romero, 2017; Hass & Kennedy, 2014). For instance, students can be observed while interacting with peers and educators at school or playing with siblings at home. This information helps to further contextualize and capture a more holistic understanding of a student's behaviors in response to changing stimuli, interpersonal interactions, and environmental settings. Additionally, observational data represents a form of nonverbal assessment that can provide critical information while minimizing potential language barriers when evaluating CLM youth.

Observational data can vary widely depending on the target of information and the degrees of formality and structure being implemented. In all forms, observational data can be extremely useful for identifying antecedents and consequences of behavior, which helps to inform case conceptualization, data interpretation, and intervention planning (Hass & Kennedy, 2014; Mash & Hunsley, 2007). To date, a dearth of research has examined multiculturally sound assessment methodology or culturally competent practices for gathering behavioral observations of CLM youth (Merrell, 2008; Okazaki & Sue, 2016). Among the scant body of literature on the topic, Fong et al. (2016) highlight the need for behavioral analysts to engage in critical self-awareness of biases and thoroughly explore the cultural norms, values, and preferences of the individuals being observed. Cultural and contextual factors can provide essential insight into underlying aspects of behavior that might be culturally bound. Last, evaluators must recognize that the presence of an observer is likely to influence, at least to some degree, the behavior of those being assessed. Such effects could be exacerbated when language barriers and/or perceived differences in racial and cultural identities exist between assessors and clients.

Tests: Standardized Measures and Rating Scales

School-based evaluators typically use a combination of broad-based and specific rating scales to evaluate SEB functioning, as both are useful for determining how SEB difficulties impact a student (Fisher et al., 2007; Geva & Weiner, 2015). When used in combination with record reviews, observations, and interviews, rating scales can provide additional data that is necessary for a student to meet disability eligibility criteria and ultimately access individualized accommodations and academic support services (Burns & Ysseldyke, 2009). The Individuals with Disabilities Education Act (IDEA) outlined 13 disability categories under which a student may receive special education services (IDEA, 2004). Although review of all 13 categories extends beyond the scope of this chapter, the following sections review the categories of Emotional Disturbance, Other Health Impairment, and the rating scales often used to determine eligibility for these disability categories.

Emotional Disturbance

Emotional Disturbance (ED) encompasses a variety of conditions that must exhibit at least one of five characteristics over time, including difficulty learning, difficulty forming/maintaining healthy relationships, abnormal behaviors or feelings, general unhappiness, and the development of physical symptoms or fear (IDEA, 2004). Students who hold a mental health diagnosis that includes these characteristics, such as anxiety or depression, may meet eligibility criteria for ED.

Broad-Based Rating Scales

Broad-based rating scales inquire about a variety of behaviors and symptoms, and offer scores on several social-emotional dimensions, making them a widely accepted component of ED evaluations. The Behavior Assessment System for Children-Third Edition (BASC-3; Reynolds & Kamphaus, 2015) and the Achenbach System of Empirically Based Assessment (ASEBA; Achenbach & Rescorla, 2001) are particularly relevant for emergent bilingual students given their large representative samples and evidence of reliability across diverse groups.

The BASC-3: the BASC-3 includes parent, teacher, and student self-report forms, which are all available in English and Spanish (Reynolds & Kamphaus, 2015). The BASC-3 was developed using a normative sample that matched the U.S. census in 2013, making this measure more representative and culturally informed than many rating scales (Edyburn et al., 2020). Further, the BASC-3 incorporates the Behavioral and Emotional Screen System (BESS; Reynolds & Kamphaus, 2015), which more specifically measures students' behavioral and emotional strengths and difficulties. The BASC-3 BESS also includes Spanish and English versions of the parent form, teacher form, and student self-report form.

ASEBA Checklists: the ASEBA checklists measure strengths, adaptive functioning, and SEB functioning in children and adults by gathering information from students, parents, and teachers (Achenbach & Rescorla, 2001). The ASEBA forms have been translated into over 110 languages and have demonstrated generalizability across 23 countries (Ivanova et al., 2007). As such, ASEBA checklists may be particularly beneficial for evaluating emergent bilingual youth provided the extant literature documenting the usefulness of these checklists in assessing CLM individuals across the lifespan (Achenbach et al., 2003).

Behavior Specific Rating Scales

Once broad areas of concern have been evaluated, behavior-specific rating scales can be useful for identifying more specific concerns that require intervention. These more targeted rating scales may be used to better understand which specific concerns, such as symptoms of anxiety, depression, or trauma, may be impacting a student's ability to access their education.

Anxiety: the Multidimensional Anxiety Scale for Children, Second Edition (MASC-2; March, 2013) and Revised Children's Manifest Anxiety Scale, Second Edition (RCMAS-2; Reynolds & Richmond, 2008) are self-report measures that assess for symptoms of anxiety in children. The MASC-2 examines emotional, physical, cognitive, and behavioral symptoms using a parent report form and a child self-report form. The RCMAS-2 differs from the MASC-2 by using a "yes" or "no" format. The RCMAS-2 has been widely used to assess symptoms of anxiety in culturally diverse youth and has been translated into Spanish, Italian, and Korean.

Depression: the Beck Depression Inventory, Second Edition (BDI-II; Beck et al., 1996) and the Children's Depression Inventory 2 (CDI 2; Kovaks, 2011) are both self-report forms used to assess symptoms of depression in children. The BDI-II focuses on the severity of physical and emotional symptoms of depression and is available in English and Spanish (García-Batista et al., 2018). The CDI 2 assesses for behavioral, affective, and cognitive symptoms of depression and is also available in English and Spanish.

Trauma: emergent bilingual students often experience the compounding stress of learning a new language, adapting to new cultural environments, and potentially lacking access to social support (Geva & Weiner, 2015). Ehntholt and Yule (2006) recommend the use of semi-structured interviews with CLM students and families to collect information about possible trauma histories. Information from interviews is highly informative, given that most standardized measures of trauma have not yet been validated with CLM populations and do not include unique traumas that may be especially relevant to the experiences of emergent bilingual students.

Other Health Impairment

Other Health Impairment (OHI) is defined as "having limited strength, vitality, or alertness, including a heightened alertness to environmental stimuli, that results in limited alertness with respect to the educational environment" (IDEA, 2004, Sec. 300.8 [c] [9]). OHI includes a variety of conditions, such as asthma, diabetes, and autism spectrum disorder. Further, approximately 66% of individuals with OHI have been diagnosed with attention-deficit/hyperactivity disorder (ADHD; Schnoes et al., 2006).

Evaluating for ADHD

The Conners Rating Scales, Third Edition (Conners 3; Conners, 2008) is widely used to assess symptoms of ADHD, including inattention, impulsivity, and executive functioning. The Conners 3 can be administered to students, as well as their caregivers and teachers, and is available in both English and Spanish. Evaluators are strongly encouraged to use the Conners 3 in conjunction with additional assessment measures and observations, especially if there are concerns about the norms being valid for a particular CLM student (Geva & Weiner, 2015).

Limitations of Standardized Measures

The measures discussed above are not meant to represent an exhaustive list of evaluation tools and may not be appropriate for every emergent bilingual student. Standardized measures have significant language demands and should not be administered to a student or family in a language they are limited in, as misunderstandings can cause inaccurate results (Geva & Weiner, 2015). Additionally, cultural differences in importance placed on various behaviors and emotions can also influence how students and families respond to standardized rating scales (Geva & Weiner, 2015). Certain factors, such as culturally relevant contributors to behaviors or symptoms that present differently in other cultures (e.g., physical manifestation or somatization of anxiety) may not be represented on typical standardized rating scales (Gajjar et al., 2000).

Ultimately, it is the ethical responsibility of the evaluator to carefully review the manuals of any standardized measures used in the SEB assessment of emergent bilingual youth to seek confirmation that the client's background is represented in the norming process and/or standardization sample. It is important to note that any identified concerns that lead to special education eligibility may be inaccurate if evaluators are not utilizing rating scales with sound reliability and validity (Raines & Crumpton, 2017).

Considerations for Interpreting Data and Providing Feedback

As is true throughout the SEB evaluation process, an ecological approach remains critically important for the interpretation of data and results (Elizalde-Utnick & Romero, 2017). Thus, all assessment data needs to be interpreted through a culturally and contextually informed lens. Evaluators must reflect on any compromises they might have made when selecting assessment tasks, as this will have important implications for interpreting data (Trent et al., 2018). Additionally, there are several cultural, linguistic, and acculturative considerations to keep in mind when data collection is complete and the evaluator is preparing to interpret results. Linguistic considerations are of particular importance, given that characteristics of acquiring a second language can often present similarly to those of a learning disability (Hoover et al., 2016). A comprehensive yet non-exhaustive list of questions to consider when beginning the interpretation process is presented in Table 11.1.

Evaluators should remain mindful of these questions and considerations when presenting SEB assessment results to students and their caregivers. Feedback sessions can run the risk of becoming one-sided, deficit-focused, and overwhelming. In effort to counter this tendency, evaluators can provide feedback in a curious and collaborative manner by acknowledging the students and caregivers as the experts of their own lives. Feedback can also be framed as an opportunity for the evaluator to continue learning about the student within their cultural and familial contexts (Trent et al., 2018). To increase collaboration, evaluators can encourage students and families to reflect back information and ask questions throughout the feedback session. Taking the time to answer questions and attend to reflections can enhance a family's understanding of the student and strengthen bonds between students and caregivers (Gart et al., 2016; Tharinger et al., 2008). During feedback sessions, evaluators should highlight any limitations of the assessment procedures and

Table 11.1 Questions to consider for culturally informed interpretation of assessment data

Variable	Questions to consider
Culture	Has the student been able to access their education historically?
	Did caregivers have access to their own education, or was it lacking due to cultural factors (e.g., having to start working at a young age)?
	Has the student had any gaps in their education?
	Is the student comfortable with individuals outside of their own culture? Are any of their thoughts, feelings, or behaviors due to a cultural mismatch?
Linguistics	Were all assessment tasks presented in the most appropriate language?
	Did the student and family confirm their understanding of assessment tasks and comfort with the language they were presented in?
	Is the student having to code-switch? How is switching back and forth between languages contributing to language confusion?
	Is the student proficient in any language? Do they have low proficiency in their first language and English due to second language acquisition?
Acculturation	How does the school system differ from the student's home culture?
	Are any of the student's SEB difficulties due to trauma or extreme stress related to cultural factors (e.g., migration)?
	Does the student feel safe at school?
	Does the student have a sense of community and social support at school? Are they being treated differently due to how they look, feel, or sound?

measurement tools and explain the possible implications of such limitations on evaluation results (Acevedo-Polakkovich et al., 2007).

Determining Eligibility

In the K-12 setting, determining eligibility for special education and related services is a **team** decision (which includes caregivers; IDEA, 2004). Additionally, eligibility is not **predetermined**, meaning the team makes a decision after the review of available data (including, if applicable, formal assessment findings; IDEA, 2004). Formal assessment findings (and any associated data that informed the assessment) will be presented by the school-based evaluator at the eligibility determination meeting, and thus the guidance outlined above is not only crucial for presenting findings to caregivers, but to the educational team as well. As a member of the team—and to ensure students' needs are being appropriately identified and referral decisions are accurately made—the school-based evaluator may also need to use various parts of the strategies outlined in this chapter to challenge other team members' interpretation of their data.

As previously mentioned, social, emotional, and behavioral difficulties are most often found eligible for special education and related services via ED or OHI. When considering eligibility under these categories, school-based evaluators should utilize the comprehensive data they have gathered to consider the impact of one's

ED Eligibility Criteria	CLM Youth	OHI Eligibility Criteria
(A) An inability to learn that cannot be explained by intellectual, sensory, or health factors.	Does the student feel safe enough to establish relationships? (B)	(i) Is due to chronic or acute health problems such as asthma, attention deficit disorder or attention deficit hyperactivity disorder, diabetes, epilepsy, a heart condition, hemophilia, lead poisoning, leukemia, nephritis, rheumatic fever, sickle cell anemia, and Tourette syndrome; and
(B) An inability to build or maintain satisfactory interpersonal relationships with peers and teachers.	Is the behavior or feeling "inappropriate" in their cultural context? (C)	
(C) Inappropriate types of behavior or feelings under normal circumstances.	Does their CLM experience include trauma? (C, D, E, i*)	
	Do they feel understood and respected at school? (B, C, D, E)	(ii) Adversely affects a child's educational performance.
(D) A general pervasive mood of unhappiness or depression.	Do their "symptoms" exist across settings? (A, B, C, D, E, i)	
(E) A tendency to develop physical symptoms or fears associated with personal or school problems.	Are there deportation-related fears for themselves and/or their families? (B, C, D, i)	*Trauma can mimic ADHD symptoms

Fig. 11.1 Bilingualism and eligibility criteria for ED and OHI

status as a bilingual student on each criterion. Though not exhaustive, Fig. 11.1 outlines this process based on IDEA (2004, Sec. 300.8) eligibility criteria for ED and OHI.

Answering "yes" to any of these questions warrants further follow-up before rendering an eligibility determination. It may be the case that Tier I or II evidence-based interventions appropriate for emergent bilingual youth should be tried before making an eligibility determination (see Chap. 6).

Like with other eligibility categories, the team will also need to consider if the bilingual student's social, emotional, and/or behavioral difficulties meet criteria for services under IDEA's (2004) 'three prongs' of eligibility. Considerations for each prong have already been outlined in this chapter, but to summarize: a) ED or OHI should only be assigned when it can be determined, via various sources of data across multiple settings, that the labels are appropriate (**prong 1**), b) the student's social, emotional, and/or behavioral difficulties are impacting their ability to meaningfully and equitably access their education (**prong 2**), and c) special education and related services are needed to support the child's needs (because, for example, Tier I and Tier II strategies have not been effective; **prong 3**).

Summary and Conclusions

SEB assessment in emergent bilingual students is quite complex, which is appropriate considering the unique needs and challenges often faced by this diverse population. From a social justice perspective, the role of the evaluator extends beyond traditional bounds to include serving as an advocate for the students being assessed.

As such, it is the evaluator's ethical responsibility to ensure that the evaluation process is culturally informed, equitable, and as bias free as possible. The first steps involve understanding and working from a culturally informed framework and using an integrated approach that includes gathering information from various sources across multiple contexts. Reliance on standardized measures alone can result in inaccurate information about and interventions for the student, which can ultimately cause harm. In addition to the critical self-awareness required of all evaluators, multicultural and bilingual assessors should remain aware of and sensitive to potential differences between their own cultural backgrounds and those of their clients, how their own experiences and biases might impact their clinical approach, and the limits of their competency and expertise (Sue, 2001).

While there is no single "blanket approach" to any SEB assessment, cultural and contextual considerations are particularly important for the evaluation of CLM students. Emergent bilingual students may differ from their monolingual English-speaking peers in areas of family educational backgrounds, acculturation, and access to social support, all of which can impact stress levels and SEB presentations in school (Elizalde-Utnick & Romero, 2017). Thus, all assessment procedures, from clinical interviews and observations to identifying measurement tools and providing feedback, should be tailored to fit the unique needs of each student being evaluated. Further, evaluators are called to critically reflect on the use of alternative or informal assessment procedures, rationality for choosing specific measures, and the appropriate use of interpreters and translated materials. Each of these culturally informed approaches represent meaningful steps towards creating more equitable and inclusive assessment services for emergent bilingual students.

References

Acevedo-Polakovich, I. D., Reynaga-Abiko, G., Garriott, P. O., Derefinko, K. J., Wimsatt, M. K., Gudonis, L. C., & Brown, T. L. (2007). Beyond instrument selection: Cultural considerations in the psychological assessment of U.S. Latinas/os. *Professional Psychology: Research and Practice, 38*(4), 375–384. https://doi.org/10.1037/0735-7028.38.4.375

Achenbach, T. M., Dumenci, L., & Rescorla, L. A. (2003). DSM-oriented and empirically based approaches to constructing scales from the same item pools. *Journal of Clinical Child and Adolescent Psychology, 32*(3), 328–340. https://doi.org/10.1207/S15374424JCCP3203_02

Achenbach, T. M., & Rescorla, L. A. (2001). *Manual for the ASEBA school-age forms & profiles*. University of Vermont, Research Center for Children, Youth, and Families.

American Psychological Association. (2002). Guidelines on multicultural education, training, research, practice, and organizational change for psychologists. *American Psychologist, 58*(5), 377–402. https://doi.org/10.1037/0003-066X.58.5.377

Beck, A. T., Steer, R. A., & Brown, G. K. (1996). Manual for the Beck depression inventory-II. Psychological Corporation.

Benard, B. (2004). Environmental protective factors. In *Resiliency: What we have learned* (pp. 43–48). WestEd.

Burns, M. K., & Ysseldyke, J. E. (2009). Reported prevalence of evidence-based instructional practices in special education. *The Journal of Special Education, 43*(1), 3–11. https://doi.org/10.1177/0022466908315563

Clauss-Ehlers, C. S., Chiriboga, D. A., Hunter, S. J., Roysircar, G., & Tummala-Narra, P. (2019). APA multicultural guidelines executive summary: Ecological approach to context, identity, and intersectionality. *American Psychologist, 74*(2), 232–244. https://doi.org/10.1037/amp0000382

Conners, C. K. (2008). *Conners* (3rd ed.). Multi-Health Systems.

Dana, R. H. (Ed.). (2000). *Handbook of cross-cultural and multicultural personality assessment.* Lawrence Erlbaum Associates Publishers.

Durlak, J. A., Weissberg, R. P., Dymnicki, A. B., Taylor, R. D., & Schellinger, K. B. (2011). The impact of enhancing students' social and emotional learning: A meta-analysis of school-based universal interventions. *Child Development, 82*(1), 405–432. https://doi.org/10.1111/j.1467-8624.2010.01564.x

Edyburn, K. L., Dowdy, E., DiStefano, C., Bertone, A., & Greer, F. (2020). Measurement invariance of the English and Spanish BASC-3 behavioral and emotional screening system parent preschool forms. *Early Childhood Research Quarterly, 51*, 307–316. https://doi.org/10.1016/j.ecresq.2019.12.002

Ehntholt, K. A., & Yule, W. (2006). Practitioner review: Assessment and treatment of refugee children and adolescents who have experienced war-related trauma. *Journal of Child Psychology and Psychiatry, and Allied Disciplines, 47*(12), 1197–1210. https://doi.org/10.1111/j.1469-7610.2006.01638.x

Elizalde-Utnick, G., & Romero, P. A. (2017). Assessment of English language learners. In E. C. Lopez, S. G. Nahari, & S. Proctor (Eds.), *Handbook of multicultural school psychology: An interdisciplinary perspective* (2nd ed., pp. 193–217). Routledge.

Farmer, R. L., Goforth, A. N., Kim, S. Y., Naser, S. C., Lockwood, A. B., & Affrunti, N. W. (2021). Status of school psychology in 2020: Part 2, professional practices in the NASP membership survey. *NASP Research Reports, 5*(3), 1–17.

Fisher, E. S., Doyon, K. E., Saldaña, E., & Allen, M. R. (2007). Comprehensive assessment of emotional disturbance: A cross-validation approach. *California School Psychologist, 12*, 47–58. https://doi.org/10.1007/BF03340931

Fong, E. H., Catagnus, R. M., Brodhead, M. T., Quigley, S., & Field, S. (2016). Developing the cultural awareness skills of behavior analysts. *Behavior Analysis in Practice, 9*, 84–94. https://doi.org/10.1007/s40617-016-0111-6

Fouad, N. A., & Arredondo, P. (2007). Becoming culturally oriented: Practical advice for psychologists and educators. *American Psychological Association.* https://doi.org/10.1037/11483-000

Gajjar, E., Humphries, T., Peterson-Badali, M., & Otsubo, H. (2000). A new scale to assess culture-specific beliefs and attitudes about epilepsy. *Epilepsy & Behavior, 1*(4), 235–255. https://doi.org/10.1006/ebeh.2000.0078

García-Batista, Z. E., Guerra-Peña, K., Cano-Vindel, A., Herrera-Martínez, S. X., & Medrano, L. A. (2018). Validity and reliability of the Beck depression inventory (BDI-II) in general and hospital population of Dominican Republic. *PLoS One, 13*(6), 1–12. https://doi.org/10.1371/journal.pone.0199750

Gart, N., Zamora, I., & Williams, M. E. (2016). Parallel models of assessment: Infant mental health and therapeutic assessment models intersect through early childhood case studies. *Infant Mental Health Journal, 37*(4), 452–465. https://doi.org/10.1002/imhj.21573

Geva, E., & Weiner, J. (2015). *Psychological assessment of culturally and linguistically diverse children: A practitioner's guide*. Springer.

Hass, M. R., & Kennedy, K. S. (2014). Integrated social-emotional assessment of the bilingual child. In A. B. Clinton (Ed.), *Assessing bilingual children in context: An integrated approach* (pp. 163–187). American Psychological Association. https://doi.org/10.1037/14320-000

Hook, J. N., Davis, D. E., Owen, J., Worthington, E. L., Jr., & Utsey, S. O. (2013). Cultural humility: Measuring openness to culturally diverse clients. *Journal of Counseling Psychology, 60*(3), 353. https://doi.org/10.1037/a0032595

Hoover, J. J., Baca, L. M., & Klingner, J. K. (2016). *Why do English learners struggle with reading? Distinguishing language acquisition from learning disabilities* (2nd ed.). Corwin Press.

Individuals with Disabilities Education Act. (2004). Publ. L. No. 108-446, 118 Stat. 2647. https://sites.ed.gov/idea/regs/b.

Ivanova, M. Y., Achenbach, T. M., Dumenci, L., Rescorla, L. A., Almqvist, F., Weintraub, S., Bilenberg, N., Bird, H., Chen, W. J., Dobrean, A., Döpfner, M., Erol, N., Fombonne, E., Fonseca, A. C., Frigerio, A., Grietens, H., Hannesdóttir, H., Kanbayashi, Y., Lambert, M., et al. (2007). Testing the 8-syndrome structure of the child behavior checklist in 30 societies. *Journal of Clinical Child and Adolescent Psychology, 36*(3), 405–417. https://doi.org/10.1080/15374410701444363

Karliner, L. S., Jacobs, E. A., Chen, A. H., & Mutha, S. (2007). Do professional interpreters improve clinical care for patients with limited English proficiency? A systematic review of the literature. *Health Services Research, 42*, 727–754. https://doi.org/10.1111/j.1475-6773.2006.00629.x

Kohn, S. W., Scorcia, D., & Esquivel, G. B. (2007). Personality and behavioral assessment: Considerations for culturally and linguistically diverse individuals. In G. B. Esquivel, E. C. Lopez, & S. G. Nahari (Eds.), *Handbook of multicultural school psychology: An interdisciplinary perspective* (pp. 289–307). Lawrence Erlbaum Associates Publishers.

Kovacs, M. (2011). Children's depression inventory 2nd edition (CDI 2). Multi-Health Systems.

March, J. S. (2013). *Multidimensional anxiety scale for children* (2nd ed.). Multi-Health Systems.

Mash, E. J., & Hunsley, J. (2007). Assessment of child and family disturbance: A developmental systems approach. In E. J. Mash & R. A. Barkley (Eds.), *Assessment of childhood disorders* (4th ed., pp. 3–52). The Guilford Press.

McClain, M. B., Shahidullah, J. D., Harris, B., McIntyre, L. L., & Azad, G. (2022). Reconceptualizing educational contexts: The imperative for interprofessional and interagency collaboration in school psychology. *School Psychology Review, 51*(6), 742–754. https://doi.org/10.1080/2372966X.2021.1949247

McLaughlin, K. A., Costello, E. J., Leblanc, W., Sampson, N. A., & Kessler, R. C. (2012). Socioeconomic status and adolescent mental disorders. *American Journal of Public Health, 102*(9), 1742–1750. https://doi.org/10.2105/AJPH.2011.300477

Merrell, K. (2008). *Behavioral, social, and emotional assessment of children and adolescents* (3rd ed.). Erlbaum.

Nagaoka, J., Farrington, C. A., Ehrlich, S. B., & Heath, R. D. (2015). Foundations for young adult success: A developmental framework. Concept paper for research and practice. University of Chicago Consortium on Chicago School Research.

National Association of School Psychologists. (2023). *The provision of school psychological services to multilingual students*. [Position Statement].

National Center for Education Statistics (NCES). (May, 2024). English learners in public schools. Retrieved from https://nces.ed.gov/programs/coe/indicator/cgf/english-learners.

Okazaki, S., & Sue, S. (2016). Methodological issues in assessment research with ethnic minorities. In A. E. Kazdin (Ed.), *Methodological issues and strategies in clinical research* (pp. 235–247). American Psychological Association. https://doi.org/10.1037/14805-015

Raines, T. C., & Crumpton, H. (2017). Social, emotional, and behavioral assessment with culturally and linguistically diverse populations. In E. C. Lopez, S. G. Nahari, & S. Proctor (Eds.), *Handbook of multicultural school psychology: An interdisciplinary perspective* (2nd ed., pp. 218–235). Routledge. https://doi.org/10.4324/9780203754948

Reynolds, C. R., & Kamphaus, R. W. (2015). *BASC-3: Behavior assessment system for children* (3rd ed.). NCS Pearson, Inc.

Reynolds, C. R., & Richmond, B. O. (2008). T*he revised children's manifest anxiety scale.* (2nd ed.) (RCMAS-2). Western Psychological Services.

Richter, A., Sjunnestrand, M., Romare Strandh, M., & Hasson, H. (2022). Implementing school-based mental health services: A scoping review of the literature summarizing the factors that affect implementation. *International Journal of Environmental Research and Public Health, 19*(6), 3489. https://doi.org/10.3390/ijerph19063489

Sattler, J. M. (2018). *Assessment of children: Cognitive foundations and applications* (6th ed.). Jerome M. Sattler, Publisher, Inc.

Schnoes, C., Reid, R., Wagner, M., & Marder, C. (2006). ADHD among students receiving special education services: A national survey. *Exceptional Children, 72*(4), 483–496. https://doi.org/10.1177/001440290607200406

Soland, J., & Sandilos, L. E. (2021). English language learners, self-efficacy, and the achievement gap: Understanding the relationship between academic and social-emotional growth. *Journal of Education for Students Placed at Risk, 26*(1), 20–44. https://doi.org/10.1080/10824669.2020.1787171

Sue, D. W. (2001). Multidimensional facets of cultural competence. *The Counseling Psychologist, 29*(6), 790–821. https://doi.org/10.1177/0011000001296002

Tharinger, D. J., Finn, S. E., Hersh, B., Wilkinson, A., Christopher, G. B., & Tran, A. (2008). Assessment feedback with parents and preadolescent children: A collaborative approach. *Professional Psychology: Research and Practice, 39*(6), 600–609. https://doi.org/10.1037/0735-7028.39.6.600

Trent, E., Zamora, I., Tyree, A., & Williams, M. E. (2018). Clinical considerations in the psychological assessment of bilingual young children. *Professional Psychology: Research and Practice, 49*(3), 234–246. https://doi.org/10.1037/pro0000195

Vega, D., Wolf, J. N., Barton, D. O., Stathatos, M., Iurino, C., & Hammer, L. (2019). Identifying the training experiences and needs of bilingual school psychologists. *Psychology in the Schools, 56*(10), 1687–1699. https://doi.org/10.1002/pits.22288

Vega, D., & Wolf, J. (2023). Best practices in assessment of Bilingual learners in schools. In *Best practices in school psychology: Vol. 1. Data-based and collaborative decision making*. (Vol. 7, pp. 163–173). NASP.

Zins, J. E., Bloodworth, M. R., Weissberg, R. P., & Walberg, H. J. (2007). The scientific base linking social and emotional learning to school success. *Journal of Educational and Psychological Consultation, 17*(2–3), 191–210. https://doi.org/10.1080/10474410701413145

Chapter 12
Assessment of Emergent Bilingual Students for an Intellectual Disability

Jesslynn Rocha Neves-McCain, Brittany St. Jean, and Tamika P. La Salle-Finley

Students with an intellectual disability (ID) comprise 6% of youth receiving special education services (U.S. Department of Education, Office of Special Education and Rehabilitative Services, Office of Special Education Programs [OSEP], 2023). Yet, students with intellectual disabilities are more likely to be emergent bilingual (EB) youth than all other students with disabilities (OSEP, 2023). The assessment and identification of intellectual disabilities have been controversial due to the disproportionate and inappropriate identification of marginalized students with ID (Vega & Wolf, 2023). Emergent bilingual youth within this demographic are especially vulnerable, given the complexities of understanding their abilities within multilingual development (Ilyes, 2020). As school psychologists critically examine the factors that have contributed to disparities in the classification of ID, it is imperative to consider the intersection of language and cultural notions about dis/ability.

J. R. Neves-McCain (✉)
Department of Counseling, School Psychology, and Sport, University of Massachusetts Boston, Boston, MA, USA
e-mail: jesslynn.neves@umb.edu

B. St. Jean
White Birch Educational Services, Department of Clinical Training, Portsmouth, NH, USA
e-mail: drbrittanystjean@whitebirchedu.com

T. P. La Salle-Finley
Department of Counseling and Psychological Services, Georgia State University, Atlanta, GA, USA
e-mail: tlasalle1@gsu.edu

D. Vega, J. N. Wolf (eds.), *Culturally and Linguistically Responsive Intervention and Assessment Practices with Emergent Bilingual Students*,
https://doi.org/10.1007/978-3-032-02084-0_12

Intellectual Disabilities in Cultural-Linguistic Context

ID is defined as "a disorder with onset during the developmental period that includes both intellectual and adaptive functioning deficits in conceptual, social, and practical domains" (Diagnostic and Statistical Manual of Mental Disorders, Fifth Edition, Text Revision [DSM-5-TR]; American Psychiatric Association [APA], 2022, p. 42). The individual's profile is qualified as mild, moderate, severe, or profound based on their level of adaptive functioning and the corresponding level of support required (APA, 2022). Educationally, a student may be classified as having an intellectual impairment if they demonstrate significantly subaverage general intellectual functioning and deficits in adaptive behavior that manifested during the developmental period, and both of which adversely affect a child's educational performance (Individuals with Disabilities Education Act [IDEA], 2004).

ID definitions, as well as approaches to intervention and education, have evolved alongside theories of intelligence, psychological assessment, and societal context. Intelligence is a European-Western conceptualization that has been used to propel eugenics theory; its problematic basis was transferred to cognitive tests that defined intelligence based on white cultural knowledge and experiences (Vega & Wolf, 2023; Yakushko, 2019). The flawed data obtained from such tests have been weaponized to exclude racially and linguistically minoritized students—especially Black students—by asserting that Black, Brown, and bilingual children are inherently ineducable (Womack et al., 2021; Yakushko, 2019). Educators have attempted to address the problem through the development and validation of culturally appropriate measures, legislation restricting the use of intelligence quotient (IQ) tests, and expansion of the factors that must be considered when assessing student abilities (Vega & Wolf, 2023). Nonetheless, racial disparities persist in the inappropriate special education referral and disproportionate identification for EB youth in the category of ID (Frey, 2019).

This chapter describes and illustrates a culturally informed approach to the assessment of ID for EB students, especially in the context of historical definitions of disability, intelligence, and thriving in society. We posit that emergent bilingualism inherently implies cultural diversity in terms of family, internationalism, immigration status, multicultural development, and much more; therefore, we discuss a linguistically and culturally sensitive approach to assessing intellectual disabilities.

Assessment of Emergent Bilingual Youth for an Intellectual Disability

Existing systematic processes for assessment of EB youth emphasize a comprehensive file review, family interview, and observations; assessment of proficiency in language one (L1; native language) and two (L2; second language); and determining an appropriate pathway for cognitive assessment based on the student's ability

(Olvera & Gómez-Cerrillo, 2014; Rhodes et al., 2005). Drawing from the previous work of scholars, the authors propose a sequential process for the assessment of ID in EB youth. This process focuses specifically on ID assessment while centering the feasibility of application within school-based contexts.

Emergent bilingual K-12 students comprise a growing and increasingly linguistically diverse population in schools nationwide (National Center for Education Statistics, 2024). Moreover, there is no official training requirement or certification for bilingual school psychologists (National Association of School Psychologists, n.d.). Yet, the solution cannot be to avoid or undermine the assessment process for EB youth. There is a distinction between *bilingual assessment,* or the use of bilingual and English measures with an examinee by a bilingual examiner, and *assessment of bilingual youth,* or the application of nondiscriminatory, culturally appropriate assessment practices to a bilingual examinee by any practitioner (Ortiz, 2009). Consistent with this perspective, the authors assert that a flexible, ecologically based approach can support both multilingual and culturally humble practitioners in enhancing their assessment of bilingual youth for an ID. Further, our recommendations are situated within education and special education law while integrating assessment focus areas recommended by the American Association on Intellectual Disabilities (2010). Table 12.1 summarizes the steps of this process.

Prevention, Intervention, and Referral

Though ID itself is a naturally occurring diversity that cannot be prevented, the premature or unwarranted referral of emergent bilingual learners for ID evaluation should be prevented via early identification, assessment, and effective intervention. At a minimum, schools are legally required to identify students as potential dual language learners, assess students' need for language-based services, develop a program that has a reasonable chance for success, ensure that necessary staff, curricular materials, and facilities are in place and used properly, develop appropriate evaluation standards, including program exit criteria, for measuring the progress of students, and assess the success of the program and modify it when needed (U.S. Department of Justice & U.S. Department of Education, 2015). This applies to both academic and environmental learning, so educational teams should consider the culturally based opportunities offered for the student to develop problem-solving and adaptive skills before assuming a special education referral is warranted.

Specifically, rather than assuming all students arrive with skills that are specific to thriving in a U.S. classroom, educators should ensure they are explicitly teaching and scaffolding skills to navigate the school setting while acknowledging that these tasks and situations may not be the adaptive focus in the home (Sternberg, 2021). For example, a student may be involved in the caregiving of a younger sibling and thrive in situations where they have a leadership role; however, this strength may not be evident if they have not had the chance to demonstrate leadership skills in the classroom. Proactive consultation with parents and families about each child's home

Table 12.1 Steps in Assessment of Emergent Bilingual Youth for an Intellectual Disability

Prevention, intervention and referral	Record and background review	Cognitive assessment	Adaptive assessment	Reporting results and deliberation	Intervention recommendations
Goal(s): 1. Prevent premature or inappropriate special education referral. 2. Establish referral question related to the presence of an ID. 3. Identify assessment, research, consultation, and/or interpreter resources required and available to carry out the evaluation.	Goal(s): 1. Determine language(s) appropriate for assessment. 2. Determine presenting problems and whether they "manifested during the developmental period" (IDEA, 2004).	Goal(s): 1. Select an appropriate approach and measure for assessment. 2. Determine whether the student exhibits "significantly subaverage general intellectual functioning" (IDEA, 2004).	Goal(s): 1. Select an appropriate approach and measure for assessment. 2. Determine whether the student exhibits "deficits in adaptive behavior" (IDEA, 2004) in multiple settings from the perspectives of multiple informants.	Goal(s): 1. Determine whether an ID is present and "adversely affects a child's educational performance". 2. Convey both ID and the student's profile, along with implications in a culturally appropriate manner.	Goal(s): 1. Provide culturally appropriate recommendations for educational programming and family-school collaboration.

navigation and responsibilities can also support educators in developing a strengths-based understanding of the assets and areas for growth that their students possess.

Additionally, the student's adjustment and mental health should be considered, especially if there has been a change in the student's cultural setting (i.e., school transfer, immigration). Academic performance tends to improve alongside the process of acculturation, or the process by which students negotiate multiple cultural identities (Sirin & Sin, 2023). Thus, students adjusting to a novel linguistic and cultural setting should not be expected to immediately reach their full scholastic or adjustment potential when navigating novel linguistic and cultural settings (Sirin & Sin, 2023). This can apply to students who have primarily spoken L1 (native language) at home and are transitioning to a setting where the dominant language is L2 (developing language), or students who have recently immigrated. Shifting to a focus on the learning trajectory creates space to weigh performance issues against true weaknesses, rerouting students toward appropriate interventions rather than inapplicable areas of suspected disability.

Without adequate time, delivery, and progress monitoring of preventive interventions for language, adaptive skills development, and acculturation, there is no basis for a special education evaluation, as an appropriate referral question cannot be developed (Geva & Wiener, 2015). However, after each of these areas has been thoroughly considered and addressed, a referral for special education assessment may be warranted in light of an EB student's weak educational progress. In the case of ID, common signs that may present at school include difficulty learning, limited social skills and interactions, impaired focus, self-injurious behavior, or emotional and behavioral dysregulation (Patel et al., 2018). Multidisciplinary assessment is also recommended, as some features of intellectual disability may be related to health, occupational functioning, motor skills, behavior, and speech (Brue & Wilmshurst, 2016).

Identification of Bilingual Resources

At the outset of a special education referral, resources for bilingual assessment should be discussed candidly. At this stage, the main questions are (1) what is the primary language of the family and, potentially, the examinee, and (2) what bilingual resources are at the disposal of the school psychologist? Through advocacy, research, and professional workgroups, bilingual school psychologists have developed some norms for bilingual school psychologists: they must be fluent in at least two languages; culturally competent in all domains of practice; trained on theories of second language acquisition; trained in the process of acculturation; and trained on how the process of second language acquisition and acculturation impact the learning process (NASP, n.d.; Sotelo-Dynega & Dixon, 2014). In the absence of a bilingual examiner, a school psychologist can work to complete a multi-method assessment in consultation with, preferably, a school psychologist with experience assessing EB students (Vega & Wolf, 2023).

Record and Background Review

After identifying the target language(s) and resources available, the evaluating school psychologist must conduct a substantial record and background review to conceptualize the case. A comprehensive review of both school and family involvement is crucial in the context of assessing an ID, given that it is a pervasive disorder that emerges in the early developmental period (APA, 2022).

Presenting Concerns

The student's presenting concerns should be refined and culturally contextualized to guide the assessment process. Distress is conceptualized distinctly based on the cultural notions regarding expression (what is problematic behavior), attribution (what causes distress), and treatments (what resolves distress; Allison & Strydom, 2009). Therefore, when an examiner solicits input from the student's educator(s) and parents/caregivers via interviews, discrepancies are expected based on distinct roles in the child's life across settings and cultural values that govern these roles. Leaning into these discrepancies can actually help identify areas of need, helpful support, and interventions (De Los Reyes et al., 2022).

For example, if self-care adaptive skills are relatively stronger in the home environment, this may be interpreted as a student thriving in a highly familiar and structured self-care environment that can be replicated in the school setting. This perspective allows a special education team to acknowledge that a student is not performing a skill in the school context *and* that they can perform the skill with a given level of support. Interpretively, this discrepancy reflects a variation in needs depending on the context and warrants corresponding intervention in the school setting (De Los Reyes et al., 2022).

The educator's perspective is framed by their expectations of a student in school, and thus problematic symptoms may be conceptualized as those that disrupt relationships with adults and peers, rule compliance, and/or attitudes toward school and learning (Musu et al., 2019). The examiner can leverage this perspective to gather information about the child's socialization, learning, ability to follow a school routine, and other school-based behaviors. At this time, the examiner should also note the classroom language of instruction, the child's preferred language of expression in and out of the classroom, and the teacher's opinion of the child's level of understanding in both L1 and L2 (Vega & Wolf, 2023). Initial support for an intellectual disability consideration may include limited independent participation in classroom routines, developmentally immature social interactions, and very slow acquisition of academic concepts across subjects despite exposure in the student's spoken languages (Patel et al., 2018).

From the parents‘role and perspective, distress may be expressed as behaviors that disrupt cultural socialization goals, including development, rule compliance, and collective family and community functioning (Runge & Soellner, 2022). In terms of family functioning and cohesion, this is an opportunity to understand the family culture, child's family role, ability to participate in routines, and relationships with family members. The examiner can also explore the types of community activities the family engages in (i.e., grocery shopping, religious services, celebrations, etc.), which vary depending on culture, and the child's ability to tolerate and integrate in these settings.

The parent/caregiver interview is especially helpful in determining the child's developmental trajectory and whether problems emerged within the developmental period. For example, in non-Western cultures, parents of a child with an intellectual disability may emphasize the caregiving required by all members of the family to support the youth in everyday activities (Lauderdale-Littin & Blacher, 2017). Other areas to consider include: gestation and birth; developmental timeline of milestones and regressions; biological family history (medical/mental health); genetic history; sensory, motor, and language development; diagnostic history; trauma history; and adjustment to L2 environment (APA, 2022; Ware et al., 2015).

Notably, the examiner may need to ask directly about co-occurring neurodevelopmental and/or medical conditions that are frequently associated with ID, including: chromosomal disorders, genetic syndromes, congenital brain malformations, neurodegenerative diseases, congenital infections, inborn errors of metabolism, and birth injury (Patel et al., 2018). Finally, though educational records reviews are described subsequently, confirming details about emergent bilingualism, home language, and other language-related history with parents/caregivers may be helpful.

Record Review

The record review includes the review of permanent products related to the child's education and is an opportunity for an objective and thorough understanding of the student's educational trajectory (Olvera & Gomez-Cerrillo, 2011). Pertinent information includes previous psychoeducational reports, individualized education programs, all schools of attendance, retention records, attendance history, truancies, grades, behavioral comments, health records, discipline records, and achievement results from state-normed tests. If the examinee has been educated in another language or country, any documents from these institutions should be translated and available to the current examiner (Allshouse, 2019). Specific evidence that may support a special education classification of ID in the record includes documentation of developmental delays, early intervention services, chronic academic underperformance, behavior problems, and previously low results of cognitive and/or adaptive assessments.

Academic History

Although the hallmarks of ID are cognitive and adaptive needs, the special education context demands consideration of educational progress and, therefore, academic assessment. The academic history of a youth with ID is often characterized by difficulty mastering skills across subject areas, weak academic stamina, and limited application of a learned skill in a novel context (Smiley et al., 2022). Though they have difficulties with higher-order thinking, students with intellectual disabilities often respond well to repeated exposure and can master skills they have been exposed to intensively (Smiley et al., 2022). The examiner should, therefore, consider how the student progressed in foundational academic skills historically and in L1 and current instructional progression in L1 and L2.

Consider the example of a first-grade EB student who speaks Spanish (L1) and English (L2), has attended 3 years of preschool conducted in Spanish, and began attending school and receiving English instruction in kindergarten. If their profile is indicative of ID, they are likely to have struggled to master pre-academic skills like color naming and counting in Spanish and to be presently struggling to master these same skills in English despite exposure throughout kindergarten and some of grade 1 (Sanchez et al., 2013). The examiner should evaluate the student's pre-academic skills in Spanish in the context of 3 years of exposure. They should also evaluate in English, in the context of over a year of exposure, as evidence of their learning process.

Language Skills

Examiners must rule out linguistic and cultural factors in student functioning prior to evaluation for a special education disability (Vega & Wolf, 2023). Therefore, a combination of norm-referenced and alternative measures is optimal to convey the child's skills and rule out other classifications that may present as cognitive limitations (Freeman & Schroeder, 2022). For example, a notable pattern among young multilingual students with ID is the acquisition of some vocabulary words in both languages but deficits in overall expressive language (Bird et al., 2016). Consultation with a speech-language pathologist can also support this process, given their expertise in language development (Vega & Wolf, 2023). The student's linguistic abilities in all languages spoken should be assessed (Kaplan et al., 2016). Direct assessment of language skills may be carried out via a number of measures: Woodcock-Muñoz Language Survey, Woodcock-Johnson Test of Oral Language (WJ-TOL), and Ortiz Picture Vocabulary Acquisition Test (PVAT). Assessment with direct measures also allows the examiner to determine the cognitive academic language proficiency (CALP), or specialized language for academic contexts in L1 and/or L2 (Cummins, 1989; Pham et al., 2017). The WJ-TOL, for example, provides CALP scores derived from performance on subtests (Pham et al., 2017). Unfortunately, direct measures are available in a limited variety of languages that may not apply to every case. As a result, additional sources of information and qualitative data may be solicited (Kaplan et al., 2016).

The EB student will often have completed an English proficiency assessment upon enrolling in school and annually as part of language-based educational programming. For example, a widely used tool is the Assessing Comprehension and Communication in English State-to-State (ACCESS) by World-Class Instructional

Design and Assessment (WIDA), a suite of summative English language proficiency tests for students in grades K-12. The ACCESS tool provides standard scores that help compare the student to EB peers and an overall WIDA index score of English language proficiency ranging from Level 1 (Entering) to Level 6 (Reaching) (WIDA, 2024). Drawing on the progression of Cummins' (1989) initial distinction of basic interpersonal communicative skills (BICS)/CALP, the WIDA ACCESS recognizes that social language is part of school learning and integrates it as part of this proficiency scale (WIDA, 2024). For example, a student at Level 1 uses minimal social and academic English with visuals, a student at Level 3 uses social English language and minimal academic language, and a student at Level 6 knows and uses social and academic language at the highest level measured by the test (WIDA, 2024).

The examiner may conduct alternative assessments in educational and home environments to offer insight into a student's language, cognitive, adaptive, and academic abilities. Observations reveal a more accurate understanding of a student's level of acculturation, including the preferred language of communication, allowing for a deeper contextual understanding of their cultural and linguistic profile (Li et al., 2013). Specifically, observations and interviews can reflect a student's BICS, or social language (Cummins, 1989). Examiners may begin with educator and parent reports of language ability; structured forms are available to assess bilingual language development (Li et al., 2013; Marian, 2007). Methods to incorporate observations or informal assessments include teacher rating scales, storytelling, story retelling, cloze techniques, and language samples (Rhodes et al., 2005). Observational rating scales of BICS/CALP are also available to support further clarification of social and language skills (Refer to Student Oral Language Observation Matrix; San Jose Area Bilingual Consortium, n.d.). Finally, if the student has not been evaluated in L1 and has primarily been educated in L2, the examiner can rely on benchmark evaluations or state standardized tests related to language development. A helpful tool to conduct and organize information related to language is the Educational File Language Review Checklist by Olvera and Gómez-Cerrillo (2014).

At the very least, a school psychologist should have meaningful scores or grades that reflect the student's performance patterns and overall proficiency in reading, writing, and language (both receptive and expressive) in at least one language of primary instruction before proceeding with the evaluation (Clark-Garcea et al., 2020). If possible, the review should include the student's progression of English language development over time (Pham et al., 2017). With this information, the examiner can determine the language(s) for direct assessment of the student.

Cognitive Assessment

The determination of an ID has traditionally hinged on the results of cognitive assessment, but more recent definitions weigh adaptive skills and the application of problem-solving skills more heavily (Fiorello & Jenkins, 2018). A contextual view of cognitive results is important because most students show varying problem-solving abilities depending on setting, and EBs experience the added layer of linguistic context that affects their performance (Thaler & Jones-Forrester, 2013). Reschly and Grimes (1990) were among the first to propose such guidelines for assessing culturally and linguistically minoritized students, emphasizing the prevention of premature or inappropriate referral through a multi-method, multi-informant assessment approach to evaluate strengths and weaknesses globally.

Other models center on the cultural loading of measures, cognitive in the context of this chapter, to inform the cultural demands bilingual students experience in assessment. The Culture-Language Test Classifications (C-LTC) and Culture-Language Interpretive Matrix (C-LIM) provide classifications for selected cognitive, special-purpose, and neuropsychological assessments (Flanagan et al., 2013). The C-LTC Framework classifies subtests as low, moderate, or high in terms of cultural loading, the cultural knowledge required to perform a task, and linguistic demand, the level of language skills required to complete a task. For example, a visual-spatial task may have low linguistic and cultural demands, while a verbal comprehension task has high cultural and linguistic demands. The C-LTC led to the development of the C-LIM Matrix, a method of organizing assessment tasks into a matrix of expected cultural and linguistic demand for EB examinees (Flanagan et al., 2013). Each should be used with further resources and clinical judgment, as the C-LIM and C-LTC methods have been critiqued due to mixed findings on the limited predictive validity of these methods on emergent bilingual students' performance on related measures (Calderón-Tena et al., 2022; McGill & Spurgin, 2016).

No single subtest score or cognitive profile will result in a definitive statement about brain function or dis/ability (McGill et al., 2018). Thus, neither the full-scale IQ score nor cognitive profile analysis should be the focal point in the overall consideration for an intellectual disability. Cognitive profile analysis, or an examination of the student's strengths and weaknesses across cognitive subdomains, is a popular method among school psychologists and can provide helpful information for intervention planning at present (Fiorello & Jenkins, 2018). However, it has been critiqued as a method for gauging long-term ability due to the limited reliability of subtest performance over time, small addition of unique information above and beyond indicators of overall intellectual ability, and weak evidence of applied utility (McGill et al., 2018). Further, the inferences that can be drawn about an examinee's underlying cognitive ability or intelligence are limited to the extent to which they have been exposed to the same language and culture to the same degree as the normative sample (Fiorello & Jenkins, 2018).

The cons of each assessment approach may seem to overshadow utility. However, cognitive assessment results can provide a meaningful hypothesis about where an individual falls relative to developmentally similar peers in a variety of problem-solving situations and, thus, how well an individual could perform in an English-speaking U.S. school with no instructional accommodations, support, or services (DiStefano et al., 2020). The full-scale IQ score is required to access services, and the strengths and weaknesses that inform interventions (Fiorello & Jenkins, 2018). A flexible mindset and assessment approach can support the process of obtaining this information in light of the potential limitations an EB student with an ID may show (Brue & Wilmshurst, 2016). With these considerations, an examiner who suspects an ID may engage in a twofold process on a case-by-case basis for an EB student: (1) determining the appropriate combination of assessment approaches to the case and (2) selecting appropriate measures. Appendix A summarizes the strengths and drawbacks of English language, translated/adapted, and nonverbal measures, as well as corresponding assessments that may be used with EB examinees in each scenario.

Assessment Approaches

In choosing a cognitive assessment approach, the examinee should remain grounded in the goal of determining whether an EB student can perform comparably to developmentally similar peers in problem-solving situations to establish subaverage general intellectual functioning, as required for special education classification. That is, an EB student should be compared in terms of what a developmentally similar EB student would be able to do (i.e., appropriate normative sample; Fiorello & Jenkins, 2018). Intellectual assessment should always be conducted in the bilingual student's most proficient language or mode of communication, and a combination of measures and methods is often most appropriate given that bilingual students do not "neatly" distribute skills across languages spoken (Paradis, 2010).

English Language Measures

English assessment is most appropriate when a student's dominant language is English (Vega & Wolf, 2023). When assessing in English, cognitive assessments that minimize language (i.e., Gc/knowledge/comprehension) and cultural load are recommended for EB youth (Fiorello & Jenkins, 2018). Most intelligence tests measure crystallized abilities acquired through formal and informal experiences and education (Sajewicz-Radtke et al., 2022). By definition, these skills are inseparable from prior learning or achievement, so they cannot be true measures of innate ability. Additionally, those with enriched backgrounds and educational experiences typically score better on crystallized measures than those from impoverished or varied backgrounds (Sajewicz-Radtke et al., 2022). Clinical judgment is required in this scenario to focus on the results with the most valid interpretation.

Therefore, the examiner may still elect to exclude subtests related to verbal comprehension, as both emerging bilingualism and intellectual disabilities can undermine performance on verbal subtests (Bedore et al., 2012; Sajewicz-Radtke et al., 2022). Evaluators may use a framework when selecting an English language assessment with reduced cultural and linguistic demands, including the Culture-Language Test Classifications (C-LTC) and the Cultural Language Interpretive Matrix (C-LIM), which are based on the CHC and Cross Battery approach (Flanagan et al., 2007, 2013; described in previous sections). Alternatively, the Luria model omits measures of crystallized abilities and focuses on cognitive processing aspects; this is one of the most popular methods of assessment among school psychologists for the assessment of culturally and linguistically minoritized students (McGill & Spurgin, 2016; Sotelo-Dynega, 2015). In this model, the examiner would administer eight core subtests, four first-order factor scores (Sequential Processing, Simultaneous Processing, Planning, and Learning), and a higher-order full-scale Mental Processing Index (MPI) meant to capture the individual's overall level of cognitive processing (McGill & Spurgin, 2016). The Kaufman Assessment Battery for Children (KABC-II), Second Edition, Normative Update, in particular, lends well to the Luria model.

The advantage of using English language measures is that most school psychologists could select a battery of assessments with which they are familiar and confident. Additionally, these measures correspond to at least one of the primary languages of instruction for the EB student. The major drawback is the limited availability of normative and validation data warranting their use with culturally and linguistically minoritized students (Ware et al., 2015). This may lead to an underestimate of the student's cognitive abilities. Additionally, the models of assessment selection and scoring involve limitations that should be clear in interpreting and reporting findings. Results obtained with an English language cognitive measure provide an index of general or overall cognitive functioning that reflects only the student's performance (1) in English, (2) in a U.S. American cultural context, and (3) in a one-to-one testing setting (DiStefano et al., 2020). This information can thus help determine what the student is capable of in an English language instructional context (e.g., general education setting) with some adult support (e.g., after-school tutoring). A low full-scale IQ or cognitive functioning score indicates concerns with the execution of problem-solving skills in this situation, which may be due to various reasons, and it is not sufficient for a classification of ID (Patel et al., 2018). An ID classification may be supported if this information is corroborated by markedly subtypical performance in other functional problem-solving situations in English and the native language. The following sections detail how to obtain further information regarding cognitive functioning.

Translated/Adapted Measures

Native language assessment is appropriate when a student's dominant language is their native language, when they have received instruction in their native language, and/or when the dominant language cannot be determined (Vega & Wolf, 2023). Translated/adapted assessments can be useful in determining whether performance is comparable across L1 and L2. A student with an intellectual disability would show similar levels of skills across both languages, whereas markedly stronger performance in L1 might indicate a different educational disability or simply a need for more time to acquire language skills (Pham et al., 2017). Technical manuals of adapted measures should be thoroughly reviewed prior to administration to evaluate psychometric properties and cultural appropriateness. Translation methods must go beyond word-for-word translation to validly capture the semantic nuances of language and culture; if not, the translated measure is inappropriate for interpretation in a cultural context (Beaton et al., 2000). For example, in a review of internationally adapted versions of the WISC-V, McGill et al. (2020) found that technical manuals were largely inconsistent in the extent of psychometric information reported to support the validity of the adapted measures. Examiners should always seek information in the technical manuals to be able to cite caveats if electing to use a translated/adapted measure.

There are limitations to the use of translated/adapted cognitive measures. Regarding verbal assessment, a translated/adapted measure does not necessarily guarantee obtaining a valid score. For EB students, verbal ability fluctuates in both languages of development over the childhood trajectory (Bedore et al., 2012). One may consider or assess aspects that relate to the examinee's direct instruction, such as vocabulary recognition. Regardless, the examiner should not assume a student can perform higher-order verbal comprehension tasks in either language if considering intellectual disability (Patel et al., 2018). Additionally, translated/adapted cognitive measures do not exist for an extensive range of languages, so they are not always an option.

Nonverbal Measures

Nonverbal measures address an overlapping issue that may be characteristic of both EB youth and students who may have an ID: limited oral expression and comprehension (Brue & Wilmshurst, 2016; Liu et al., 2015). Since the assessment of intellectual disability should be centered on the student's ability, the decision to omit verbal intelligence measures is highly warranted in the case of EB students and/or students who are judged not to be able to perform on the available measure of verbal ability. This approach is most beneficial when a student shows limited expression at school and/or home, or when their expression in the intended language of evaluation is significantly limited (Liu et al., 2015).

Nonverbal measures also lend well to assessing students who may have an intellectual impairment that affects their testing stamina, as they typically have reduced demands and administration times (Brue & Wilmshurst, 2016). On the other hand, there are potential challenges associated with relying solely on nonverbal assessments. A major drawback is the limitation of the scope of a nonverbal assessment (Sotelo-Dynega, 2015). Though a full-scale IQ or other broad composite of intellectual functioning is obtained from a nonverbal measure, this is not a pattern of abilities across areas. Additionally, nonverbal measures may require a high level of sustained attention or manipulation of materials that is challenging for students with intellectual disability (DiStefano et al., 2020). Finally, tests are never truly nonverbal, given the high degree of receptive language that many nonverbal assessments require (Ortiz et al., 2011). The assessment process may be undermined if students cannot understand or respond to the examiner or the testing environment. The examiner may elect to perform additional measures or subtests to probe a broad range of abilities.

Assessment Selection

Appropriate assessment selection allows an examiner to obtain a full-scale IQ for service eligibility along with a profile of strengths and weaknesses that can be integrated into service recommendations that meet individual needs (i.e., visual, verbal, auditory, working memory, processing, etc.). After considering a psychometric approach that matches the EB learner's profile, the selection of assessments should include the appropriate areas for assessment, bilingual resources, and available assessment materials. For the determination of an ID, a global intellectual impairment must be evidenced; this includes weaknesses in reasoning, problem solving, planning, abstract thinking, judgment, and learning from experience (Sajewicz-Radtke et al., 2022). Thus, the examiner may select assessment tests or subtests that specifically assess fluid reasoning, visual-spatial reasoning, memory, executive functioning, and/or general knowledge. While a broad range of assessments can yield the most information, examiners should be mindful that students with ID may not be able to sustain prolonged assessment procedures, and therefore, the minimum testing required should be conducted (DiStefano et al., 2020). Alternative methods of assessing these areas can be considered to reduce demands while maintaining the integrity of the evaluation, such as executive functioning rating scales for individuals with ID (Freeman & Schroeder, 2022) and cognitive ability checklists (Stephenson et al., 2024). With these added sources, examiners may prioritize the assessment of areas that are especially pertinent to the classification of ID (e.g., fluid reasoning, visual-spatial tasks) for direct assessment. Thompson et al. (2018) provide guidance and recommendations for accommodations and modifications in assessing individuals with intellectual disability.

Next, the range of possible assessments to incorporate is naturally the broadest when a bilingual examiner is available: translated/adapted measures, nonverbal measures, and/or English measures. Without a bilingual examiner, nonverbal and English language measures can be considered. Finally, logistical aspects determine the materials and resources available to the examiner; some districts offer limited or outdated tests and may require borrowing measures from colleagues (Brue & Wilmshurst, 2016). A case for the purchase of new tests can also be made to the district, given the examinees' right to an evaluation that is both non-discriminatory and conducted in their native language (IDEA, 2004). It is not recommended to use outdated tests (i.e., a test that was not recently normed and does not account for the longitudinal rise in average IQ) in any case, as results may be inflated and inaccurate (Brue & Wilmshurst, 2016).

Adaptive Assessment

Adaptive behavior generally refers to the capacity to meet one's daily functional needs based on age and the culture in which the individual lives (Fiorello & Jenkins, 2018). Some definitions of adaptive functioning specify the use of global adaptive behavior composite scores, whereas others specify the use of adaptive domains (i.e., conceptual, social, and practical) or adaptive skill areas (i.e., self-care, community, safety, etc.). Yet, norm-referenced, standardized measures (i.e., rating scales) of adaptive functioning are not recommended as the sole source of information when evaluating the adaptive skills of culturally and linguistically minoritized students, given the cultural context of adaptive skills that has been discussed (Blatchley & Lau, 2010).

Like intelligence tests, adaptive measures were also conceived within Western culture and are difficult to translate and adapt for use with culturally and linguistically minoritized populations (Oakland et al., 2013). Cultural nuances such as opportunities, expectations, standards, and the developmental trajectories for adaptive skills must be considered in order to validly assess adaptive functioning. The examiner may instead include three common methods of adaptive assessment—interviews, observations, and adaptive scales—to provide a comprehensive evaluation (Colorado Department of Education, 2013). This multi-informant, multi-method assessment of adaptive functioning is essential to establish the pervasiveness of functioning weaknesses while practicing from an ecological and culturally informed approach (Fiorello & Jenkins, 2018).

Observations

Direct observation of the examinee in the school environment provides an opportunity for a clinically informed assessment of a student's adaptive behavior (Moynahan, 2018). Conducting multiple observations in a variety of school settings, such as the classroom, lunch, or recess, can offer the maximum opportunities for the student to showcase their adaptive skills. It is also recommended to record peer functioning to gather evidence of differences in adaptive functioning compared to developmentally similar peers (Colorado Department of Education, 2013). Target behaviors of observation should be consistent with the adaptive domains (i.e., conceptual, social, and practical) but may be tailored for the school-based observation setting; the examiner should also focus on the student's level of independence in these skills to inform any potentially required educational supports (Brue & Wilmshurst, 2016).

To illustrate, conceptual skills to observe may include the effectiveness of verbal and written communication, number sense, application of basic academic skills, communication of needs, and task initiation and monitoring. Social skills can be evaluated in terms of the EB child's interactions in *any* verbal or nonverbal language and may include initiation of conversations with peers, back-and-forth dialogue, emotional reciprocity, appropriateness of social and emotional reactions, enjoying individual games or activities, and following norms in group games or play. Practical skills to observe may include awareness of surroundings, engagement in familiar classroom routines, rule-following, responsiveness to safety announcements or procedures, responsible use of materials, caring for personal belongings and area, personal hygiene, and self-help. To promote consistency and fairness across evaluations, the examiner may encourage their educational setting to adopt an internally or externally developed observation tool (See Systematic Observation for Adaptive Behavior; Tennessee Department of Education, 2018).

Interviews

Interviews are conducted directly with teachers and parents/caregivers and are preferred to rating scales given their potential for individualization and cultural framing of adaptive behavior (Tassé et al., 2012). Because each culture features its own priorities and developmental milestones, the examiner should evaluate whether the student has had adequate opportunities to learn and apply adaptive skills that are relevant in a U.S. American classroom (Fiorello & Jenkins). For example, a teacher can describe the cultural expectations of students by describing a typical day in the classroom, the required level of independence in a variety of adaptive skills, and what a successful student in their classroom might look like. Teachers should also describe opportunities to develop adaptive skills in the classroom, as direct instruction of adaptive skills reduces acculturative stress for students from culturally minoritized backgrounds (Guerrero et al., 2013). This cultural context, in addition to comparing classroom and home adaptive expectations, can reduce the likelihood of conflating a lack of learning opportunities with student inability (Sternberg, 2021). For school-based interviews, information should be solicited across settings, including general education, special education, and language-based instruction, to compare the child to developmentally and linguistically similar peers. Considering adaptive domains of functioning and their application in the classroom, questions may address strengths and weaknesses in the student's participation in classroom activities, response to instruction, academic performance, learning style, level of engagement, and supports that are helpful in the classroom.

In the parent/caregiver interview, the examiner should arrange for an interpreter and administer any additional standardized adaptive measures during the same meeting, as described in the subsequent section. To establish the cultural context surrounding adaptive behavior, the examiner can ask about typical expectations of a youth that is the examinee's age (both within the family and broader culture), what types of activities the family participates in at home and in the community, the family's vision of success for the youth now and in the future, and expected level of independence at various stages of development (Allshouse, 2019). Considering adaptive domains of functioning and their application in the home and community, questions may address strengths and weaknesses in the student's communication in both L1 and L2; relationships with others in the family; independent leisure activities; ability to participate in family events; navigation of new situations or settings; ability to complete basic chores or errands; self-care; and contribution to a shared living environment.

Rating Scales

Because of the cultural nuances surrounding adaptive functioning, we recommend using measures that include or lend well to an interview (Fiorello & Jenkins, 2018). The adaptive measure can be administered directly with the family/caregiver with an interpreter so linguistic and cultural gaps in understanding the items can be clarified in the moment. Further, the examiner can directly ask if items apply or do not apply based on cultural norms.

A measure that can provide quantitative scores with qualitative interview data includes the Vineland Adaptive Behavior Scales, Third Edition (Vineland-3; Harrison & Oakland, 2015). The Vineland-3 is an adaptive measure of behavior that yields a composite of overall adaptive functioning and domain scores in the areas of Communication, Daily Living Skills, Socialization, and Maladaptive Behavior (optional). Teacher and Parent/Caregiver rating forms are meant to be completed by individuals who interact with the student daily, either in the school or home environment, depending on their role. The particular advantage of the Vineland-3 in assessing EB youth is the inclusion of an Interview Form, which allows examiners to introduce and probe items in an accessible manner so that they are best understood by informants. Examiners may also tailor their open-ended questions and probes, a tool that can be useful in working with diverse families and interpreters. Additionally, the Vineland-3 is available for purchase in English and Spanish but has also been adapted in several international contexts (Pepperdine & McCrimmon, 2018).

The examiner may still strive to integrate culturally appropriate practices if working with a measure of adaptive functioning limited to ratings. Examiners may opt for an administration format more suitable for linguistically minoritized students. For example, the Scales of Independent Behavior-Revised (SBI-R) includes both an extended version and a short form, which assesses primary adaptive behavior and may be suitable for students with limited U.S. cultural exposure (Bruininks et al., 1996; Allshouse, 2019). They may also opt to administer the scale as an interview directly with the family and/or an interpreter to enhance communication or ask additional, culturally relevant questions.

Reporting Results and Deliberation

In written and oral discussions of evaluation results, school psychologists should be candid about the fact that there is no valid assessment process for emergent bilingual youth navigating multiple linguistic settings (Bailey et al., 2020). Strategies may fall outside of standardization procedures but be helpful to evaluators and appropriate based on clinical judgment. For example, working with interpreters and/or limit testing may be particularly useful in the present context. Any time nonstandardized test procedures are considered, examiners must weigh the costs and benefits of each approach, disclose the use of such methods candidly in results reporting, and be frank about the limitations of the evaluation (Ortiz, 2018). They may preface a report or discussion with a disclaimer such as, "The assessments used as part of this evaluation were not normed or standardized under the conditions of this evaluation. Although evaluation conditions were not optimal, the professional judgment of these evaluators is that the results obtained may be an approximate representation of the student's current functioning and are offered to assist in educational programming."

Conversations about ID can be distressing for families due to both the stigma regarding ID and its lifelong implications for developmental and independent functioning (Patel et al., 2018). The added layer of cultural notions regarding ID can exacerbate stress, miscommunications, and discord among members of the planning and placement team. Practitioners should be prepared to be warm, empathic, and patient when reporting results and answering questions (Brue & Wilmshurst, 2016). Logistically, an interpreter should be present to ensure clear communication of assessment results; even a bilingual school psychologist is not a certified interpreter and cannot be responsible for the specialized work of interpreting. Ample time should be scheduled for the evaluation review meeting, with further avenues for communication clearly conveyed to the family.

For the deliberation of ID, the team will engage in a discussion of the student's intellectual functioning, adaptive skills, acculturation, and level of support that may be required based on all results of the evaluation (IDEA, 2004). Table 12.2 summarizes guiding questions for this discussion based on the evaluation process that has been presented, as well as evidence that may be considered for each as support of an intellectual disability. A classification of ID may be supported if there is evidence of support required in multiple areas assessed, specifically due to significantly delayed skills compared to developmentally similar peers.

Intervention Recommendations

The ultimate aim of this assessment process is to plan culturally appropriate, highly effective educational programming for the student. Though a full review of intervention practices exceeds the aim and scope of this chapter, the authors offer some general considerations for practitioners as a starting point to examine their current practices. Rivera et al. (2016) developed a culturally responsive framework emphasizing the following evidence-based components: (1) universal design for learning, (2) safe environment, (3) systematic and explicit instruction, (4) integrating cultural information, (5) primary language support, (6) multiple opportunities to respond, (7) technology, and (8) self-determination (Refer to Rivera et al., 2016 and Rivera et al., 2019).

The family may also benefit from psychoeducation and contact information for the many resources available to individuals with intellectual and developmental disabilities, including the Social Security Administration, Department of Developmental Services, Department of Mental Health, and state and local level resources. These

Table 12.2 Guidance for Deliberating Intellectual Disability in Emergent Bilingual Youth

Question	Evidence supporting intellectual disability (ID)
Are there health or developmental conditions/diagnoses relevant to intellectual disability?	• Medical conditions/diagnoses that are often comorbid with ID. • Developmental delays in the early years across multiple areas.
What are the language skills of the student in L1 and L2?	• Late onset of language in early years. • Currently limited oral expression comprehension in either L1 or L2. • Slow L2 acquisition despite direct, high-quality instruction for a prolonged period.
What is the educational history of the student in terms of development and skills acquisition?	• Early intervention services received. • Solid mastery of foundational academic or problem-solving skills that have been repeatedly taught. • Substantially below grade level performance across subjects historically and currently. • Limited response to tiered interventions for grade-level material. • Difficulty sustaining attention or stamina in academic tasks.
Do the problem-solving skills of the student compare to those of a developmentally, culturally, and linguistically comparable student?	• FSIQ or general cognitive ability well below average (≤ 2 SD below average). • Difficulty with higher-order or complex thinking and concept acquisition. Evidence beyond cognitive assessment: • Difficulty generalizing learned skills in new problem-solving or environmental circumstances.
Do the adaptive skills of the student compare to those of a developmentally, culturally, and linguistically comparable student?	Evidence beyond cognitive assessment: • Adaptive skills that are markedly below what is expected in light of the student's cultural background. – Self-care. – Health and safety. – Social participation. – Community navigation. – Understanding rules and norms. • Adaptive weaknesses are observed in multiple contexts. • Marked difference between functioning in highly familiar environments (e.g., home, classroom) versus new or unpredictable settings (e.g., broader school, community).

(continued)

Table 12.2 (continued)

Question	Evidence supporting intellectual disability (ID)
What are the implications for school functioning?	• The student requires moderate, frequent, or continuous adult support to engage in school learning and routines: – Classroom instruction. – Group assignments. – Independent assignments. – Assessments/quizzes/exams. – Transitions. – Safety procedures. – Lunch/recess. • To engage in the school day, the student requires highly structured activities with a greater level of adult direction and feedback than typical peers.

(American Psychiatric Association, 2022; Boat et al., 2015; DiStefano et al., 2020; Patel et al., 2018)

should be presented with information regarding accessibility for immigrants with a range of authorization statuses.

Conclusion

This chapter has presented a flexible, ecologically based approach that can support multilingual and culturally humble practitioners to enhance their assessment of bilingual youth for an ID. Our aim was to contribute to the many existing models of assessment for emergent bilingual youth, specifically for the consideration of intellectual disability, as we collectively work toward valid methods for assessing EB youth with disabilities. Still, the importance of professional development in culturally responsive assessment for school psychologists cannot be overstated, as the assessment processes for students suspected of an ID and who are EB are suggested to be flexible. Clinical judgment will develop through independent learning (e.g., reading and research, attendance at conferences, training dedicated to the assessment of culturally and linguistically minoritized students), supervision, consultation, and experience. Though the assessment of disabilities in EB youth is not a perfect science, we hope that this work supports educators to refer, assess, identify, and support emergent bilingual youth with intellectual disabilities.

Appendix A

Measure Selection for Cognitive Assessment of ID in EB Youth

	Strengths	*Limitations*	*Assessments*
English language measures	• Appropriate for EB students who have been instructed and schooled primarily in English. • Accessible to the broadest range of U.S. based, culturally humble school psychologists in terms of competency. • Lend to assessment models such as C-LIM, C-LTC, Luria method to reduce cultural loading and bias.	• Not always normed or validated for use with culturally and linguistically minoritized students. • Validity undermined when applied with flexibility/reduced demands, which are commonly needed for students with intellectual disabilities.	• Wechsler Intelligence scale for children, fifth edition (WISC-V). • Wechsler preschool and primary scales of intelligence, fourth edition (WPPSI-IV). • Wechsler adult Intelligence scale, fourth edition (WAIS-IV). • Woodcock Johnson tests of cognitive abilities, fourth edition (WJ cog-IV). • Kaufman assessment battery for children, second edition normative update-II NU. • Differential ability scales, second edition (DAS-II). • Naglieri cognitive Assessment system (CAS).

	Strengths	*Limitations*	*Assessments*
Translated/ adapted measures	• Appropriate for EB students who have been instructed and schooled primarily OR socialized in a language other than English. • Accessible to culturally humble, qualified bilingual school psychologists in terms of competency. • Allows comparison of performance across L1 and L2. • Lend to assessment models such as C-LIM, C-LTC, Luria method to reduce cultural loading and bias.	• Normative sample may be culturally incompatible with an EB student in the U.S.A (i.e., measure validated in a foreign nation but EB student has not lived there). • Psychometric properties of such measures often weak. • Limited availability of measures in a broad range of languages.	• Wechsler Intelligence scale for children, fifth edition, Spanish (WISC-V Spanish). • Wechsler adult Intelligence scale, fourth edition, Spanish (WAIS-IV Spanish). • Kaufman assessment battery for children, second edition normative update-II NU, Spanish. • Stanford Binet Intelligence scales, fifth edition, Spanish (SB-5 Spanish). • Woodcock Johnson Batería IV Pruebas de Habilidades Cognitivas (Batería IV).
Nonverbal measures	• Appropriate for EB students who have been instructed in any language. • Appropriate for verbal/oral expression weaknesses that can be observed in EB students and students with ID. • Accessible to all culturally humble, qualified school psychologists in terms of competency. • Reduces expressive language demands.	• Substantially limit the scope of assessment. • May require attention and fine motor manipulation of materials that is incompatible with an intellectual disability profile. • Not entirely "nonverbal" due to receptive language demands.	• Test of nonverbal intelligence, fourth edition (TONI-4). • Universal nonverbal Intelligence test, second edition (UNIT-2). • Leiter international performance scale-revised. • Kaufman assessment battery for children, second edition, normative update-II NU.

*list of assessments is not exhaustive and centers measures commonly used with culturally and linguistically minoritized students and students with intellectual disabilities

References

Allison, L., & Strydom, A. (2009). Intellectual disability across cultures. *Psychiatry, 8*(9), 355–357. https://doi.org/10.1016/j.mppsy.2009.06.008

Allshouse, K. (2019, February). *Best practice guidelines for diagnosing intellectual disability in people with cultural and linguistic differences.* Vermont Developmental Disabilities Service Department. https://ddsd.vermont.gov/sites/ddsd/files/documents/Best%20Practice%20Guidelines%20for%20Diagnosing%20ID%20in%20People%20wiith%20Cultural%20and%20Linguistic%20Differences.pdf

American Psychiatric Association. (2022). *Diagnostic and statistical manual of mental disorders* (5th ed., rev. ed.). https://doi.org/10.1176/appi.books.9780890425787.

Bailey, C., Venta, A., & Langley, H. (2020). The bilingual [dis] advantage. *Language and Cognition, 12*(2), 225–281. https://doi.org/10.1017/langcog.2019.43.

Beaton, D. E., Bombardier, C., Guillemin, F., & Ferraz, M. B. (2000). Guidelines for the process of cross-cultural adaptation of self-report measures. *Spine, 25*(24), 3186–3191. https://doi.org/10.1097/00007632-200012150-00014

Bedore, L. M., Pena, E. D., Summers, C. L., Boerger, K. M., Resendiz, M. D., Greene, K., Bohman, T. M., & Gillam, R. B. (2012). The measure matters: Language dominance profiles across measures in Spanish–English bilingual children. *Bilingualism: Language and Cognition, 15*(3), 616–629. https://doi.org/10.1017/s1366728912000090

Bird, E. K. R., Genesee, F., & Verhoeven, L. (2016). Bilingualism in children with developmental disorders: A narrative review. Journal of communication disorders, 63, 1-14. https://doi.org/10.1016/j.jcomdis.2016.07.003

Blatchley, L., & Lau, M. Y. (2010). Culturally competent assessment of English language learners for special education services. *Communiqué*, 1–8.

Boat, T. F., Wu, J. T., & National Academies of Sciences, Engineering, and Medicine. (2015). Clinical characteristics of intellectual disabilities. In *Mental disorders and disabilities among low-income children.* National Academies Press (US). https://www.ncbi.nlm.nih.gov/books/NBK332882/doi:10.17226/21780

Brue, A. W., & Wilmshurst, L. (2016). In A. S. Kaufman & N. L. Kaufman (Eds.), *Essentials of intellectual disability assessment and identification* (pp. 156–157). Wiley.

Bruininks, R., Woodcock, R. W., Weatherman, R. F., & Hill, B. K. (1996). *Scales of independent behavior–revised (SIB-R).* Riverside Publishing.

Calderón-Tena, C. O., Styck, K. M., Vega, D., & Kranzler, J. H. (2022). Evaluating cultural and linguistic load of IQ scores for English language learners. *International Journal of School & Educational Psychology, 10*(1), 46–62. https://doi.org/10.1080/21683603.2020.1803164

Clark-Garcea, B., Shore, D., Lukes, M., & Sharp-Ross, M. (2020). Long-term English learners: Current research, policy, and practice. *TESOL Journal, 11*(1), 1–15. https://doi.org/10.1002/tesj.452

Colorado Department of Education. (2013, September). *Guidelines for the determination of eligibility for a child with an intellectual disability or multiple disabilities.* https://www.cde.state.co.us/cdesped/guideliensfordeterminationeligibility_id_md

Cummins, J. (1989). *Empowering minority students.* California Association for Bilingual Students.

De Los Reyes, A., Talbott, E., Power, T. J., Michel, J. J., Cook, C. R., Racz, S. J., & Fitzpatrick, O. (2022). The needs-to-goals gap: How informant discrepancies in youth mental health assessments impact service delivery. *Clinical Psychology Review, 92.* https://doi.org/10.1016/j.cpr.2021.102114

DiStefano, C., Sadhwani, A., & Wheeler, A. C. (2020). Comprehensive assessment of individuals with significant levels of intellectual disability: Challenges, strategies, and future directions. *American Journal on Intellectual and Developmental Disabilities, 125*(6), 434–448. https://doi.org/10.1352/1944-7558-125.6.434

Fiorello, C. A., & Jenkins, T. K. (2018). Best practices in intellectual disability identification. *Communiqué, 46*(5).

Flanagan, D. P., Ortiz, S. O., & Alfonso, V. C. (2013). In A. S. Kaufman & N. L. Kaufman (Eds.), *Essentials of cross-battery assessment* (3rd ed., pp. 287–350). Wiley.

Flanagan, D. P., Ortiz, S. O., & Alfonso, V. C. (2007). *Essentials of cross-battery assessment* (2nd ed.). Wiley.

Freeman, M. R., & Schroeder, S. R. (2022). Assessing language skills in bilingual children: Current trends in research and practice. *Journal of Child Science, 12*(01), e33–e46.

Frey, J. R. (2019). Assessment for special education: Diagnosis and placement. *The Annals of the American Academy of Political and Social Science, 683*(1), 149–161. https://doi.org/10.1177/0002716219841352

Geva, E., & Wiener, J. (2015). *Psychological assessment of culturally and linguistically diverse children and adolescents*. Springer.

Guerrero, A. D., Fuller, B., Chu, L., Kim, A., Franke, T., Bridges, M., & Kuo, A. (2013). Early growth of Mexican–American children: Lagging in preliteracy skills but not social development. *Maternal and Child Health Journal, 17*(9), 1701–1711. https://doi.org/10.1007/s10995-012-1184-7

Harrison, P., & Oakland, T. (2015). *Adaptive behavior assessment system, Third edition (ABAS-3) Manual*. Pearson.

Ilyes, E. (2020). Psychology's eugenic history and the invention of intellectual disability. *Social and Personality Psychology Compass, 14*(7). https://doi.org/10.1111/spc3.12537

Individuals With Disabilities Education Act (IDEA), 20 U.S.C. § 1400. (2004). https://www.law.cornell.edu/uscode/text/20/1400

Kaplan, I., Stolk, Y., Valibhoy, M., Tucker, A., & Baker, J. (2016). Cognitive assessment of refugee children: Effects of trauma and new language acquisition. *Transcultural Psychiatry, 53*(1), 81–109. https://doi.org/10.1177/1363461515612933

Lauderdale-Littin, S., & Blacher, J. (2017). Young adults with severe intellectual disability: Culture, parent, and sibling impact. *Journal of Intellectual & Developmental Disability, 42*(3), 230–239.

Li, P., Zhang, F., Tsai, E., & Puls, B. (2013). Language history questionnaire (LHQ 2.0): A new dynamic web-based research tool. *Bilingualism: Language and Cognition, 17*(3), 673–680. https://doi.org/10.1017/s1366728913000606

Liu, K. K., Thurlow, M. L., & Quenemoen, R. F. (2015). *Instructing and assessing English learners with significant cognitive disabilities*. University of Minnesota, National Center on Educational Outcomes.

Marian, B., & Kaushanskaya. (2007). The language experience and proficiency questionnaire (LEAP-Q): Assessing language profiles in bilinguals and multilinguals. *Journal of Speech Language and Hearing Research, 50*(4), 940–967. https://bilingualism.soc.northwestern.edu/wp-content/uploads/2017/01/LEAP-Q_Child_pencil.pdf

McGill, R. J., Dombrowski, S. C., & Canivez, G. L. (2018). Cognitive profile analysis in school psychology: History, issues, and continued concerns. *Journal of School Psychology, 71*, 108–121. https://doi.org/10.1016/j.jsp.2018.10.007

McGill, R. J., & Spurgin, A. R. (2016). Assessing the incremental value of KABC-II Luria model scores in predicting achievement: What do they tell us beyond the MPI? *Psychology in the Schools, 53*(7), 677–689. https://doi.org/10.1002/pits.21940

McGill, R. J., Ward, T. J., & Canivez, G. L. (2020). Use of translated and adapted versions of the WISC-V: Caveat emptor. *School Psychology International, 41*(3), 276–294. https://doi.org/10.1177/0143034320903790

Moynahan, K. C. (2018). *Adaptive behavior assessment of ethnically different children referred for special education services* [doctoral dissertation, Walden University]. Scholar Works. https://scholarworks.waldenu.edu/dissertations/4748/.

Musu, L., Zhang, A., Wang, K., Zhang, J., & Oudekerk, B. A. (2019). *Indicators of school crime and safety: 2018*. National Center for Education Statistics, U.S. Department of Education, and Bureau of Justice Statistics, Office of Justice Programs,U.S. Department of Justice. https://nces.ed.gov/pubs2019/2019047.pdf

National Association of School Psychologists. (n.d.). *Bilingual school psychology certification*. Retrieved from https://www.nasponline.org/resources-and-publications/resources-and-podcasts/diversity-and-social-justice/cultural-responsiveness/bilingual-school-psychology-certification

National Center for Education Statistics. (2024). English learners in public schools. *Condition of education*. U.S. Department of Education, Institute of Education Sciences. Retrieved [28 Jan 2025], from https://nces.ed.gov/programs/coe/indicator/cgf

Oakland, T., Iliescu, D., Chen, H. Y., & Chen, J. H. (2013). Cross-national assessment of adaptive behavior in three countries. *Journal of Psychoeducational Assessment, 31*(5), 435–447. https://doi.org/10.1177/0734282912469492

Office of Special Education Programs. (2023, September 27). *OSEP fast facts: Children identified with ID*. Retrieved from https://sites.ed.gov/idea/osep-fast-facts-children-identified-with-intellectual-disability/

Office of Special Education Programs. (2022, April). *OSEP fast facts: Students with disabilities who are english learners (ELs) served under IDEA Part B*. Retrieved from https://sites.ed.gov/idea/osep-fast-facts-students-with-disabilities-english-learners

Olvera, P., & Gomez-Cerrillo, L. (2011). A bilingual (English & Spanish) psychoeducational assessment MODEL grounded in Cattell-horn Carroll (CHC) theory: A cross-battery approach. *Contemporary School Psychology, 15*, 117–127. https://doi.org/10.1007/BF03340968

Olvera, P., & Gómez-Cerrillo, L. (2014). Integrated intellectual assessment of the bilingual student. In A. B. Clinton (Ed.), *Assessing bilingual children in context: An integrated approach* (pp. 109–135). American Psychological Association. https://doi.org/10.1037/14320-006

Ortiz, S. O. (2009). Bilingual-multicultural assessment with the WISC-IV. In D. P. Flanagan, S. O. Ortiz, V. C. Alfonso, & N. L. Kaufman (Eds.), *Essentials of cross-battery assessment* (3rd ed., pp. 295–309). Wiley.

Ortiz, S. O. (2018). Chapter 13: Procedures for conducting intellectual assessments of english learners. In *Minnesota Department of Education The English Learner (EL) Companion to Promoting Fair Special Education Evaluations* (pp. 196–238). https://education.mn.gov/MDE/dse/sped/div/el/MDE087755#:~:text=The%20English%20Learner%20Companion%20to,with%20actual%20or%20suspected%20disabilities

Ortiz, A. A., Robertson, P. M., Wilkinson, C. Y., Liu, Y.-J., McGhee, B. D., & Kushner, M. I. (2011). The role of bilingual education teachers in preventing inappropriate referrals of ells to special education: Implications for response to intervention. *Bilingual Research Journal, 34*(3), 316–333. https://doi.org/10.1080/15235882.2011.628608

Paradis, J. (2010). The interface between bilingual development and specific language impairment. *Applied PsychoLinguistics, 31*(2), 227–252. https://doi.org/10.1017/S0142716409990373

Patel, D., Apple, R., Kanungo, S., & Akkal, A. (2018). Narrative review of intellectual disability: Definitions, evaluation and principles of treatment. *Pediatric Medicine, 1*. https://doi.org/10.21037/pm.2018.12.02

Pham, A. V., Castro-Olivo, S., Chun, H., & Goforth, A. N. (2017). Cognitive abilities in bilinguals in L1 and L2. *Psychology of Bilingualism: The Cognitive and Emotional World of Bilinguals, 269-291*. https://doi.org/10.1007/978-3-319-64099-0_12

Pepperdine, C. R., & McCrimmon, A. W. (2018). Test review: Vineland adaptive behavior scales, (Vineland-3) by sparrow.

Reschly, D. J., & Grimes, J. P. (1990). Best practices in intellectual assessment. In A. Thomas & J. Grimes (Eds.), *Best practices in school psychology* (pp. 425–439). National Association of School Psychologists.

Rhodes, R. L., Ochoa, S. H., & Ortiz, S. O. (2005). *Assessing culturally and linguistically diverse students: A practical guide*. Guilford.

Rivera, C. J., Baker, J., Tucktuck, M. N., Rüdenauer, H., & Atwell, N. (2019). Research-based practices for emergent bilinguals with moderate intellectual disability: A review of literature. *Journal of Latinos and Education, 20*(4), 412–426. https://doi.org/10.1080/15348431.2019.1609478

Rivera, C. J., Jimenez, B. A., Baker, J. N., Spies, T., Mims, P. J., & Courtade, G. (2016). A culturally and linguistically responsive framework for improving academic and postsecondary outcomes of students with moderate or severe intellectual disability. *Research, Advocacy, and Practice for Complex and Chronic Conditions, 35*(2), 23–48. https://doi.org/10.14434/pders.v35i2.22171

Runge, R. A., & Soellner, R. (2022). Cultural bias in parent reports: The role of socialization goals when parents report on their child's problem behavior. *Child Psychiatry & Human Development, 55*(4), 1020–1030. https://doi.org/10.1007/s10578-022-01464-y

Sajewicz-Radtke, U., Jurek, P., Olech, M., Łada-Maśko, A. B., Jankowska, A. M., & Radtke, B. M. (2022). Heterogeneity of cognitive profiles in children and adolescents with mild intellectual disability (MID). *International Journal of Environmental Research and Public Health, 19*(12), 7230. https://doi.org/10.3390/ijerph19127230

San Jose Area Bilingual Consortium. (n.d.). Student oral language observation matrix (SOLOM). https://www.cal.org/twi/EvalToolkit/appendix/solom.pdf

Sanchez, S. V., Rodriguez, B. J., Soto-Huerta, M. E., Villarreal, F. C., Guerra, N. S., & Flores, B. B. (2013). A case for multidimensional bilingual assessment. *Language Assessment Quarterly, 10*(2), 160–177. https://doi.org/10.1080/15434303.2013.769544

Sirin, S. R., & Sin, E. J. (2023). Meta-analysis on the relation between acculturation and academic performance: Testing the immigrant paradox. *Educational Research Review, 39*. https://doi.org/10.1016/j.edurev.2023.100526

Smiley, L. R., Richards, S. B., & Taylor, R. (2022). *Exceptional students: Preparing teachers for the 21st century* (4th ed.). McGraw Hill.

Sotelo-Dynega, M. (2015). What is a bilingual school psychologist? A national survey of the credentialing bodies of school psychologists: Implications for the assessment of bilinguals. *Journal of Psychoeducational Assessment, 33*(3), 247–258. https://doi.org/10.1177/0734282914550811

Sotelo-Dynega, M., & Dixon, S. G. (2014). Cognitive assessment practices: A survey of school psychologists. *Psychology in the Schools, 51*(10), 1031–1045. https://doi.org/10.1002/pits.21802

Stephenson, K. G., Vargo, K. C., Cacciato, N. M., Albright, C. M., & Kryszak, E. M. (2024). Developmental assessment in children at higher likelihood for developmental delays: Comparison of parent report and direct assessment. *Journal of Autism and Developmental Disorders, 1*(11). https://doi.org/10.1007/s10803-024-06420-4

Sternberg, R. J. (2021). Adaptive intelligence: Intelligence is not a personal trait but rather a person× task× situation interaction. *Journal of Intelligence, 9*(4), 58. https://doi.org/10.3390/jintelligence9040058

Tassé, M. J., Schalock, R. L., Balboni, G., Bersani, H., Jr., Borthwick-Duffy, S. A., Spreat, S., Thissen, D., Widaman, K. F., & Zhang, D. (2012). The construct of adaptive behavior: Its conceptualization, measurement, and use in the field of intellectual disability. *American Journal on Intellectual and Developmental Disabilities, 117*(4), 291–303. https://doi.org/10.1352/1944-7558-117.4.291

Tennessee Department of Education. (2018, November). *Functional delay evaluation guidance.* https://www.tn.gov/content/dam/tn/education/special-education/eligibility/se_functional_delay_evaluation_guidance.pdf

Thaler, N. S., & Jones-Forrester, S. (2013). IQ testing and the Hispanic client. In L. T. Benuto (Ed.), *Guide to psychological assessment with Hispanics* (pp. 81–98). Springer. https://doi.org/10.1007/978-1-4614-4412-1_6

Thompson, T., Coleman, J. M., Riley, K., Snider, L. A., Howard, L. J., Sansone, S. M., & Hessl, D. (2018). Standardized assessment accommodations for individuals with intellectual disability. *Contemporary School Psychology, 22*, 443–457.

U.S. Department of Education, Office of Special Education and Rehabilitative Services, Office of Special Education Programs (2024). 45th annual report to congress on the implementation of the individuals with disabilities education act, 2023.

U.S. Department of Justice & U.S. Department of Education (2015). *Ensuring english learner students can participate meaningfully and equally in educational programs.* https://www2.ed.gov/about/offices/list/ocr/docs/dcl-factsheet-el-students-201501.pdf

Vega, D., & Wolf, J. N. (2023). Best practices in assessment of bilingual learners in schools. In P. Harrison, S. Proctor, & A. Thomas (Eds.), *Best practices in school psychology* (Vol. 1, 7th ed., pp. 163–174). National Association of School Psychologists.

Ware, J., Lye, C. B., & Kyffin, F. (2015). Bilingualism and students (learners) with intellectual disability: A review. *Journal of Policy and Practice in Intellectual Disabilities, 12*(3), 220–231. https://doi.org/10.1111/jppi.12124

WIDA. (2024). *ACCESS for ELLs interpretive guide for score reports grades K-12.* Board of Regents of the University of Wisconsin System.

Womack, T. A., Anazagasty, J. M., Vega, D., & Johnson, A. H. (2021). Interrogating cognitive assessment using a critical study of whiteness lens. In *Critical theories for school psychology and counseling* (pp. 144–158). Routledge.

Yakushko, O. (2019). Eugenics and its evolution in the history of Western psychology: A critical archival review. *Psychotherapy and Politics International, 17*(2). https://doi.org/10.1002/ppi.1495

Chapter 13
Assessing Emergent Bilingual Students for Speech-Language Impairments and Collaboration with School Psychologists

Trianna K. Oglivie and Genesis D. Arizmendi

As school systems continue to serve increasingly diverse student populations, the need for targeted support for emergent bilingual (EB) students becomes more pressing. Children whose first language is Spanish and second language is English make up 76.4% of EBs (National Center for Education Statistics [NCES], 2024). A challenge that these children face is that they often display difficulties in school because of the additional cognitive load of learning a new language, all while learning the expectations, routines, and academic demands of a subtractive (i.e., English-only development to subtract/replace home language development) school environment (e.g., Valenzuela, 2010). Assessing EB students for speech-language impairments requires careful consideration of both linguistic and cultural factors. Recognizing the intersectional nature of an EB student's needs, collaboration between speech-language pathologists (SLPs) and school psychologists (SPs) in the schools plays a pivotal role in effectively serving EB students.

This chapter focuses on effective strategies for identifying speech-language impairments in EB students. First, the chapter begins with an overview of EB students in the public school system. Next, a discussion on speech-language pathology and the role of SLPs within the school system is presented. The chapter then provides detailed information on the nondiscriminatory approaches and procedures utilized to conduct speech and language evaluations for students who speak more than one language. Lastly, approaches to collaboration between SLPs and SPs are

T. K. Oglivie (✉)
Department of Speech, Language, and Hearing Sciences, University of Arizona, Tucson, AZ, USA
e-mail: triannao@arizona.edu

G. D. Arizmendi
Department of Speech, Language, and Hearing Sciences and Cognitive Science Program, College of Science, University of Arizona, Tucson, AZ, USA
e-mail: genesis@arizona.edu

D. Vega, J. N. Wolf (eds.), *Culturally and Linguistically Responsive Intervention and Assessment Practices with Emergent Bilingual Students*,
https://doi.org/10.1007/978-3-032-02084-0_13

presented. By understanding the nature of bilingualism, special education practitioners can pursue accurate identification and promote appropriate services and support for EB students within the U.S. public school system.

Emergent Bilingual Students

Many terms are used to label bilingual learners who enter the school system and require assistance in developing their English language skills for access to the general curriculum (Kanno et al., 2024). The term *emergent bilingual* was coined to focus on the valuable skills and lived experiences these students possess as they engage in learning multiple languages (Garcia, 2009). This term is used in contrast to other terms that convey ideas of deficit and/or center monolingual English language skills for students who are developing English alongside their home language(s) (e.g., *English language learner, English learner,* or *Limited English Proficiency*; Garcia, 2009). The intentional use of the term *emergent bilingual* also serves to recognize and support the use and development of a student's home language as they develop.

Emergent bilingual students represent 10.6% of public school students within the U.S. (NCES, 2024). The current national data on EB students identified with an educational disability is a cause for concern. In Fall 2021, 15.8% of EB students were identified as students with disabilities (NCES, 2024). This lies in contrast to 14.7% of students proficient in English who were identified as students with disabilities in the public school system (NCES, 2024). While this data suggests overrepresentation for EB students in special education, there is also data that points to an underrepresentation and inconsistent/shifting representation when examining enrollment across grades and qualification categories (Artiles et al., 2005; Mancilla-Martinez et al., 2023; Morgan et al., 2015; Sullivan, 2011). The overall picture is one of disproportionate representation of EB students within the special education system. Disproportionate representation refers to the unequal identification of specific groups in programs or categories relative to their proportion in the general population. This manifests as either overrepresentation, where EB students are identified for special education services at comparably higher rates (sometimes twice as likely), or under-representation, where EB students are identified at comparably lower rates (sometimes rarely at all) than their English proficient peers (e.g., Artiles et al., 2005; De Valenzuela et al., 2006; Harris et al., 2015; Morgan et al., 2015; Morgan et al., 2018; Sullivan, 2011). Overall, disproportionate representation has negative consequences and leads to inequities. Over-identification leads to EB students being removed from the general education curriculum and not receiving the instruction necessary to meet their learning potential. Under-identification leads to EB students' needs being overlooked, their language proficiency being blamed for difficulties, and ultimately, them not receiving the necessary support to access and make progress in the general curriculum.

EB students are at a heightened risk of misidentification (over- and under-identification) within public school systems due to several interrelated factors. First, mismatches between the student's linguistic and cultural backgrounds and those of the dominant school environment can lead to misunderstandings or misinterpretations of their abilities (e.g., Crago et al., 1997; Freeman & Schroeder, 2022; Peña et al., 2023; Carter et al., 2005; Peña & Halle, 2011). These mismatches often exacerbate challenges in accurately identifying whether a student's difficulties stem from typical second-language acquisition processes or an underlying brain-based language learning disorder (e.g., De Lamo White & Jin, 2011; Freeman & Schroeder, 2022; Peña et al., 2023). Furthermore, the scarcity of formalized assessment tools designed specifically for bilingual populations, coupled with the frequent use of inappropriate or non-normed tools, contributes to inaccurate evaluations (Barragan et al., 2018; Bedore & Peña, 2008; Freeman & Schroeder, 2022; Restrepo, 1998; Restrepo & Silverman, 2001). Lastly, many professionals working within these systems lack adequate training and familiarity with bilingual language development, further complicating their ability to effectively distinguish between typical development or disorder in the presence of language differences (Arias & Friberg, 2017; De Lamo White & Jin, 2011; Freeman & Schroeder, 2022). Together, these factors create a systemic vulnerability to misidentifying EB students within the school system.

As a team member in the educational decision-making process, SLPs play a vital role in addressing the complexities associated with identifying the presence or absence of speech-language impairment in EB students. In collaboration with other educational team members, SLPs are tasked with providing nondiscriminatory progress monitoring and assessment practices for all children, including those from culturally and linguistically minoritized populations, like EB students. The next section will discuss the general role of SLPs as well as the speech and language evaluation process for EB students.

The Speech-Language Pathologist: Not 'Just' Speech

SLPs are licensed healthcare professionals who specialize in preventing, diagnosing, and treating communication and swallowing disorders (ASHA, 2016a, 2016b). SLPs' work spans multiple areas, including speech (the physical production of sounds), language (how words are understood and used), voice (quality, pitch, loudness of voice production), fluency (such as stuttering), and social communication skills (how and why we use language to communicate) (ASHA, 2016a, 2016b). SLPs also address swallowing disorders, known as dysphagia (ASHA, 2016a, 2016b). SLPs work with a wide range of individuals, from infants who need supports with feeding, children with speech and/or language delays, to adults recovering from stroke, traumatic brain injuries, or other conditions that affect communication (ASHA, 2016a, 2016b). They play an essential role in helping individuals improve their ability to communicate effectively, whether in school, social settings, or professional environments.

In school settings, SLPs also specialize in the prevention, assessment, and treatment of communication and swallowing disorders in preschool through high school settings (ASHA, 2010). Guided by federal and state mandates, as well as district policies, school-based SLPs address a wide range of challenges (e.g., speech sound disorders, fluency disorders, language-based learning disabilities, social communication challenges, voice disorders, and more) that impact both academic and functional student success (ASHA, 2010; Ireland et al., 2020). As a member of a public school's special education team, school-based SLPs adhere to the federal regulations in the Individuals with Disability Education Act (IDEA) to ensure students with disabilities have a free appropriate education (ASHA, 2010; Ireland et al., 2020). Under IDEA (2004), SLPs use their specialized skills to evaluate students who are suspected of having a speech or language impairment. When an evaluation is complete, SLPs, along with other members of the education team, participate in the special education eligibility decision-making process. If the student qualifies for special education and requires speech and/or language services, SLPs provide intervention services as special education or a related service for the student to make progress in the general education curriculum.

SLPs' expertise extends beyond common perceptions of "speech" to include *all* aspects of language development—phonology (how sounds pattern in words), morphology (how words are structured), semantics (the meaning of words), syntax (how words are structured within sentences), and pragmatics (understanding and using social aspects of language) (ASHA, 2010, 2016a, 2016b). These five language areas develop in spoken language (listening and speaking) and written language (reading and writing). SLPs support students in understanding and using language, whether through learning vocabulary, constructing oral or written sentences, comprehending spoken or written language, or organizing their thoughts. They also address social communication, helping students navigate the social rules of language, such as turn-taking, recognizing social cues, and adapting communication to different contexts.

SLPs further support students with cognitive-communication challenges, such as memory, attention, or problem-solving difficulties, often associated with brain injuries or learning disabilities (ASHA, 2010, 2016a, 2016b). They assist students with fluency issues, such as stuttering, and provide strategies to improve speech smoothness (ASHA, 2010, 2016a, 2016b). Voice disorders, swallowing difficulties (dysphagia), and augmentative and alternative communication (AAC) needs are also within their scope, ensuring students can safely eat, communicate effectively, or use tools like communication devices to functionally participate in the school environment (ASHA, 2010, 2016a, 2016b). For students with hearing loss, SLPs support the development of speech, language, and alternative communication strategies (ASHA, 2010, 2016a, 2016b). By addressing diverse communication needs and collaborating across cultural and linguistic contexts, school-based SLPs play a critical role in helping students achieve academic and functional success.

SLPs are commonly referred to as "speech teachers" in the school environment. However, as discussed above, the role of school-based SLPs extends far beyond the commonly held perception of addressing speech sound production. In addition, "speech teacher" limits a general understanding of the myriad of ways SLPs support learning within the school environment. We encourage readers to use "speech and language" when referring to SLPs. While helping students articulate sounds clearly is part of their work, SLPs are critical collaborators in fostering language and communication skills that underpin nearly all aspects of learning and social interaction.

Their expertise ensures that students not only develop the skills necessary to succeed academically but also gain the communication tools they need to navigate their educational environment, advocate for themselves, and participate fully in their communities. For other educators and professionals, recognizing the multifaceted work of SLPs is key to building collaborative, interdisciplinary approaches that benefit all students. Indeed, SLPs can also serve as consultants to other educational practitioners by drawing upon their expertise in language development and the impact language development has on students in the educational environment (ASHA, 2010). This includes the role of language in learning and performance on assessment. Understanding the expertise that our educational teams are equipped with helps all team members recognize how they may collaborate and work together to meet the needs of our students.

Assessment Process Fundamentals

Key to the special education process is the accurate identification of students with and without disabilities. IDEA (2004) provides educational teams with general requirements for administering special education evaluations. Included in these requirements are guidelines for the evaluation of students from culturally and linguistically minoritized backgrounds. Section 300.304(b)(1–2) of Part B of IDEA states multiple technically sound assessment tools and strategies must be used to collect information on the student's developmental, functional, and academic performance. For students from culturally and linguistically minoritized backgrounds, like EB students, IDEA (2004) Part B 300.304(c)(1)(i-ii) specifies that assessment and evaluation materials "(a)re…not to be discriminatory on a racial or cultural basis" and must be "provided and administered in the child's native language or other mode of communication." Testing materials are to be "in the form most likely to yield accurate information on what the child knows and can do academically, developmentally, and functionally" (IDEA Part B Sect. 300.304 (c) (1)(ii)).

The focus on accurate information is critical. To ensure the assessment process and any evaluation materials yield accurate information, SLPs and other special education practitioners must engage in a critical analysis of their beliefs and practices when working with culturally and linguistically minoritized students. Part of this critical analysis involves practitioners identifying and challenging misconceptions about bilingualism before engaging in the evaluation process. Indeed, there are a variety of misconceptions about bilingual language development that are perpetuated among medical professionals, educators, and the general public that are false and can lead to negative ramifications for EB students and their families. See Table 13.1 for a list of common misconceptions on bilingual language development (Insert Table 13.1 about here). Prior to engaging in assessment processes, each practitioner should participate in a critical inquiry stance (Brea Spahn & Vaz Bauler, 2022). A critical inquiry stance requires team members to name biases and misconceptions, disrupt those biases (challenge biases through questioning and evidence),

Table 13.1 Common Beliefs About Bilingual Language Development and Evidence Debunking Them

Beliefs	True or False	Supporting Evidence
Bilingualism causes language delays.	**False**	Research shows bilingual children reach language milestones at the same rate as monolingual children (e.g., Peña et al., 2023).
Children will confuse the two languages.	**False**	The majority of the world speaks more than one language. Code-switching is a natural part of bilingual development and is a sign of linguistic competence developing across both languages, not as a sign of confusion or limited skills (e.g., Genesee et al., 2004).
It's better to wait until a child is proficient in one language before introducing another.	**False**	Simultaneous bilingualism (learning more than one language at the same time in early development) does not negatively affect development; early exposure can enhance cognitive flexibility (e.g., Bialystok, 2001).
Bilingualism increases the risk of speech or language disorders.	**False**	Speech and language disorders occur at the same rate in monolingual and bilingual children (e.g., Hambly et al., 2013; Peña et al., 2023).
Using a language other than English at home will slow academic success in school.	**False**	The home language is a foundation for language development in the second language, maintenance of the home language supports cognitive, linguistic, and social-emotional development, which is critical for academic achievement (Cummins, 2000).
Bilingual children will never be as fluent as monolinguals in either language.	**False**	Bilinguals are not two monolinguals in one. Many bilinguals achieve high proficiency in both languages, with fluency levels depending on exposure and use (e.g., Grosjean, 1989; Kohnert et al., 2020).
Bilingualism leads to lower intelligence.	**False**	Studies consistently show bilingualism enhances executive functioning and cognitive skills (e.g., Bialystok, 2011).
If a child struggles in one language, the other language should be abandoned.	**False**	Continuing to develop both languages strengthens overall language ability and prevents loss of the home language (e.g., Paradis, 2011).

reframe perspectives through new knowledge and training, and reflect and act in ways that represent the reframing to remove biases (Brea Spahn & Vaz Bauler, 2022). This allows each practitioner to begin the process with a stance toward equity when engaging in the assessment of EB students.

Student Background in Assessment

To accurately evaluate EB students, it is essential to consider their knowledge and abilities across all of their languages. Second language acquisition is not a uniform process. Factors such as when a child starts learning their languages (age of acquisition) and how (simultaneously or sequentially), opportunities in exposure and use of their languages, and the features of language pairings greatly impact an EB student's acquisition of each of their languages (e.g., Bosch & Ramon-Casas, 2014; Gampe et al., 2021). In terms of language pairings, there may be similarities and shared features (e.g., phonemes, syntax, cognates, etc.) between language pairings that may accelerate the development of those language features (e.g., Spanish and English share words with similar spellings and meanings, like *elefante* and elephant) (Fabiano-Smith & Goldstein, 2010; Lubliner & Hiebert, 2011; Paradis & Genesee, 1996; Squires et al., 2020). Alternatively, there may be unshared features between languages that do not allow for acceleration (e.g., Korean uses a subject-object-verb sentence structure, whereas English uses a subject-verb-object) (Fabiano-Smith & Goldstein, 2010; Paradis & Genesee, 1996; Squires et al., 2020). As such, typical bilingual language acquisition is variable based on the unique language experiences of the student.

EB students often exhibit language skills that vary across contexts and languages as well. For example, a student may excel in conversational skills in their home language, but struggle with academic vocabulary in English, or vice versa. Evaluators must consider the interaction between languages by using culturally and linguistically appropriate and valid assessments. This includes employing bilingual assessment tools and procedures, conducting observations of skills across various contexts, and collaborating with families, interpreters, or bilingual practitioners when necessary (Freeman & Schroeder, 2022; McLeod & Verdon, 2017; Castilla-Earls et al., 2020). Additionally, evaluators should consider the influence of sociocultural factors, such as family background and educational experiences, that shape language development.

A comprehensive assessment that incorporates all a student's linguistic resources provides a more complete understanding of their skills and abilities. Assessing skills in only one language (e.g., English-only testing) risks underestimating their competencies and increases the likelihood of misidentification—whether as having a disability when they do not or failing to identify a legitimate need for support (e.g., assuming they just require more time to learn English) (Barragan et al., 2018; Castilla-Earls et al., 2020; Freeman & Schroeder, 2022; Peña et al., 2023). Such misidentifications can have far-reaching consequences and negatively affect the student's social-emotional and academic outcomes, as well as misallocating critical resources within the school system.

Valid and Reliable Tools in Assessment

Educational practitioners must also recognize the systemic biases that can arise in traditional assessment practices (Nair et al., 2023). Tools developed for monolingual English speakers often fail to capture the linguistic diversity of EB students, leading to an overemphasis on deficits rather than strengths (Barragan et al., 2018; Castilla-Earls et al., 2020; Freeman & Schroeder, 2022; Peña et al., 2023). By adopting an asset-based approach that values bilingualism as a strength and norm, practitioners can better distinguish between language variety and a language-based disorder. This approach not only leads toward equitable identification but also promotes interventions that support the student's full linguistic and academic potential (e.g., Arizmendi et al., 2021). In order to do so, practitioners must recognize the limitations of current assessment practices and the tools that are used to determine the presence or absence of an underlying brain-based language-learning disorder or disability.

One way of recognizing these limitations is by understanding the psychometric properties of diagnostic instruments for language and learning disorders, which are particularly critical when evaluating culturally and linguistically minoritized populations. *Sensitivity* refers to the ability to correctly identify those with disorders, and *specificity* refers to the ability to correctly identify those without disorders (Plante & Vance, 1994). These two psychometric properties are often compromised when tests are administered to students from linguistic backgrounds that differ from the norming population (Peña et al., 2014). This concern is especially salient when considering dialectal and regional variations within the same language. For instance, when Spanish language assessments normed on peninsular Spanish speakers are administered to U.S. students who speak Mexican Spanish, both sensitivity and specificity may be adversely affected, potentially leading to misidentification of language disorders (Bedore & Peña, 2008; Gutiérrez-Clellen & Simon-Cereijido, 2010). This misalignment between test content and students' linguistic background and varieties can result in *false positives*, where typical language variation is mistaken for disorder, or *false negatives*, where genuine language impairments are missed due to inappropriate linguistic benchmarks (Dollaghan & Horner, 2011). In sum, standardized tests often fail to account for linguistic variation, which carries different linguistic rules and properties that may lead to the identification of more 'errors,' further complicating the inappropriate practice of comparing EB students to monolingual students.

These psychometric limitations underscore the need for assessment tools and practices that account for the linguistic diversity within language communities rather than treating languages as monolithic entities. However, accessing normative data on EB typical language development can be difficult to gather at a large scale because of the varied language experiences students come with. The heterogeneous nature of bilingual language development and the variety of linguistic backgrounds make the development of norm-referenced, standardized assessments challenging.

In the school setting, SLPs and other education professionals tend to rely heavily on scores from formal standardized assessments for special education evaluations (Castilla-Earls et al., 2020; Fulcher-Rood et al., 2018; Harris et al., 2015). Reporting scores from norm-referenced, standardized assessments that match a student's demographics may be an appropriate source of data in the special education qualification process. However, if a student's demographics, including language background and experience, do not match the normative data of a particular assessment, reporting scores is inappropriate and invalid. Unfortunately, most norm-referenced, standardized assessment tools in speech-language pathology are designed for monolingual English-speaking students who use Standard American English. This is no different from assessments that exist in other disciplines. There are few norm-referenced, standardized assessment tools that match the language background and experiences of EB students represented among most commercially available assessments that also hold strong psychometric properties, such as sensitivity and specificity. As a result, EB students are compared to monolingual English speakers or monolingual speakers of their home language (e.g., monolingual Spanish speakers). We encourage the reader to review and interrogate the manuals for commonly used measures that they use to qualify students for special education services and try to identify: 1) the norming population, 2) the geography of the norming population, 3) the socioeconomic status of the norming population, 4) whether sensitivity and/or specificity is reported (Plante & Vance, 1994 recommend that tools have a sensitivity and specificity of 80% or above for diagnostic accuracy) to better understand the biases that may arise from using such measure in the evaluation process.

Ultimately, identifying impairment can be more difficult because different rates and processes of language acquisition may be mistaken for signs of language disorder and/or learning disabilities. Identification is further complicated in educational systems that prioritize models of monolingual language acquisition and encourage subtractive language environments. In these environments, students face negative socio-political pressures for using their home language and may automatically be viewed by educational teams as deficient (Flores & Rosa, 2015).

Guiding Principles in *EB* Assessment Processes

For bilingually developing students, the evaluation process differs from that of a monolingual English-speaking student, and understanding and applying key guiding principles to the assessment process can lead to more appropriate approaches to diagnostic accuracy. First, when a speech and/or language impairment is present, evidence of the impairment will appear across both of the student's languages. If a student demonstrates developmentally appropriate linguistic skills in one of their languages, difficulties that the student may be experiencing in the classroom may be due to limitations in the current acquisition of the school language. This should signal that the student needs more supports in the acquisition of English and could benefit from English as a Second Language (ESL) educational programming and instructional approaches that support the acquisition of English in the classroom (refer to Chaps. 2 and 8 for a review of these approaches). In this case, ESL and special education services may both be indicated to support the EB student's needs within the school system. Importantly, the EB students' skills are examined in both of their languages to characterize their language-learning abilities.

Another guiding principle is the knowledge that an EB student's languages interact. SLPs and other special education practitioners must be aware of how features from one language may transfer or influence features in the other language and vice versa. Called cross-linguistic interactions, linguistic transfers between languages are rule-based patterns that are typical of bilingual language development

(Fabiano-Smith & Goldstein, 2010; Potapova & Pruitt-Lord, 2020). For example, a bilingual Spanish-English speaking student may say "bacuum" for "vacuum" because Spanish does not have the "v" sound. Conversely, this child may also use an English "r" sound in the word "rojo" for the Spanish trill "r" because English does not have the Spanish trill "r." These are examples of possible linguistic interactions for an EB student who speaks Spanish and English. However, without the knowledge of language interaction and examination of language features across an EB student's languages, the pattern may look like disorder or language confusion. For SLPs and other educational practitioners, knowledge of cross-linguistic interaction is necessary for avoiding misidentification.

Components of EB Speech and Language Assessments

With an understanding of the fundamentals of the EB assessment process, we now discuss the components of an EB speech and language assessment. Basic components of a speech and language evaluation are completed, including collecting information on the student's medical, educational, and developmental history, assessing their hearing status, and examining the structure and function of their oral mechanism. In addition, the SLP moves on to characterizing the student's speech and language skills using formal and informal assessments. For EB students, Castilla-Earls et al. (2020) advocate for gathering multiple pieces of assessment data for diagnostic decision-making. Specifically, informal tools (i.e., language experience questionnaires, reports on speech and language concerns, speech and language sample analysis in both languages, and learning potential tasks) and, if available, appropriate formal assessment tools (i.e., standardized tests) are recommended to guide a process of converging evidence to identify the presence or absence of impairment. Assessment practices for a nondiscriminatory comprehensive speech and language assessment are described in the section below.

Language Background Questionnaires and Interviews

One of the first steps in the speech and language assessment process is understanding the student's language background, experiences, and environments. While this assessment process is similarly completed for monolingual English students (i.e., speech and language milestones, regional-geographical language variety, caregiver and teacher concerns, and family history of speech and language and academic problems, etc.), the language questionnaires and interviews for EB students are more complex and dynamic. As Grosjean (1989) observes, "the bilingual is not the sum of two complete or incomplete monolinguals; rather, he or she has a unique and specific linguistic configuration" (p.3). This has important implications for how bilingualism is considered. Comparing bilinguals to monolinguals leads to erroneous conclusions about the skills of bilinguals because it assumes that monolingualism is the norm. Instead, bilinguals are unique in their language experiences, and how, when, and where they use language impacts their language development. It will look different from monolingual students. However, this difference is not the sole indicator of impairment, nor does it place a student at greater risk for impairment. Impairment can exist in difference, but difference in and of itself is not impairment (e.g., Oetting, 2018).

To characterize an EB's language experiences, the SLP gains information through questionnaires and interviews with the student, their caregivers, and their teachers. This process begins with an understanding that bilingual language use is dynamic and changes across an EB student's life experiences (e.g., summer vacation may increase home language use and exposure, sociopolitical laws and policies may impact feelings around language and identity impacting home language use, etc.). Reports on when, where, how, and with whom the student uses their languages across their present and past environments provide important contextual information on language use and development. Several questionnaires are available to support this step, including the Language Experience and Proficiency Questionnaire (LEAP-Q; Marian et al., 2007), the Alberta Language and Development Questionnaire (ALDeQ; Paradis et al., 2010), and the Alberta Language Environment Questionnaire (ALEQ; Paradis et al., 2020). These sample informal tools are freely available and can be used to characterize development in multiple languages (e.g., the LEAP-Q is available in 42 languages).

In addition to gathering data on language background and experiences, the SLP obtains information on communication strengths and concerns from the perspective of the student, parent/caregiver, and teachers. Depending on their age, students may be able to provide insights on their linguistic experiences, language, and learning strengths and challenges, and describe supports that help them communicate and learn across their different environments.

In terms of caregivers, research has identified caregiver reports as a particularly sensitive tool for identifying speech and/or language concerns for EB students (Restrepo, 1998). Crowley (2014) provides a sample of "critical questions" that may be utilized for this step. These questions include asking caregivers to detail their concerns, share how their student compares to typical developing siblings, provide examples of when their student communicates best, and identify when the student experiences communication breakdowns. Asking caregivers these questions provides descriptive information about the student's functional communication skills in various settings.

Gathering information from teachers (general education and ESL teachers) on classroom performance and curriculum-based measures, including pre-referral interventions, also supports an understanding of the student's learning. This includes talking to the teacher about the student's strengths and challenges within the classroom, reviewing the student's work, discussing the types of supports used during instruction, examining the use of differentiated instruction, and identifying if any progress has been made (e.g., Crowley, 2014). This information provides insight into the student's classroom learning experience and teachers' perspectives to use in understanding their speech and language abilities.

Information from the student, caregivers, and teachers is important for understanding the language-learning experiences and communicative strengths and challenges the student experiences across various settings and perspectives. This information provides the SLP and educational team with a preview of what skills may be present across and within their languages. In addition, this data can be used to identify any potential speech and/or language concerns that should be addressed during the evaluation.

Collecting and Analyzing Speech and Language Samples

Another important component of speech and language evaluations is collecting and analyzing speech and language samples in each of the EB student's languages. SLPs collect single-word speech samples and connected speech and language samples (spoken and written, if possible) to examine the contextualized communication skills of the student. Speech and language samples allow SLPs to analyze multiple aspects of communication, including phonology, morphology, syntax, semantics, and pragmatics, as well as fluency, voice, and articulation. By observing how students construct sentences, organize their thoughts, or respond to conversational prompts, they can identify patterns and challenges that might not surface in formal, standardized testing in the languages that the student speaks. In addition, these skills are representative of general educational curriculum tasks (i.e., ecologically valid) and can be compared to curriculum-based materials.

Several tools are available for the collection and analysis of speech and language samples. Elicitation tools include single-word lists and connected speech assessments like those from *Multilingual Children's Speech* (McLeod, 2024), wordless picture books from libraries and/or picture story cards to gather narrative language samples in multiple languages (see examples from *School-Age Language Assessment Measures* from Crowley & Baigorri, 2015), and generic prompts to gather written language samples (e.g., What is your favorite thing to do after school?). After transcribing samples, SLPs can perform their own analysis or use available computer software programs (see Pezold et al., 2020) to complete the analysis. SLPs should engage interpreters and/or translators to support elicitation, transcription, and analysis for languages they do not speak and/or read for this process (see Alani et al., 2024 for guidance on the use of interpretation and translation services within speech-language pathology).

Dynamic Assessment

Dynamic assessment is a highly effective approach for evaluating the skills of EB students, offering a more equitable alternative to traditional standardized assessments (Lidz & Peña, 1996; Peña et al., 2001). Unlike static measures, which capture performance at a single point in time, dynamic assessment focuses on the *process of learning* and the student's ability to respond to instruction or prompts. This approach evaluates a child's potential for growth, rather than relying on prior knowledge, making it particularly suitable for distinguishing between language and learning varieties and true language and learning disorders in bilingual populations. Dynamic assessment typically follows a test-teach-retest model, allowing evaluators to observe how a student learns new concepts and whether they can apply these concepts with support that is reduced gradually. Narrative assessment and even standardized assessment tools (used in a non-standard way) can be utilized in dynamic assessment tasks. The SLP characterizes the type and quantity of supports the student needs for their learning. Similar to SLPs, other educational team members (school psychologists and teachers) may use curriculum-based measures in a dynamic way to assess student learning abilities. In addition, researchers in speech-language pathology have designed procedures for ways to conduct dynamic assessment for language testing (e.g., Kapantzoglou et al., 2012; Laurie & Pesco, 2023; Orellana et al., 2019; Petersen et al., 2024).

For EB students, dynamic assessment is critical because it accounts for their unique language-learning trajectories and minimizes cultural and linguistic biases inherent in standardized testing (Peña et al., 2007). This approach provides insight into the student's zone of proximal development (Vygotsky, 1978) and their capacity to acquire and apply new skills, even when faced with limited exposure to English. For example, dynamic assessment can be used to evaluate a bilingual student's ability to learn new vocabulary. The evaluator may first test the student's baseline knowledge of specific words, provide a brief teaching session in which the words are explained and practiced in both the first (L1) and second language (L2), and then retest to see how well the student has learned and retained the new words. If the student demonstrates significant improvement with teaching and minimal repetition, this suggests that their challenges are likely due to limited exposure to the language and concepts, rather than an underlying brain-based language disorder or learning disability. Conversely, if the student struggles to acquire the new vocabulary even with support, this may indicate a more fundamental difficulty with learning that warrants further investigation. This process not only highlights how well the student can respond to instruction but also provides insight into effective strategies for teaching and intervention. For example, the evaluator may notice that using visuals and increased repetition in L1 supports their vocabulary acquisition, which can inform special educational programming and instructional approaches. This type of dynamic, responsive evaluation underscores the importance of school psychologists and speech-language pathologists working together to ensure assessments are accurate and culturally responsive.

Selecting and Administering Standardized Assessments

Norm-referenced and criterion-referenced tests are two types of standardized assessment tools that may be considered in evaluating EB students' speech and language skills. Norm-referenced tests compare a student's performance to that of a representative sample of the population, while criterion-referenced tests compare a student's performance to a predetermined standard. These tools provide a standard score that is used to interpret the student's performance in reference to the normative sample. They are frequently used in the school setting to support qualification decisions. Norm-referenced and criterion-referenced assessments used for diagnostic decision-making must be carefully selected. As discussed previously, selected diagnostic assessments must be appropriate for the EB student and have appropriate sensitivity and specificity. If a student's cultural and linguistic background does not match the normative sample of a selected tool, the student's score should not be used for identification purposes as it can lead to misidentification. As EB students are a heterogeneous group of students who have differing backgrounds in terms of their language experiences and language development, there are limited assessments in which they match the normative sample. Instead of obtaining and using standard scores, norm-referenced and criterion-referenced tests can be used to describe what the EB student knows in different content areas and support dynamic assessment tasks to characterize the student's learning abilities.

Collaboration between School Psychologists and Speech-Language Pathologists

School psychologists (SPs) and SLPs share similarities in their roles and responsibilities within the school system. SPs and SLPs are both responsible for prevention, assessment, and intervention activities for children suspected of or identified with a disability within the school system. They also gather and analyze data, provide consultation, and collaborate with students, their families, and their teachers to provide services and programming to support student success within the general education curriculum. Despite these similarities, SLPs and SPs rarely engage in collaborative practices (Dunsmuir et al., 2006). Large caseloads, the amount of legal paperwork requirements/of interprofessional training opportunities, and limited knowledge of team member roles and practices interfere with attempts to engage in collaboration. However, the benefits of engaging in collaborative practices, particularly when working with EB students, have the potential to provide more accurate assessment results and programming for students, leading to better outcomes for EB students with and without disabilities. This section of the chapter will suggest ways for SPs and SLPs to collaborate when assessing EB students. Table 13.2 offers general ways for SPs and SLPs to successfully collaborate in the evaluation of EB students to increase accuracy in the assessment process.

In the evaluation process, SPs and SLPs often overlap in their assessment of a student's cognitive-linguistic skills and abilities. Specifically, SPs and SLPs overlap in assessing a student's receptive and expressive semantic and morphosyntactic skills (e.g., semantic relationships, academic vocabulary, ability to answer questions, ability to follow directions, etc.). They also overlap in assessing a student's

Table 13.2 Strategies to Improve Collaboration Between School Psychologists and Speech-Language Pathologists (based on Mitchell et al., 2020)

Collaboration Component	Examples of Implementation
Establish a commitment for Collaboration and training	• Get to know the practitioners at your site. • Ask practitioners about their roles and responsibilities. • Recommend relevant chapters from this book to get the educational team on the same page on concepts related to considerations in assessing bilingual students. • Establish norms for collaboration.
Advocate for and implement collaborative meetings	• Discuss the importance of and reasons for collaborative planning time with school administration and the team. • Identify a regular, dedicated collaborative meeting time where educational team members can discuss and prepare for cases. • Create team standards for working on special education referrals and evaluations for students. • Plan and participate in trainings on increasing culturally responsive practices, including nondiscriminatory assessment approaches and sharing new learning that challenges biases in educational systems.
Design a collaborative evaluation plan	• Design a plan that includes roles and responsibilities for all aspects of the assessment process. • After collecting and reviewing information from the pre-referral team, request trained interpreters, translators, and/or consultants for the assessment process. • Consider the different measures that will be needed for a given student's evaluation. • If using standardized assessments, review the appropriateness of the measures for the student's background and the ability for the test to accurately distinguish disorder (i.e., *sensitivity and specificity*). • Decide which team member will conduct specific measure(s). • If possible, establish a timeline for when measures will be completed to determine if there is a need for additional measures.
Share evaluation data throughout process	• As data is collected, ensure there is a mechanism to share results throughout the evaluation process instead of only at a review of results meeting. • Sharing results throughout the process may inform other team members about a student's strengths and needs that have not been accounted for in the original evaluation plan.

phonological and orthographic processing (e.g., phonological awareness tasks, non-word and real word repetition, spelling, and reading tasks, etc.), language organization and inferencing skills (e.g., narrative and expositive macrostructure comprehension and production), and language-mediated cognitive tasks (e.g., problem-solving and decision-making). Lastly, both SPs and SLPs' assessment tasks overlap in assessing a student's receptive and expressive pragmatic language skills (e.g., theory of mind, non-verbal communication, and contextual language tasks). While these overlaps occur, SPs and SLPs each focus on distinct areas and purposes in the assessment process. That is, a SLP is the expert in how the development of speech, language, and communication may impact academics and learning.

In contrast, a SP is the expert in understanding the underlying cognitive, socio-emotional, behavioral, and adaptive skills that impact academics and learning. These lenses impact the interpretation of findings on similar assessment processes and domains examined, including oral and written language abilities, executive functions, and memory.

While some academic, cognitive, and social-emotional assessments administered by SPs may not directly test 'language' skills, they often require the student to utilize their linguistic skills and abilities to successfully participate in the assessment tasks. These tasks may broadly include areas of language comprehension and language production. It is the case that language appears throughout the administration of the majority of assessments. Therefore, an understanding of an EB student's language skills and abilities is necessary for accurate assessment across multiple domains. For example, even mathematics-based assessments often incorporate linguistically dense word problems that require students to use and comprehend language to access and solve mathematics problems (e.g., Arizmendi et al., 2021; refer to Chap. 8, for review). Indeed, the majority of assessments assume typical language development and may not consider the underlying language-based skills needed to accomplish a specific task. This impacts students who have an underlying brain-based language learning disorder, such as Developmental Language Disorder, who are also learning a second language. These assumptions rooted in typical development of language in assessment, along with assumptions rooted in monolingual norms and limited control for the complexity of language (e.g., frequency and complexity of words in items, length of utterances in the instruction), may lead students who are developing a second language to have poor performance on the measures. Therefore, SLPs and SPs can make their assessment plan known with each other to prevent reduplicated efforts in assessment that can invalidate results and confer findings with each other to better understand the nature of the difficulties. SLPs and SPs may work together to answer questions like: are difficulties due to limitations in working memory? Are difficulties manifesting because of the cognitive load of the second language without reducing the linguistic load? Are they related most to social environments (i.e., bullying and depression) that lead to difficulties in sustaining attention in class and impact learning? These discussions are grounded in the understanding that the domains tested are deeply interconnected to each other, while also recognizing the distinct areas of expertise in the assessment process that can inform diagnosis, and the best supports and accommodations for a student to reach their full potential.

If SPs and SLPs work in isolation during the assessment process, they may face situations where they are testing students in the same content areas, using similar testing tools, or using inappropriate tests and procedures based on the student's cultural and linguistic background. This results in lost time and resources. In addition, the potential for duplication of testing procedures may invalidate results due to practice effects (a student's familiarity with the task that leads to improved performance). It may also lead to confusion regarding results if SPs and SLPs have not had an opportunity to decipher differences in performance on similar measures.

Collaboration between SLPs, SPs, and other special education team members addresses the numerous challenges that arise from working in isolation. This collaboration is critical for increasing the accuracy of assessment practices for EB students suspected of having a disability. As mentioned previously, assessment of EB students is more complicated due to the heterogenous nature of EB students' backgrounds and experiences (both linguistically and culturally), the presence of cultural and linguistic mismatches between the student's home and school environment, the paucity of norm-referenced and standardized assessments for bilingual populations, and educational professionals' bias and potential lack of knowledge and training on bilingual service provision. Special education team members, including SPs and SLPs, should develop collaborative practices to address these assessment challenges.

Interprofessional Practice

Interprofessional practice (IPP) is a framework for building special education team collaboration to support the assessment of EB students. As defined by ASHA (2016a, 2016b), IPP is a service-delivery model where "two or more professionals collaborate together, without any perceived hierarchy, and with full understanding of each other's roles and responsibilities to improve the client's outcomes and care" (p. 4). In the school setting, IPP requires special education team members, each with their own expertise and specialized training, to work together to accurately serve students with disabilities. Importantly, IPP is not working in parallel whereby special education team members conduct their assessment and intervention activities in isolation (Giess & Serianni, 2018). While this may be considered multidisciplinary, it is not collaborative. Unfortunately, working in isolation is common practice among many special education teams. For example, SPs and SLPs may plan and administer their evaluations independently. This includes SPs and SLPs separately contacting caregivers and teachers to gather similar data, administering similar or even the same assessments, and reporting evaluation results without making connections across the data. This lack of collaboration is often evident in results meetings where SPs and SLPs provide isolated results (i.e., the SLP will now share the results of their testing, the SP will now share the results of their testing, etc.). The evaluation practices and the special education meetings themselves provide evidence of the lack of collaboration in the assessment process (Giess & Serianni, 2018).

Instead of working in isolation, SPs and SLPs have an opportunity to create and model IPP on their special education teams. As discussed above, EB student assessments provide a unique and necessary opportunity to do so. While all teams may approach steps to collaboration differently, key aspects of IPP should be defined and discussed at the beginning of the IPP process. SPs and SLPs can facilitate the beginning of the process by: (1) leading discussions to determine how the team will communicate (e.g., timing, methods, decisions on common language, etc.), (2) creating opportunities for each team member to educate other team members on their individual roles and responsibilities, and (3) leading discussions to determine the team's values, ethics, and culture of teamwork (Giess & Serianni, 2018). Important to this process is intentionally setting aside a time and place to foster and plan for collaboration. Practically, this means a regularly scheduled time and location to meet, creating specific plans that map out how IPP will occur for student cases, and determining a timeline and processes that provide accountability for the implementation of the IPP plan.

When designing a specific IPP plan, SPs and SLPs may create their own plan or use sample rubrics, like The Interprofessional Practice (IPP) Case Rubric (ASHA, n.d.). SPs, SLPs, and other special education team members should outline specifically how the team will gather the following information: (1) the EB student's case history, (2) specific information on the EB student's cultural and linguistic background and experiences (linguistic questionnaires), (3) information on the EB student's strengths and challenges from the perspective of caregivers, teachers, and other professionals (e.g., physician), (4) the EB student's performance on curriculum-based measures and pre-referral intervention data, and (5) any additional documentation and other information needed by a team member. Assigned team members should be responsible for gathering background information from the unique sources (e.g., caregivers, teachers, physicians, files, etc.) and sharing it with the entire team. This avoids duplication of efforts and limits potential confusion caused by multiple team members contacting caregivers during the process.

When gathering the EB student's background information, team members may need to coordinate the use of trained interpreters, translators, and/or consultants for the assessment process (see Alani et al., 2024 for guidance on using interpreters and/or translators). After gathering and reviewing the EB student's background information, the team can design an assessment plan that delineates evaluation roles and responsibilities (Giess & Serianni, 2018). At this stage, SLPs and SPs should review overlapping assessment domains and consider how differences in culture and language may influence those domains. Next, they should decide how different domains will be assessed, select psychometrically sound assessment tools and tasks, and make plans for observing the student across different school settings. This collaboration avoids duplication and saves resources. For example, if the team determines an assessment of an EB student's phonological processing is necessary, the SLP and SP may identify tasks across the student's languages (e.g., nonword repetition, spelling, and reading tasks in English and Spanish) and decide the logistics of who, when, and how those tasks will be administered and analyzed.

SPs and SLPs may also determine a sequential order for assessment administration and analysis. This can inform decisions on upcoming assessment tasks. For example, an SLP may first administer and analyze an EB student's performance on a dynamic assessment vocabulary task and narrative language tasks in Spanish and English. The SLPs' data can inform the SP on the student's response to mediated learning experiences (e.g., learning effort, attention, strategy use, beneficial supports, socio-emotional responses, etc.) and provide detailed information on the student's English and Spanish language skills (macrostructure, and microstructure). The SP can use this data to adjust their administration of future academic assessment tasks. In addition, the team may decide to revise the assessment plan to accommodate new information on the student's language and learning abilities. Collaborative assessment planning, including sequential ordering of assessments and sharing of data during the assessment process, has the benefit of improving the overall effectiveness and efficiency of an EB student's special education assessment. It allows for improved assessment plans (e.g., adjustment to the administration and selection of assessments), removes duplication of efforts, and saves time and resources for team members during the assessment process.

The IPP framework also provides guidance for team members as they make decisions regarding special education qualification for EB students. At the completion of data collection and analysis, team members should gather to review information from all the assessment sources. Recall that the IPP definition states that team members should engage "without any perceived hierarchy" (ASHA, 2016a, 2016b, p. 4). Instead of one or two team members making decisions based on their independent testing (e.g., working in isolation), the IPP framework empowers all team members to arrive at a collective decision, reviewing and discussing their view of the data from their specialized roles. This type of collaboration supports a holistic picture of the EB student's skills and abilities. The result is a more accurate determination as to whether the EB student presents with a true language-based learning disability or simply requires additional supports (e.g., dual-language supports, differentiated instruction, etc.) that are available in the general education curriculum. Prior to and throughout the assessment process, there are many more ways that SPs and SLPs can implement IPP to support improved outcomes for EB students with and without disabilities. Table 13.2 provides a list of recommendations for SPs and SLPs to consider as they endeavor to improve collaboration within special education teams. With these recommendations in mind, SLPs and SPs are better equipped to enhance collaboration and create more individualized support plans that lead to stronger educational outcomes for EB students.

Conclusions

Understanding bilingual language development and utilizing valid and reliable assessment practices results in increased accuracy in identifying EB students with and without disability. As members of special educational teams, SLPs have expertise in speech and language development and play an important role in characterizing the language-learning abilities of EB students during the special education evaluation process. Key features in speech and language evaluations include challenging misconceptions associated with bilingualism, understanding the unique language background and experiences of EB students, evaluating speech and language skills in both of the student's languages, and using a variety of valid and reliable evaluation tools to accurately identify if a student does or does not have a disability. Lastly, as the EB evaluation process may be more complex, require more resources, and rely less on standardized assessment scores, collaboration between SLPs and SPs is crucial to ensuring more accurate and thorough evaluations for EB students.

References

Alani, S., Boyer, V. E., Harden, A., Franca, M., Stierwalt, J. A. G., & Pegoraro-Krook, M. (2024). Guidance on the effective collaboration with interpreters and translators in speech-language pathology. *Perspectives of the ASHA Special Interest Groups, 9*(3), 795–803. https://doi.org/10.1044/2024_PERSP-23-00143

American Speech-Language Hearing Association. (n.d.). *Interprofessional education/interprofessional practice (IPE/IPP). The IPP case rubric.* Retrieved from https://www.asha.org/Practice/The-IPP-Case-Rubric/

American Speech-Language-Hearing Association. (2010). *Roles and responsibilities of speech-language pathologists in schools [Professional Issues Statement].* Retrieved from https://www.asha.org/policy

American Speech-Language-Hearing Association. (2016a). *Interprofessional education and interprofessional practice in communication sciences and disorders: An introduction and cased-based examples of implementation in education and health care settings.* Retrieved from http://www.asha.org/uploadedFiles/IPE-IPP-Reader-eBook.pdf

American Speech-Language-Hearing Association. (2016b). *Scope of practice in speech-language pathology*. https://www.asha.org/siteassets/publications/sp2016-00343.pdf

Arias, G., & Friberg, J. (2017). Bilingual language assessment: Contemporary versus recommended practice in American schools. *Language, Speech, and Hearing Services in Schools, 48*(1), 1–15. https://doi.org/10.1044/2016_LSHSS-15-009

Arizmendi, G. D., Li, J. T., Van Horn, M. L., Petcu, S. D., & Swanson, H. L. (2021). Language–focused interventions on math performance for English learners: A selective meta–analysis of the literature. *Learning Disabilities Research & Practice, 36*(1), 56–75. https://doi.org/10.1111/ldrp.12239

Artiles, A. J., Rueda, R., Salazar, J. J., & Higareda, I. (2005). Within-group diversity in minority disproportionate representation: English language learners in urban school districts. *Exceptional Children, 71*(3), 283–300. https://doi.org/10.1177/001440290507100305

Barragan, B., Castilla-Earls, A., Martinez-Nieto, L., Restrepo, M. A., & Gray, S. (2018). Performance of low-income dual language learners attending English-only schools on the Clinical Evaluation of Language Fundamentals–Fourth Edition, Spanish. *Language, Speech, and Hearing Services in Schools, 49*(2), 292–305. https://doi.org/10.1044/2017_LSHSS-17-00

Bedore, L. M., & Peña, E. D. (2008). Assessment of bilingual children for identification of language impairment: Current findings and implications for practice. *International Journal of Bilingual Education and Bilingualism, 11*(1), 1–29. https://doi.org/10.2167/beb392.0

Bialystok, E. (2001). *Bilingualism in development: Language, literacy, and cognition.* Cambridge University Press. https://doi.org/10.1017/CBO9780511605963

Bialystok, E. (2011). Reshaping the mind: The benefits of bilingualism. *Canadian Journal of Experimental Psychology, 65*(4), 229–235. https://doi.org/10.1037/a0025406

Bosch, L., & Ramon-Casas, M. (2014). First translation equivalents in bilingual toddlers' expressive vocabulary. *International Journal of Behavioral Development, 38*(4), 317–322. https://doi.org/10.1177/0165025414532559

Brea Spahn, M., & Vaz Bauler, C. (2022). Where do you anchor your beliefs? An invitation to interrogate dominant ideologies of language and languaging in speech-language pathology. *Language, Speech, and Hearing Services in Schools, 54*(3), 675–687. https://doi.org/10.1044/2023_LSHSS-22-0013

Carter, J. A., Lees, J. A., Murira, G. M., Gona, J., Neville, B. G. R., & Newton, C. R. J. C. (2005). Issues in the development of cross-cultural assessments of speech and language for children. *International Journal of Language & Communication Disorders, 40*(4), 385–401. https://doi.org/10.1080/13682820500057301

Castilla-Earls, A., Bedore, L., Rojas, R., Fabiano-Smith, L., Pruitt-Lord, S., Restrepo, M. A., & Peña, E. (2020). Beyond scores: Using converging evidence to determine speech and language services eligibility for dual language learners. *American Journal of Speech-Language Pathology, 29*(3), 1116–1132. https://doi.org/10.1044/2020_AJSLP-19-00177

Crago, M. B., Eriks-Brophy, A., Pesco, D., & McAlpine, L. (1997). Culturally based miscommunication in classroom interaction. *Language, Speech, and Hearing Services in Schools, 28*(3), 245–254. https://doi.org/10.1044/0161-1461.2803.245

Crowley, C. (2014). *Parent/caregiver critical questions and the teacher interview*. Leadersproject.org. https://www.leadersproject.org/2015/03/18/the-critical-questions/

Crowley, C., & Baigorri, M. (2015). *School-age language assessment measures*. https://www.leadersproject.org/disability-evaluation/school-age-language-assessment-measures-slam/

Cummins, J. (2000). Language, power, and pedagogy: Bilingual children in the crossfire. *Multilingual Matters*. https://doi.org/10.21832/9781853596773

De Lamo White, C., & Jin, L. (2011). Evaluation of speech and language assessment approaches with bilingual children. *International Journal of Language & Communication Disorders, 46*(6), 613–627. https://doi.org/10.1111/j.1460-6984.2011.00049.x

De Valenzuela, J. S., Copeland, S. R., Qi, C. H., & Park, M. (2006). Examining educational equity: Revisiting the disproportionate representation of minority students in special education. *Exceptional Children, 72*(4), 425–441. https://doi.org/10.1177/001440290607200040

Dollaghan, C. A., & Horner, E. A. (2011). Bilingual language assessment: A meta-analysis of diagnostic accuracy. *Journal of Speech, Language, and Hearing Research, 54*(4), 1077–1088. https://doi.org/10.1044/1092-4388(2010/10-0093)

Dunsmuir, S., Clifford, V., & Took, S. (2006). Collaboration between educational psychologists and speech and language therapists: Barriers and opportunities. *Educational Psychology in Practice, 22*(02), 125–140. https://doi.org/10.1080/02667360600668246

Fabiano-Smith, L., & Goldstein, B. A. (2010). Phonological acquisition in bilingual Spanish-English speaking children. *Journal of Speech, Language, and Hearing Research, 53*(1), 160–178. https://doi.org/10.1044/1092-4388(2009/07-0064)

Flores, N., & Rosa, J. (2015). Undoing appropriateness: Raciolinguistic ideologies and language diversity in education. *Harvard Educational Review, 85*(2), 149–171. https://doi.org/10.17763/0017-8055.85.2.149

Freeman, M. R., & Schroeder, S. R. (2022). Assessing language skills in bilingual children: Current trends in research and practice. *Journal of Child Science, 12*(01), e33–e46. https://doi.org/10.1055/s-0042-1743575

Fulcher-Rood, K., Castilla-Earls, A. P., & Higginbotham, J. (2018). School-based speech-language pathologists' perspectives on diagnostic decision making. *American Journal of Speech-Language Pathology, 27*(2), 796–812. https://doi.org/10.1044/2018_ajslp-16-0121

Gampe, A., Quick, A. E., & Daum, M. M. (2021). Does linguistic similarity affect early simultaneous bilingual language acquisition? *Journal of Language Contact, 13*(3), 482–500. https://doi.org/10.1163/19552629-13030001

Garcia, O. (2009). Emergent bilinguals and TESOL: What's in a name? *TESOL Quarterly, 43*(2), 322–326. https://doi.org/10.1002/j.1545-7249.2009.tb00172.x

Giess, S., & Serianni, R. (2018). Interprofessional practice in schools. *Perspectives of the ASHA Special Interest Groups, 3*(16), 88–94. https://doi.org/10.1044/persp3.SIG16.88

Genesee, F., Paradis, J., & Crago, M. B. (2004). In H. Paul (Ed.), *Dual language development and disorders: A handbook on bilingualism and second language learning*. Brookes Publishing.

Grosjean, F. (1989). Neurolinguists, beware! The bilingual is not two monolinguals in one person. *Brain and Language, 36*(1), 3–15. https://doi.org/10.1016/0093-934X(89)90048-5

Gutiérrez-Clellen, V. F., & Simon-Cereijido, G. (2010). Using language sampling in clinical assessments with bilingual children: Challenges and future directions. *Seminars in Speech and Language, 31*(4), 234–245. https://doi.org/10.1055/s-0029-1241722

Harris, B., Sullivan, A. L., Oades-Sese, G. V., & Sotelo-Dynega, M. (2015). Culturally and linguistically responsive practices in psychoeducational reports for English language learners. *Journal of Applied School Psychology, 31*(2), 141–166. https://doi.org/10.1080/15377903.2014.1002144

Hambly, H., Wren, Y., McLeod, S., & Roulstone, S. (2013). The influence of bilingualism on speech production: A systematic review. *International Journal of Language & Communication Disorders, 48*(1), 1–24. https://doi.org/10.1111/j.1460-6984.2012.00178.x

Individuals with Disabilities Education Act. (2004). 20 U.S.C. §§ 1400 et. seq.

Ireland, M., McLeod, S., Farquharson, K., & Crowe, K. (2020). Evaluating children in US public schools with speech sound disorders: Considering federal and state laws, guidance, and research. *Topics in Language Disorders, 40*(4), 326–340. https://doi.org/10.1097/TLD.0000000000000226

Kanno, Y., Rios-Aguilar, C., & Bunch, G. C. (2024). English learners? Emergent bilinguals? Multilingual learners?: Goals, contexts, and consequences in labeling students. *TESOL Journal, 15*(3), e797. https://doi.org/10.1002/tesj.797

Kapantzoglou, M., Restrepo, M. A., & Thompson, M. S. (2012). Dynamic assessment of word learning skills: Identifying language impairment in bilingual children. *Language, Speech, and Hearing Services in Schools, 43*(1), 81–96. https://doi.org/10.1044/0161-1461(2011/10-009

Kohnert, K., Ebert, K. D., & Pham, G. T. (2020). *Language disorders in bilingual children and adults* (Vol. 1). Plural Publishing.

Laurie, A., & Pesco, D. (2023). Curriculum-based dynamic assessment of narratives for bilingual Filipino children. *Language, Speech, and Hearing Services in Schools, 54*(2), 489–503. https://doi.org/10.1044/2022_LSHSS-22-00

Lidz, C. S., & Peña, E. D. (1996). Dynamic assessment: The model, its relevance as a nonbiased approach, and its application to Latino American preschool children. *Language, Speech, and Hearing Services in Schools, 40*(1), 53–65. https://doi.org/10.1044/0161-1461.2704.367

Lubliner, S., & Hiebert, E. H. (2011). An analysis of English–Spanish cognates as a source of general academic language. *Bilingual Research Journal, 34*(1), 76–93. https://doi.org/10.1080/15235882.2011.568589

Mancilla-Martinez, J., Oh, M. H., Luk, G., & Rollins, A. (2023). Special education representation trends vary by language status: Evidence of underrepresentation in Tennessee. *Journal of Learning Disabilities, 00222194231178285*. https://doi.org/10.1177/00222194231178285

Marian, V., Blumenfeld, H. K., & Kaushanskaya, M. (2007). The language experience and proficiency questionnaire (LEAP-Q): Assessing language profiles in bilinguals and multilinguals. *Journal of Speech, Language, and Hearing Research, 50*(4), 940–967. https://doi.org/10.1044/1092-4388(2007/067

McLeod, S., & Verdon, S. (2017). Tutorial: Speech assessment for multilingual children who do not speak the same language (s) as the speech-language pathologist. *American Journal of Speech-Language Pathology, 26*(3), 691–708. https://doi.org/10.1044/2017_AJSLP-15-0161

McLeod, S. (2024). *Multilingual children's speech*. Charles Sturt University. http://www.csu.edu.au/research/multilingual-speech/

Mitchell, M. P., Ehren, B. J., & Towson, J. A. (2020). Collaboration in schools: Let's define it. *Perspectives of the ASHA Special Interest Groups, 5*(3), 732–751. https://doi.org/10.1044/2020_PERSP-19-00125

Morgan, P. L., Farkas, G., Cook, M., Strassfeld, N. M., Hillemeier, M. M., Pun, W. H., Wang, Y., & Schussler, D. L. (2018). Are Hispanic, Asian, native American, or language-minority children overrepresented in special education? *Exceptional Children, 84*(3), 261–279. https://doi.org/10.1177/0014402917748303

Morgan, P. L., Farkas, G., Hillemeier, M. M., Mattison, R., Maczuga, S., Li, H., & Cook, M. (2015). Minorities are disproportionately underrepresented in special education: Longitudinal evidence across five disability conditions. *Educational Researcher, 44*(5), 278–292. https://doi.org/10.3102/0013189X15591157

Nair, V. K., Farah, W., & Cushing, I. (2023). A critical analysis of standardized testing in speech and language therapy. *Language, Speech, and Hearing Services in Schools, 54*(3), 781–793. https://doi.org/10.1044/2023_LSHSS-22-0014

National Center for Education Statistics. (2024). *English learners in public schools. Condition of Education.* U.S. Department of Education, National Center for Education Statistics. https://nces.ed.gov/programs/coe/indicator/cgf

Oetting, J. B. (2018). Prologue: Toward accurate identification of developmental language disorder within linguistically diverse schools. *Language, Speech, and Hearing Services in Schools, 49*(2), 213–217. https://doi.org/10.1044/2018_LSHSS-CLSLD-17-0156

Orellana, C. I., Wada, R., & Gillam, R. B. (2019). The use of dynamic assessment for the diagnosis of language disorders in bilingual children: A meta-analysis. *American Journal of Speech-Language Pathology, 28*(3), 1298–1317. https://doi.org/10.1044/2019_AJSLP-18-0202

Paradis, J. (2011). Individual differences in child English second language acquisition: Comparing child-internal and child-external factors. *Linguistic Approaches to Bilingualism, 1*(3), 213–237. https://doi.org/10.1075/lab.1.3.01par

Paradis, J., Emmerzael, K., & Duncan, T. S. (2010). *Alberta language and development questionnaire (ALDeQ)* [Database record]. APA PsycTests. https://doi.org/10.1037/t85853-000

Paradis, J., & Genesee, F. (1996). Syntactic acquisition in bilingual children: Autonomous or interdependent? *Studies in Second Language Acquisition, 18*(1), 1–25. https://doi.org/10.1017/S0272263100014662

Paradis, J., Soto-Corominas, A., Chen, X., & Gottardo, A. (2020). How language environment, age, and cognitive capacity support the bilingual development of Syrian refugee children recently arrived in Canada. *Applied Psycholinguistics., 41*(6), 1255–1281. https://doi.org/10.1017/S014271642000017X

Peña, E. D., Bedore, L. M., & Vargas, A. G. (2023). Exploring assumptions of the bilingual delay in children with and without developmental language disorder. *Journal of Speech, Language, and Hearing Research, 66*(12), 4739–4755. https://doi.org/10.1044/2023_JSLHR-23-0011

Peña, E. D., & Halle, T. G. (2011). Assessing preschool dual language learners: Traveling a multiforked road. *Child Development Perspectives, 5*(1), 28–32. https://doi.org/10.1111/j.1750-8606.2010.00143.x

Peña, E. D., Gillam, R. B., & Bedore, L. M. (2014). Dynamic assessment of narrative ability in English accurately identifies language impairment in English language learners. *Journal of Speech, Language, and Hearing Research, 57*(6), 2208–2220. https://doi.org/10.1044/2014_JSLHR-L-13-0151

Peña, E. D., Iglesias, A., & Lidz, C. S. (2001). Reducing test bias through dynamic assessment of children's word learning ability. *American Journal of Speech-Language Pathology, 10*(2), 138–154. https://doi.org/10.1044/1058-0360(2001/014)

Peña, E. D., Reséndiz, M., & Gillam, R. B. (2007). Dynamic assessment of school-age children's narrative ability: An experimental investigation of classification accuracy. *Journal of Speech, Language, and Hearing Research, 50*(3), 703–719. https://doi.org/10.1044/1092-4388(2006/074)

Petersen, D. B., Konishi-Therkildsen, A., Clark, K. D., DeRobles, A. K., Frahm, A. E., Jones, K., Lettich, C., & Spencer, T. D. (2024). Accurately identifying language disorders in school-age children using dynamic assessment of narrative language. *Journal of Speech, Language, and Hearing Research, 67*(12), 4765–4782. https://doi.org/10.1044/2024_JSLHR-23-0059

Pezold, M. J., Imgrund, C. M., & Storkel, H. L. (2020). Using computer programs for language sample analysis. *Language, Speech, and Hearing Services in the Schools, 51*(1), 103–114. https://doi.org/10.1044/2019_LSHSS-18-0144

Plante, E., & Vance, R. (1994). Selection of preschool language tests: A data-based approach. *Language, Speech, and Hearing Services in Schools, 25*(1), 15–24. https://doi.org/10.1044/0161-1461.2501.15

Potapova, I., & Pruitt-Lord, S. L. (2020). Towards understanding the bilingual profile in typical and atypical language development: A tutorial. *International Journal of Speech-Language Pathology, 22*(1), 106–116. https://doi.org/10.1080/17549507.2019.1598492

Restrepo, M. A. (1998). Identifiers of predominantly Spanish-speaking children with language impairment. *Journal of Speech, Language, and Hearing Research, 41*(6), 1398–1411. https://doi.org/10.1044/jslhr.4106.1398

Restrepo, M. A., & Silverman, S. W. (2001). Validity of the Spanish preschool language scale-3 for use with bilingual children. *American Journal of Speech-Language Pathology, 10*(4), 382–393. https://doi.org/10.1044/1058-0360(2001/032)

Squires, L. R., Ohlfest, S. J., Santoro, K. E., & Roberts, J. L. (2020). Factors influencing cognate performance for young multilingual children's vocabulary: A research synthesis. *American Journal of Speech-Language Pathology, 29*(4), 2170–2188. https://doi.org/10.1044/2020_AJSLP-19-00167

Sullivan, A. L. (2011). Disproportionality in special education identification and placement of English language learners. *Exceptional Children, 77*(3), 317–334. https://doi.org/10.1177/001440291107700304

Valenzuela, A. (2010). *Subtractive schooling: U.S.-Mexican youth and the politics of caring (10th anniversary ed.)*. State University of New York Press.

Vygotsky, L. S. (1978). *Mind in society: The development of higher psychological processes*. Harvard University Press.

Chapter 14
Culturally and Linguistically Responsive Autism Identification Among Multilingual Youth

Bryn Harris and Jingyi Yang

Multilingual students currently comprise 10.6% of U.S. public school enrollment, which is an increase from 2011 (9.4%; NCES, 2024). There is substantial variation in multilingual enrollment by state, ranging from 0.8 to 20.2%. Most multilingual students live in cities, are enrolled in lower grades, and speak Spanish (76%). In terms of racial/ethnic identity, 77.9% of multilingual students identify as Hispanic/Latine followed by 9.7% Asian, 6.1% White, 4.2% Black, 0.8% two or more races, 0.7% American Indian/Alaska Native, and 0.6% Pacific Islander (NCES, 2024). A total of 15.8% of the multilingual student enrollment is identified as a student with a disability, compared to 14.7% of the total public school enrollment that is identified as a student with a disability (NCES, 2024). In addition, the majority (56%) of children of immigrants speak English proficiently, as well as at least one other language in the home setting (Woods & Hanson, 2016). Although these statistics give a broad understanding of some of the demographic characteristics of multilingual learners, there is a great variation among local contexts and patterns of mobility and immigration.

Per the Every Student Succeeds Act (ESSA, 2015) from the U.S. Department of Education, every state and district must have a process for determining that eligible children receive and benefit from English language acquisition supports. The first step in this determination is by completing the Home Language Survey, typically provided to the family during the school enrollment process and updated on a yearly

B. Harris (✉)
School of Education & Human Development, University of Colorado Denver, Denver, CO, USA
e-mail: bryn.harris@ucdenver.edu

J. Yang
Department of Psychology, University of South Carolina, Columbia, SC, USA
e-mail: jingyiy@email.sc.edu

D. Vega, J. N. Wolf (eds.), *Culturally and Linguistically Responsive Intervention and Assessment Practices with Emergent Bilingual Students*,
https://doi.org/10.1007/978-3-032-02084-0_14

basis. The Home Language Survey often involves questions about a student's language(s) exposure and background, although there is substantial variability in the content of these surveys (Bailey & Kelly, 2010). Per the ESSA (2015), if the home language survey indicates that a language other than English is spoken at home, the school district has 30 days to administer an English language proficiency assessment. Each state can determine the type of English language proficiency assessment that will be required by each school district (U.S. Department of Education, 2016). The most common assessment is the WIDA ACCESS, created by the University of Wisconsin-Madison WIDA Consortium. A total of 41 states and the District of Columbia, Puerto Rico, and the Northern Mariana Islands participate in this consortium. The WIDA ACCESS evaluates a student's English skills in the areas of listening, reading, speaking, and writing. WIDA has created an alternate ACCESS assessment for children with significant cognitive delays, although no research has been conducted to date that analyzes the performance of children with autism or other disabilities on the WIDA ACCESS (2025). The results of the English language proficiency assessment are used to determine a student's appropriate language supports. Families can determine participation in English language supports, and districts must establish criteria for exiting such supports once English proficiency is achieved (U.S. Department of Education, 2016).

Autism Prevalence

The most recent Centers for Disease Control and Prevention (CDC) Autism and Developmental Disabilities Monitoring Network (ADDM) surveillance summary reported the overall prevalence of autism was 1 in 36 children, aged 8 years, with a male-to-female prevalence ratio of 3.8 (Maenner et al., 2023). The report noted variations in prevalence per 1000 children among different racial and ethnic groups, finding that White children (24.3) for the first time had a lower prevalence compared to American Indian or Alaska Native (26.5), Black (29.3), Hispanic (31.6), and Asian or Pacific Islander (33.4) children. The overall median age of autism identification is 49 months (4.1 years; Maenner et al., 2023), and the age of receiving the identification was found to be consistent across racial and ethnic groups (Pham et al., 2022). The ADDM Network prevalence data includes both autism clinical diagnoses as well special education identification rates for numerous states in the U.S. In school settings specifically, special education disproportionality varies by race and ethnicity. For example, the disproportionate overrepresentation of Black and Indigenous students is common among the categories of emotional disability (ED) and intellectual disability (ID; Bal et al., 2019). Among Asian students, autism is the most common category of special education eligibility, although, for other racial groups, a specific learning disability is the most commonly identified special education category (Sullivan et al., 2020). These brief examples demonstrate the complexity and intersectionality of special education identification and the potential considerations related to race, ethnicity, language, and identity in autism identification.

The most recent ADDM Network analysis indicates that professionals may be more likely to identify autism among children from minoritized populations; however, more research is needed to understand these recent demographic shifts in autism identification by race and ethnicity (and other demographic variables). Prior to 2016, there was a persistent trend of racial disparities in autism identification among White children, particularly those from middle to high socio-economic backgrounds. This group was the most likely to receive an autism diagnosis and gain access to services at a younger age (Wiggins et al., 2020; Xu et al., 2018). A consistent observed disparity in the ADDM data is that Black children are more likely to be identified with intellectual disability as well as autism (Maenner et al., 2023). Additional disparities occur, as Black children are also more likely to receive a delayed identification of autism (Constantino et al., 2020). Black and Latine youth are also more likely to receive a diagnosis of a disruptive behavior disorder and less likely to receive a diagnosis of ADHD (Fadus et al., 2020). These disparities cannot be primarily explained by genetic factors, indicating that reasons for disparities are multifactorial and may be influenced by sociodemographic factors, language and cultural barriers, and provider knowledge of autism (Aylward et al., 2021). This disparity is particularly concerning as there are significant implications of a delayed or lack of autism identification. Early intervention programs are positively associated with language, cognitive, and adaptive functioning improvements, particularly at younger ages (Makrygianni & Reed, 2010). Children who are identified with autism later are less likely to receive autism-related therapy (including school-based services) and more likely to take psychotropic medications (Zuckerman et al., 2017). Despite the evidence base for the provision of some psychotropic medications among children with autism, disparities exist as Black and Latine children are less likely to receive psychotropic medications to treat mental health concerns, Latine children are more likely to receive antipsychotic drugs (including higher metabolic side effects), and children in immigrant families are less likely to receive psychotropic medications for mental health challenges. These medication disparities may influence behaviors in school and home contexts, reduce intervention effectiveness, or contribute to problematic medication side effects (Shahidullah et al., 2023).

There have been differing findings regarding the prevalence of autism among immigrant populations in the U.S. Some studies (e.g., Becerra et al., 2014; Magnusson et al., 2012) found a greater prevalence or risk of autism among children born to immigrant parents. Lee et al. (2021) have hypothesized that the contributing factors may include nutrition and vitamin insufficiency or stress and trauma from migration (Lee et al., 2021). Other studies found that there is a lower prevalence or risk for autism among children of immigrant parents, or that the relative risk is similar to children of non-immigrant parents (Augereau et al., 2020).

Autism prevalence rates among specific populations may provide more insights into disparities that may contribute to autism identification and services. In Austria, children from immigrant backgrounds received an autism diagnosis 13 months prior to children who were not immigrants (Primo et al., 2020). Somali children born outside Minnesota received a comprehensive diagnostic evaluation for autism at 5.8 years of age, which is 2 years later than children from White backgrounds (Hall-Lande et al., 2021). The influence of language acquisition and multilingualism is rarely studied in autism research, leading to many questions about needed considerations pertaining to language and culture. However, research has continuously demonstrated that immigrant families face additional challenges when accessing health care for their children (Abdullahi et al., 2018). There have been numerous reasons for these challenges pertaining to access, including awareness of health care policies, knowledge of systems of care, availability of information in native languages, providers fluent in the family's native language, and limited financial resources (Rivard et al., 2019).

Disparities in Autism Identification Among Multilingual Children and Families

Limited research has been conducted investigating family language use (e.g., multilingualism, monolingualism in a language other than English) and its impact on potential autism identification disparities. Currently, 12 million children residing in the U.S. speak a language other than English at home (Anne E. Casey Foundation, 2024). When using national prevalence data, this equates to about 1 in 4 multilingual children that could be identified with autism. In the U.S., we do not have robust data regarding autism prevalence among multilingual populations. Multilingual populations are a heterogeneous group, representing immense diversity regarding their language histories, current language use, instructional experiences in languages, and life experiences that contribute to language exposure and use. Inclusion of such information is often not included in psychological reports or family interviews, making research on this topic challenging.

Some research has investigated cultural factors with particular populations but often excludes measures of language use. For example, Zuckerman et al. (2014) found that Latine families with children who had been identified with autism reported having limited information on autism, increased stigma of the disability in their culture, and increased dismissal of parent concern by providers. This study also found that Latine families had an increased perception of mistrust in the medical system (Zuckerman et al., 2014).

Voelkel et al. (2013) found that Latine individuals with a perceived high level of acculturation (they defined this as effective English communication and endorsing mainstream ideas related to U.S. current events), reported higher understanding of autism, greater ease in accessing autism care, and improved access to receiving autism treatment compared with Latine individuals with low levels of acculturation. This demonstrates systemic barriers that may favor families with higher English language proficiency and similarity to mainstream U.S. culture, thus creating additional access barriers and inequities for families that may not align in these ways. In another study, Vanegas (2021) investigated potential disparities in autism identification services among children of immigrant mothers and mothers who do not identify as immigrants. Although not all immigrants are multilingual, this study provides some novel information regarding the influence of multilingualism in a sample of families receiving an autism evaluation. The author found that children of immigrants had a lower age of autism diagnosis if they were raised in a multilingual household as opposed to those that resided in a monolingual household where a language other than English is spoken. This indicates that multilingualism may influence autism identification practices or that identification processes may be more accessible to multilingual families with some level of English fluency. Families with proficiency in other languages will face inequity in service provision and potentially a delay in autism identification. If a child had a diagnosis other than autism, children of immigrants were also more likely to receive a delayed autism identification. These findings may relate to service access among immigrant families. For example, parents may receive limited (if any) information about educational and health systems in their native language. This may influence their understanding of autism identification services, accessing more comprehensive evaluation services, or second opinions. Immigrant families may also rely on public insurance or not have medical insurance, influencing their access to comprehensive autism evaluations due to structural inequities and racism that contribute to oppressive and discriminatory health access (Vanegas, 2021).

Multilingualism and Autism

Numerous research studies have refuted the notion that speaking multiple languages may "confuse" children who have autism (e.g., Bialystok & Werker, 2017). Available research does not indicate that being exposed to more than one language has adverse effects on the communication skills of autistic children (Gilhuber et al., 2023; Trelles & Castro, 2019). A recent systematic review of 22 studies found that bilingualism does not have negative effects on the language and communication skills of autistic children (Gilhuber et al., 2023). The benefits of multilingualism span cognitive (e.g., improved executive functioning), educational (e.g., higher levels of abstract thought and reasoning), sociocultural (e.g., increased empathy development), and economic (e.g., greater job prospects) areas and should be seen as an asset (Office of English Language Acquisition, 2024). For children with autism, relationships with caregivers are an important factor in improving outcomes; thus, maintaining communication with caregivers is critical (Drysdale et al., 2015). Multilingualism can assist with maintaining relationships with family members and elders, continuing important family traditions, and facilitating religious and spiritual rituals (Nolte et al., 2021). Despite substantial research indicating the numerous benefits of multilingualism, families still receive recommendations that suggest the opposite (Gilhuber et al., 2023). Even when parents report positive attitudes towards maintaining bilingualism regarding their child with autism, multiple factors may ultimately influence their decision regarding maintaining the native language, including the severity of autism, advice received from trusted sources, and their perceived importance of learning English (Howard et al., 2021).

School-based research among children has also demonstrated positive outcomes of multilingualism among children identified with autism. A qualitative study by Howard et al. (2019) investigated the perceived benefits of being multilingual according to adolescents identified with autism between the ages of 7 and 14. The adolescents educated in multilingual settings perceived their multilingualism to be more positive than adolescents educated in monolingual contexts, indicating the impacts of multilingual language environments on identity. Nolte et al. (2021) surveyed multilingual adults identified with autism and asked questions about their childhood and educational experiences related to multilingualism. The participants reported that bilingualism supported their relationships with family and friends; increased access to hobbies, education, and employment opportunities; provided them with feelings of increased self-efficacy; improved self-confidence and assurance regarding social interactions; and assisted with a stronger understanding of themselves and others. Lim and Charlop (2018) found that interventions for children identified with autism had stronger outcomes when the intervention was provided in their heritage language. Although there are limitations to providing multilingual services in school settings due to provider language fluency and school-based language acquisition programming, incorporating the native language into school-based services can be beneficial; however, it is currently rarely conducted (Lim & Charlop, 2018). Providers should consider advocacy and awareness-building regarding the benefits of multilingualism and the provision of multilingual services as one of their key, critical roles.

Cultural Considerations Pertaining to Multilingual Families with Autism

Culture and language are intersectional, complex phenomena that influence behaviors, values, and ideals (Birukou et al., 2013). As culture is often expressed through language, these two concepts are aligned and important to consider when conducting an autism evaluation. A defining feature of culture is how people communicate and interact with each other (Rathje, 2009), which is also a core aspect of the assessment of social communication within an autism evaluation. Nonverbal communication, such as gesturing, differs across cultures, with cultures pointing with their fingers, nose, and lips. Nonverbal communication, such as eye contact, may also vary by culture, given cultural expectations for how individuals sustain eye contact with adults (Golson et al., 2021). For example, reduced eye contact may be a sign of respect in Native American and East Asian cultures (Akechi et al., 2013; Uono &

Hietanen, 2015). School psychologists must consider the impact of various cultural considerations on the interpretation of autism assessment data.

School psychologists should also be aware of cultural differences regarding first concerns for autism. Families may be more concerned about their child's language delays based on cultural expectations of typically developing behaviors. For example, White caregivers may be more concerned about their child's language delays and verbal communication (Matson et al., 2017), while Latine caregivers may be more concerned about their child's emotional regulation (Ratto et al., 2016). Blacher et al. (2014) found that mothers who identify as Latine and Black report fewer concerns about their child's autism-specific behaviors than White parents. Black parents were least likely to report concerns about social behaviors and restricted and repetitive behaviors, as compared to similar behaviors when reported by White parents (Blacher et al., 2014). These differences in reported concerns may impact the likelihood of obtaining a comprehensive autism evaluation as well as accessing valuable early intervention services.

The stigma of having a child with a disability varies culturally and should be considered an important factor when determining the impact of emotions, social support, and mental health symptoms of caregivers. For example, some families of East Asian descent report feeling shame regarding having a child with a disability based on hurtful comments received by family members and the community. Mothers of children with autism also report experiencing emotions such as shock, fear, despair, and depression following an autism identification (Kim et al., 2024). Some mothers may blame themselves for the child's disability, given their role in pregnancy and caretaking (Kim et al., 2021). Some families report initially denying the autism diagnosis, which may delay important early intervention services (Kim et al., 2024). These considerations may impact a family's openness to an autism evaluation and identification.

A family's understanding of autism may also be culturally derived. Families report that their immigration status and limited understanding of the services in the U.S. impacted accessing medical services, and this led to anxiety and stress for mothers. Different identification results between countries are another area of stress for mothers (Lee & Zhu, 2021). Cultural differences in the educational and medical systems of origin and the U.S. may also pose challenges for families. Families report having difficulty navigating these systems, participating in services, and being advocates for their children based on their unfamiliarity with the U.S. systems. Chinese parents reported feeling intimidated by the U.S. educational system, referring to it as too big and complicated (Hauwadhanasuk, 2020). These diverse cultural considerations will impact autism service provision, access, identification, and acceptance of the identification.

Assessment of Multilingual Children for Autism

Although there have been some positive trends in earlier and more culturally responsive autism identification practices in the U.S., disparities continue to exist and can contribute to misidentification or delayed autism identification. Utilizing culturally and linguistically responsive practices will ultimately increase understanding and family engagement in future services, thus improving the outcomes of the assessment processes. Below, we outline the main components of autism identification practices and how providers can integrate culturally and linguistically responsive practices when assessing multilingual students for autism. While this chapter focuses on the assessment of autism, providers should also consider the presence of aligned disabilities and health challenges that may share symptoms with autism (e.g., anxiety, sleep disorders, attentional concerns, trauma).

Interviews

Given the limitations of traditional standardized testing of autism among multilingual populations, providers will benefit from conducting a comprehensive family interview process that foundationally focuses on relationship-building with families, as well as obtaining important information about cultural and linguistic considerations throughout. Obtaining information from families is crucial to evaluating culturally and linguistically minoritized students for autism, particularly given the identification requirements pertaining to language development. Ideally, existing information will be collected prior to the interview and integrated to avoid redundancy.

During the family interview, school psychologists should first focus on obtaining information about a child's strengths and a family's hopes and dreams for their child (Mapp & Kuttner, 2013). Throughout the interview, providers can assure families that aspects of their cultural and linguistic identity are assets and are important aspects of a child's identity. School psychologists can learn strengths and concerns from the family perspective, understand the family's perception of developmental differences, and examine challenges displayed in the home or other settings. Interviewers will also want to get a detailed history about language exposure and history that spans home and educational settings. If the student has resided and received education in another country, in addition to asking about these experiences, school psychologists can gather language proficiency information and determine current linguistic abilities in all languages (Monsrud et al., 2019).

If the student had received an early or other intervention service, it is important to learn about the language(s) the interventionist used and how well the student responded to the service. It is also important to consider the family composition when determining who to invite to the interview. People should be invited to the family interview depending on their relationship with the child, which may not align with traditional roles (e.g., grandparent, older sibling).

Additional questions should be integrated depending on the experiences of the family. For newly immigrated families, Elizalde-Utnick and Romero (2017) recommend qualitatively assessing the family and the student's level of acculturation and the utilized acculturation strategies (i.e., integration, assimilation, separation, or marginalization). The authors also suggested collecting information regarding the community's culture(s) and demographics, the alignment level between family and community culture, and the opportunities and supports using the primary and secondary languages in the community (Elizalde-Utnick & Romero, 2017). Additionally, the authors recommended looking up specific interview questions in Rhodes et al. (2005) and lists of acculturation instruments reviewed and outlined by Taras (2007), Collier et al. (2007) as well as Romero and Branscome (2014). See Dennison et al. (2019) for additional interview questions related to distinguishing differences in patterns of communication and behaviors among multilingual learners.

Conducting interviews with multiple different people (i.e., caregivers, teachers, and the student) will add important pieces of contextual information to the evaluation. Through a teacher interview, school psychologists learn about the student's academic and behavioral strengths and concerns from the teacher's perspective. Teachers should consider using peer comparisons of students (i.e., multilingual students with those from a similar cultural and linguistic background), given the challenge of comparing multilingual children to their monolingual peers. English language acquisition teachers are especially beneficial informants, given their expertise in language acquisition and their training and experience teaching multilingual students. Physical education teachers may also provide unique perspectives, given the setting that focuses on group dynamics and traditionally noisy environments. Caregivers such as those in daycare settings or after-school programs may also give unique perspectives, given the differential expectations in these settings. School psychologists should also consider interviewing students themselves since they are the ones who navigate day-to-day life and experience social-emotional difficulties firsthand. For multilingual learners, providers might integrate questions that assess whether the student perceives their language proficiency as hindering social functioning, how their social motivation intersects with the use of language, and any social challenges they hope to overcome.

The method and environment of the interview should also be considered prior to the interview. Families may have demands on their time that need to be considered when scheduling an interview. For example, families may have other children to care for, job demands, or transportation challenges. Schools should recognize these potential barriers and modify traditional practices to accommodate the needs of families. This may include offering a meeting at a more convenient location (e.g., a local library), in-home meetings, transportation support (e.g., providing public transportation passes), and welcoming siblings and other family members or advocates to all meetings. Multilingual families will also commonly benefit from interpretation services during interviews; thus, readers are encouraged to review Chap. 9, which focuses on this topic.

Many school districts send an electronic interview form for families to complete prior to a family meeting. School psychologists must consider how this information will be understood and completed for multilingual families. For example, families with limited English proficiency may understandably struggle to answer questions, and the data collected may be limited in scope. Alternatively, families may ask children or others with advanced English proficiency to complete the forms, which may also lead to concerns regarding the validity of the information collected by the informant and their relationship and knowledge of the targeted information. All forms and communication provided to the family should be translated into the family's native language. School psychologists need to consider that some families may be asked to complete forms provided at an advanced reading level (including in their native language) and may also not provide valid information depending on the reading abilities of families. Families can be offered the option to conduct an interview in person through an oral interview process, which is also ideal for relationship building, although, in some situations, it may not be conducted in a standardized format. Providers must document any changes to standardization and consider whether reporting scores is appropriate, given their alignment with the standardization sample. Structured interviews may also limit relationship building, and a more casual conversation that covers important concepts may feel more appropriate to some families and provide more robust information for school teams.

Record Review

Family advocacy and relationship building are integral to robust services for multilingual children with autism. When school professionals request educational or health records, some families may be unsure about the need for requested documents and information or how they will be utilized. It is important to remind families of their rights (e.g., U.S. Department of Education Dear Colleague Letter, 2025) as well as provide information about educational services and disability identification more broadly.

One of the most important considerations pertaining to record keeping is the need to ensure robust documentation of communication and share this communication with the necessary providers. Schools often have multiple providers that are working with families, and these providers must have methods for efficiently sharing necessary family information to optimize educational services. In addition, other school services (e.g., multi-tiered system of supports processes and intervention data, English language acquisition plans, gifted and talented identification information) should be collected, shared, and disseminated appropriately.

Immigrant multilingual children and families may have educational or health records from other countries. These records will likely need to be translated into English and can provide helpful information regarding prior services and facilitate potential transitions to school services in the U.S. Obtaining these records and translating them appropriately will provide greater context to support a child's educational experience. It is critical to review all documents that are relevant to the student's development before the interview. For multilingual students, it is particularly imperative to review information regarding their language proficiency and language environment(s) through all possible sources (e.g., Home Language Survey, assessments of language proficiency, portfolios, and writing or work samples in English and in their native language). The home language survey often provides school psychologists with information such as the primary language usage in the home, the student's preferred language across settings, as well as the history of language acquisition. This information will help school psychologists understand the language profile of the students and their families, which can help determine methods for evaluation planning as well as beneficial interpreter and translator collaborations.

School Observation

School observation is an essential component of the autism evaluation and will offer a plethora of qualitative and quantitative data regarding the student's language development and behavioral and social-emotional functioning. To evaluate a multilingual student who is suspected of autism, school psychologists should not only record symptoms that may align with an identification of autism but also pay attention to the student's use of native language and English in social and academically demanding situations (Elizalde-Utnick & Romero, 2017). Compared to clinical settings, observation conducted in school offers more opportunities to observe the student in different contexts, including formal (e.g., classroom) and informal settings (e.g., playground, cafeteria), as well as social interaction with peers, teachers, and other adults. During observations, school psychologists can record information such as verbal (e.g., speech) and nonverbal communicative behaviors (e.g., eye contact, use of gestures and body language, and facial expressions). When the student is engaging with peers, school psychologists can document the pattern and quality of social-emotional reciprocity, such as initiating conversation with others, maintaining a reciprocal conversation, and responding to others' leads or prompts appropriately. Additional information about restricted and repetitive behaviors (e.g., fixated interests, repetitive motor movements, and insistence on sameness) and sensory interests (e.g., hyper- or hypo-reactivity to pain, temperature, and light) should be kept on file and can often be collected regardless of language ability. See Dennison et al. (2019) for more observational strategies related to distinguishing differences in patterns of communication and behaviors among multilingual learners.

Autism-Specific Rating Scales and Tools

Autism assessment falls into two main categories: screening and diagnostic/identification tools. There are two steps involved in developmental screening: (1) screening for general developmental progress (e.g., the Ages and Stages Questionnaire, Third Edition [ASQ-3; Squires & Bricker, 2009]) and (2) if indicators were found after the general screening or parents raised autism-related concerns, administration of a specific autism screening tool (e.g., the Modified Checklist for Autism in Toddlers—Revised with Follow-Up [M-CHAT-R; Robins et al., 2014]) is administered to collect more in-depth information about parental concerns. If a child is identified as at-risk by the autism screening tool, it is recommended that they are referred to specialists (e.g., psychologists or developmental pediatricians) for further evaluation. While a child is waiting to receive a comprehensive autism evaluation or following this process, they can be referred to local early intervention providers (if under age 3) or local school districts (if age 3 and above) to receive an educational determination of a disability (Schwartz & Davis, 2014). An educational determination of autism is led by a team of school professionals and the student's caregivers to determine eligibility for special education services. When assessing for the educational identification of autism, school professionals must demonstrate significant educational impact of the disability. For this reason, not all children who have a medical diagnosis of autism will qualify with an educational identification of autism.

Developmental screening is an essential component of early autism identification, which allows providers and caregivers to monitor the child's development and centers the discussion on potential developmental concerns. With more efforts put into developmental screening and early intervention (EI) referral, 63% of pediatricians reported using autism screening tools, and on average, 59% of their at-risk patients received EI referrals in 2016, which is about three times, and one and a half times, respectively, higher compared to 2002 (Lipkin et al., 2020). Considering these positive trends and better alignment with the recommended practices from the American Academy of Pediatrics that all children should be screened for autism at ages 18 and 24 months (Hyman et al., 2020), disparities in autism identification across racial and ethnic groups have seemed to reduce over time (Maenner et al., 2023; Pham et al., 2022). Despite the increased prevalence of autism identification among minoritized groups, the misuse of screening tools and lack of awareness of the impact of language and cultural differences on children and youth development may impact misidentification or delayed identification (Harris et al., 2014).

In a recent review, Morgan et al. (2023) evaluated the role of the use of the Spanish language in the autism screening process. Their systematic review found limited research on this topic and an extremely small amount of Spanish-translated resources for autism screening in Spanish. Although some assessments underwent a rigorous and culturally-informed translation process, this was not the norm. In addition, methods for translation of autism screeners varied, and the important aspect of test adaptation was not employed by multiple test publishers or authors. Due to limited information provided by test publishers and authors, multiple assessments did not have sufficient psychometric information. Thus, limited information is available about their potential appropriateness for Latine populations. The authors concluded that language and sociocultural differences impacted communication within healthcare settings and could ultimately impact disability identification and services (Morgan et al., 2023). Autism screeners available in languages other than English and Spanish are extremely limited, although more autism screeners are translated into other languages than diagnostic autism-specific identification tools (Harris et al., 2014).

Diagnostic Autism-Specific Identification Tools

Comprehensive assessments of autism are recommended but under-practiced at school. A study found that less than 25% of school psychologists conducting autism evaluations use a comprehensive developmental approach. The comprehensive approach for autism identification assesses multiple domains of a student's functioning (e.g., cognitive, language, adaptive behaviors, core autism symptoms) using rating scales and autism diagnostic tools. Instruments that are commonly used in comprehensive autism evaluation practices include: rating scales (e.g., Autism Spectrum Rating Scale [ASRS], Gilliam Autism Rating Scale, Third Edition [GARS-3]), structured interviews (e.g., Autism Diagnostic Interview-Revised [ADI-R], Monteiro Interview Guidelines for Diagnosing the Autism Spectrum, Second Edition [MIGDAS-2]), and direct observational instruments (e.g., Childhood Autism Rating Scale, Second Edition [CARS-2], Autism Diagnostic Observation Schedule, Second Edition [ADOS-2]; Harris & McClain, 2024). Although many instruments have diversified their norming samples and included culturally diverse populations in recent years, only two of them included multilingual learners (i.e., M-CHAT and SCQ; Harris et al., 2014). The M-CHAT is normed for children 18–30 months of age, thus school psychologists rarely evaluate children in this age range and might have limited use for this assessment. The SCQ is available for children 4 years and older, although there are some considerations for school psychologists. First, the SCQ is for parent respondents only and is considered an autism screener, not a diagnostic assessment. The SCQ has been translated into multiple languages, although it has not been normed in these languages. For a more comprehensive review of autism-specific measures, please see Harris and McClain (2024). There is extremely limited research that has been conducted on the use of comprehensive autism-specific tools with multilingual populations (Harris & McClain, 2024).

During the evaluation process, it is a common practice to collect information through parent-report measures, although this experience can be challenging for families from culturally and linguistically minoritized backgrounds. Literature indicates that the level of acculturation and language proficiency plays a role in autism identification. For example, in a study conducted in Latine communities, participants with low levels of acculturation (as defined by the authors) on average demonstrated less knowledge about autism and perceived more barriers in accessing resources and healthcare services than their counterparts with higher reported acculturation levels (Voelkel et al., 2013). Language barriers reportedly had the same adverse impacts regarding finding resources and navigating the healthcare service system. Studies on Asian families found caregivers who have emerging English proficiency had difficulty understanding the terminology used by medical professionals, question their qualification for enrolling in public services, and lack knowledge about how to interact with medical professionals (Cho et al. 2000; Kim et al., 2021; Wang & Casillas, 2013; You & Rosenkoetter, 2014).

To reduce the impact of language barriers in the autism screening and diagnostic assessment processes and make tools more accessible to multilingual respondents, some tools are translated and administered in the respondent's native or preferred language. In a study conducted by Morgan et al. (2023), the authors systematically reviewed 22 studies from six countries (e.g., United States, Latin America, and European countries) to strengthen the understanding of autism screening practices in the Spanish language and evaluate the cultural context of autism identification measures. Although each translated measure comes with unique weaknesses when evaluating multilingual populations, with careful and appropriate administration, many of them showed strong discriminant validity to differentiate individuals with autism from typically developing peers. The authors found that using a translated version of autism instruments not only increases validity in assessing culturally and linguistically minoritized individuals but also fosters confidence in responding. For example, researchers asked fluent speakers of either English, Mandarin, or Bahasa Malaysia (the official language of Malaysia) to complete a translated autism measure in their native language. The researchers found that when the participants were provided the measure in their native language, they expressed more confidence in their answers, and they were more likely to respond with strong and explicit answers (Chee & de Vries, 2022). Translation methods themselves were also found to influence participant responses. DuBay et al. (2022) studied 380 Spanish-speaking caregivers in the United States. The participants were randomly assigned to complete an autism screening tool that had been translated via a forward-back Spanish translation method or an autism screening tool that had undergone rigorous translation methods with cultural adaptation. The authors found that the two tools were psychometrically dissimilar, which indicates that caregivers interpreted and responded to the same questions differently, depending on the screening tool they completed. Specifically, they found that participants of the forward-back translation group were more likely to choose extreme responses (either "always" or "never") than the cultural adaptation methods group. This study highlights the psychometric complexity of translation methods and their impact on participant responses.

Assessing Social Communication

Differences in social communication and social interaction are a defining feature of autism identification. However, when school psychologists assess multilingual students, they may find it hard to discern whether social differences are a core feature of autism or an indication of language proficiency. The American Speech-Language-Hearing Association's (ASHA, 2004) guidelines for the assessment of bilingual children state that, in addition to language use, language proficiency should be measured in each language. Assessing social communication using a two-language approach has been found to provide a more accurate reflection of language skills than single-language assessments (e.g., Core et al., 2013; Peña et al., 2016). In typical language development for multilingual children, children are expected to have a smaller vocabulary in each language, but the sum of the two should equal or surpass a monolingual speaker (Herrera & Murry, 2011). In addition, since multilingual children are exposed to more than one language, the speech complexity of a second language may be different from their first language. When multilingual children speak their second language, they may use less advanced sentence structure or have more grammatical errors in their speech. Moreover, speech characteristics such as using a flat tone may be displayed in students with autism and also found in multilingual students whose native language is syllable-timed rather than stress-timed. For example, students whose first language is Chinese may exhibit irregular rhythm and less varied intonation when speaking English (Wu, 2019). Therefore, it is beneficial to assess communication in the native language as well as the second language and note the discrepancy in language acquisition between the two, as well as the specific characteristics (i.e., intonation, volume, rhythm, and rate) of their speech. A disability will not occur in only one language, and a comprehensive evaluation will aim to understand the whole child—including a holistic view of their language abilities.

There are numerous examples of social communication characteristics that must be considered with culture and language when interpreting autism assessment data. For example, idiosyncratic speech can be found in both students with autism and multilingual learners, although the nature and quality of this speech will be distinct. Multilingual students may mix up pronouns and generate novel words or phrases (also referred to as "interlanguage"; Ellis, 2008) as a normative part of their language acquisition processes (Dennison et al., 2019). Bilingual students without autism may use these stereotyped phrases less repetitively, in a more flexible manner, and are understandable within the context. Nonverbal communication can vary greatly by culture, which can be challenging for school psychologists to assess and interpret. Golson et al. (2021) summarized cultural differences in social communication and interaction and noted that different cultures may have preferences in eye contact, interpersonal space during interaction, and gestures. For example, compared to using the index finger to gesture "pointing," some other cultures also point with their lips, nose, and chin (Golson et al., 2021). An international study revealed that people from individualistic cultures (e.g., United States, Denmark, Australia) were found to be more emotionally expressive than the collectivism group (e.g., Indonesia, Hong Kong, Russia; Matsumoto et al., 2008). Engaging in social communication can be challenging for both multilingual children with autism and multilingual children who are being asked to speak in a language of emerging proficiency. Multilingual children, as well as children with autism, can be timid in social situations, offer limited information when questioned, or ask minimal follow-up questions. These are all common communication characteristics of multilingual learners (Dennison et al., 2019). It is important to collect social communication data across settings, conduct the assessment in the student's native and second languages involving interpreters who share similar cultural backgrounds, and have extensive input from families to understand the student's quality of social communication and language history.

Implications for Practice

There are numerous implications for practice when conducting culturally and linguistically responsive autism assessments. First, it is important to engage in interprofessional collaboration, as this can improve numerous outcomes for multilingual learners (McClain et al., 2021). School psychologists are required to participate in multidisciplinary collaboration per IDEA, although interprofessional collaboration expands beyond multidisciplinary collaboration to include other service providers in health and community contexts. Given the commonly aligned challenges with autism (e.g., nutrition, sleep), interprofessional collaboration aims to better align and reinforce the various services to maximize various outcomes for the children and family (McClain et al., 2021). School psychologists can consider collaborating with various healthcare providers such as family navigators, interventionists, providers, and specialists. There are various other community partners that are strong collaborators, such as early intervention staff, community providers, agencies, and advocacy groups. School psychologists should also have a strong understanding of professional associations and their family advocacy resources, as well as community resources such as support groups and family meet-ups. Families should be seen as central to all collaboration efforts, and promoting their engagement through relationship-building and promoting the assets of multilingualism will be beneficial.

In the school context in particular, when assessing a multilingual child for autism, school psychologists will benefit from increasing their collaboration with English language acquisition teachers and speech-language pathologists in particular. English language acquisition teachers develop language development plans and regularly compare peers with similar language histories. Speech-language pathologists generally have the most training pertaining to language acquisition compared to other school staff and can strongly inform linguistically responsive assessment techniques. Many schools often employ a community liaison position who may have a strong relationship with the family and should be considered part of the multidisciplinary team.

Given the limitations of using standardized tools to evaluate for autism, obtaining significant qualitative information should be a strong focus for school psychologists. The most important aspect of the assessment process is the family interview. For multilingual learners, a comprehensive family interview that covers cultural and linguistic contexts must be robust and will inform future assessment practices. When conducting assessments with families, school psychologists can consider asking them if assessment materials recognize and align with their culture and language, as well as their experiences. During the interview process with multilingual families, it is likely that school psychologists will collaborate with interpreters. Please see Chap. 9 for a comprehensive review of important considerations when working with interpreters.

School psychologists should also consider how data is interpreted throughout the assessment process. For example, school psychologists must consider the potential impacts of culture and language throughout the assessment selection process. It is more important that school psychologists understand the characteristics of autism and not rely on particular scores for potential identification. If using standardized scores, school psychologists should consider if cultural or linguistic aspects could have influenced these scores and how the information should be interpreted if so. For the multilingual population, it is possible that the use of standardized scores is not preferable or accurate, and other ratings are superior (e.g., using the confidence interval or qualitative ranges (i.e., above average). In an autism evaluation, providing standard scores in a psychoeducational report is not required for identification, and school psychologists must consider the implications of providing standard scores when their validity is in question.

Implications for Training

The most recent NASP membership survey of school psychologists indicated that 92% of participants reported they are monolingual. A total of 12% of participants reported that they provide services in a second language, and a total of 24 unique languages were reported (Goforth et al., 2021). Although the percentage of bilingual school psychologists has increased over the past decades, the vast majority of school psychologists continue to be monolingual and do not reflect the linguistic diversity of the U.S.

The age of children evaluated by school psychologists may influence their knowledge of autism. School psychologists who work with younger children (i.e., 3–5 years) reported having more autism assessment experience than those who worked with children at older ages (Aiello et al., 2017). Researchers gave school psychology graduate students the Autism Spectrum Knowledge Scale Professional Version (ASKSP) to obtain autism knowledge and were asked about their self-perceived autism knowledge and clinical skill competencies with children and families with autism. The results demonstrate that, in general, graduate students have many limitations regarding autism knowledge and self-perceived competencies.

The researchers found a positive trend toward obtaining more knowledge and competencies throughout their graduate program, although there are multiple areas where increased training and professional development are needed, most notably in the area of providing assessment and intervention services to culturally and linguistically minoritized populations with autism (Harris et al., 2020).

There continue to be few training programs for bilingual school psychologists, although these programs have been increasing in numbers over the past two decades in particular. To provide culturally and linguistically responsive services, bilingual school psychologists must receive training in the provision of bilingual school psychology services. We acknowledge that bilingual school psychologists should have advanced training related to concepts such as language acquisition, family partnerships, and equitable assessment interpretation, and not solely a command of another language. More training for graduate students and practicing school psychologists is needed to improve access to bilingual school psychology services (Harris et al., 2021).

School psychology graduate programs should integrate more content pertaining to autism, particularly given the increasing prevalence of the disability. More professional learning opportunities on this topic should also be provided to practicing school psychologists. These training opportunities must integrate information pertaining to cultural and linguistically responsive autism assessment among multilingual learners and their families. School districts can evaluate their interpretation and translation processes and current practices for family-centered communication to improve equitable practices. Most importantly, school psychologists must be trained to view their role as a family advocate for all populations, and that advancing equity is foundational to the role of the school psychologist.

References

Abdullahi, I., Leonard, H., Cherian, S., Mutch, R., Glasson, E. J., de Klerk, N., & Downs, J. (2018). The risk of neurodevelopmental disabilities in children of immigrant and refugee parents: Current knowledge and directions for future research. *Review Journal of Autism and Developmental Disorders, 5*, 29–42.

Aiello, R., Ruble, L., & Esler, A. (2017). National study of school psychologists' use of evidence-based assessment in autism spectrum disorder. *Journal of Applied School Psychology, 33*(1), 67–88. https://doi.org/10.1080/15377903.2016.1236307

Akechi, H., Kikuchi, Y., Tojo, Y., Osanai, H., & Hasegawa, T. (2013). Brief report: Pointing cues facilitate word learning in children with autism spectrum disorder. *Journal of Autism and Developmental Disorders, 43*, 230–235.

American Speech-Language-Hearing Association. (2004). Preferred practice patterns for the profession of speech-language pathology. https://doi.org/10.1044/policy.PP2004-00191.

Anne E. Casey Foundation. (2024). Children who speak a language other than English at home in United States. Retrieved from https://datacenter.aecf.org/data/tables/81-children-who-speak-a-language-other-than-english-at-home#detailed/1/any/false/2545,1095,2048,1729,37,871,870,573,869,36/any/396,397.

Augereau, N., Lagdas, I., Kermarrec, S., Gicquel, L., Martin, V., Xavier, J., Cohen, D., Bouvet, M., Rolland, A. C., & Tordjman, S. (2020). Premigration social adversity and autism spectrum disorder. *BJPsych Open, 6*(5), e92. https://doi.org/10.1192/bjo.2020.56

Aylward, B. S., Gal-Szabo, D. E., & Taraman, S. (2021). Racial, ethnic, and sociodemographic disparities in diagnosis of children with autism spectrum disorder. *Journal of Developmental and Behavioral Pediatrics, 42*(8), 682–689. https://doi.org/10.1097/DBP.0000000000000996

Bailey, A. L., & Kelly, K. R. (2010). The use and validity of home language surveys in state English language proficiency assessment systems: A review and issues perspective. *Evaluating the Validity of English Language Proficiency Assessment*. EVEA. Retrieved from https://edcount.com/wp-content/uploads/2020/10/Bailey-Kelly-HLS-EVEA-white-paper-July-2010-revised-Jan-2011and-Sept-2011.pdf

Bal, A., Betters-Bubon, J., & Fish, R. E. (2019). A multilevel analysis of statewide disproportionality in exclusionary discipline and the identification of emotional disturbance. *Education and Urban Society, 51*(2), 247–268.

Becerra, T. A., von Ehrenstein, O. S., Heck, J. E., Olsen, J., Arah, O. A., Jeste, S. S., Rodriguez, M., & Ritz, B. (2014). Autism spectrum disorders and race, ethnicity, and nativity: A population-based study. *Pediatrics, 134*(1), e63–e71.

Bialystok, E., & Werker, J. F. (2017). The systematic effects of bilingualism on children's development. *Developmental Science, 20*(1). https://doi.org/10.1111/desc.12535

Birukou, A., Blanzieri, E., Giorgini, P., & Giunchiglia, F. (2013). A formal definition of culture. *Models for Intercultural Collaboration and Negotiation*, 1–26.

Blacher, J., Cohen, S. R., & Azad, G. (2014). In the eye of the beholder: Reports of autism symptoms by Anglo and Latino mothers. *Research in Autism Spectrum Disorders, 8*(12), 1648–1656.

Chee, Z. J., & De Vries, M. (2022). Language matters: The autism-spectrum quotient in English, Mandarin and Bahasa Malaysia. *Journal of Autism and Developmental Disorders, 52*(9), 3814–3824. https://doi.org/10.1007/s10803-021-05253-9

Cho, S. -J., Singer, G. H. S., & Brenner, M. (Betsy). (2000). Adaptation and accommodation to young children with disabilities: A comparison of Korean and Korean American parents. *Topics in Early Childhood Special Education, 20*(4), 236–249.

Collier, C., Brice, A. E., & Oades-Sese, G. V. (2007). Assessment of acculturation. In G. B. Esquivel, E. C. Lopez, & S. Nahari (Eds.), *Handbook of multicultural school psychology: An interdisciplinary perspective* (pp. 353–380). Lawrence Erlbaum.

Constantino, J. N., Abbacchi, A. M., Saulnier, C., Klaiman, C., Mandell, D. S., Zhang, Y., Hawks, Z., Bates, J., Klin, A., Shattuck, P., Molholm, S., Fitzgerald, R., Roux, A., Lowe, J. K., & Geschwind, D. H. (2020). Timing of the diagnosis of autism in African American children. *Pediatrics, 146*(3), 1–9.

Core, C., Hoff, E., Rumiche, R., & Señor, M. (2013). Total and conceptual vocabulary in Spanish-English bilinguals from 22 to 30 months: Implications for assessment. *Journal of Speech, Language, and Hearing Research, 56*(5), 1637–1649. https://doi.org/10.1044/1092-4388(2013/11-0044)

Dennison, A., Hall, S. P., Leal, J., & Madres, D. A. (2019). ASD or ELL? Distinguishing differences in patterns of communication and behavior. *Contemporary School Psychology, 23*(1), 57–67. https://doi.org/10.1007/s40688-018-0206-x

Drysdale, H., van der Meer, L., & Kagohara, D. (2015). Children with autism spectrum disorder from bilingual families: A systematic review. *Review Journal of Autism and Developmental Disorders, 2*, 26–38.

DuBay, M., Sideris, J., & Rouch, E. (2022). Is traditional back translation enough? Comparison of translation methodology for an ASD screening tool. *Autism Research, 15*(10), 1868–1882. https://doi.org/10.1002/aur.2783

Elizalde-Utnick, G., & Romero, P. A. (2017). Assessment of English language learners. In E. C. Lopez, S. G. Nahari, & S. Proctor (Eds.), *Handbook of multicultural school psychology: An interdisciplinary perspective* (2nd ed.). Routledge. https://doi.org/10.4324/9780203754948

Ellis, N. C. (2008). The dynamics of second language emergence: Cycles of language use, language change, and language acquisition. *The Modern Language Journal, 92*(2), 232–249.
Every Student Succeeds Act, 20 U.S.C. § 6301. (2015). Retrieved from https://www.congress.gov/bill/114th-congress/senate-bill/1177.
Fadus, M. C., Ginsburg, K. R., Sobowale, K., Halliday-Boykins, C. A., Bryant, B. E., Gray, K. M., & Squeglia, L. M. (2020). Unconscious bias and the diagnosis of disruptive behavior disorders and ADHD in African American and Hispanic youth. *Academic Psychiatry: The Journal of the American Association of Directors of Psychiatric Residency Training and the Association for Academic Psychiatry, 44*(1), 95–102. https://doi.org/10.1007/s40596-019-01127-6
Gilhuber, C. S., Raulston, T. J., & Galley, K. (2023). Language and communication skills in multilingual children on the autism spectrum: A systematic review. *Autism, 27*(6), 1516–1531.
Goforth, A. N., Farmer, R. L., Kim, S. Y., Naser, S. C., Lockwood, A. B., & Affrunti, N. W. (2021). Status of school psychology in 2020: Part 1, demographics of the NASP membership survey. *NASP Research Reports, 5*(2), 1–17.
Golson, M. E., Haverkamp, C. R., McClain, M. B., Schwartz, S. E., Ha, J., Harris, B., & Benallie, K. J. (2021). Influences of student race/ethnicity and gender on autism special education classification considerations. *Autism, 26*(6), 1423–1435. https://doi.org/10.1177/13623613211050440
Hall-Lande, J., Esler, A. N., Hewitt, A., & Gunty, A. L. (2021). Age of initial identification of autism spectrum disorder in a diverse urban sample. *Journal of Autism and Developmental Disorders, 51*(3), 798–803. https://doi.org/10.1007/s10803-018-3763-y
Harris, B., Barton, E. E., & Albert, C. (2014). Evaluating autism diagnostic and screening tools for cultural and linguistic responsiveness. *Journal of Autism and Developmental Disorders, 44*(6), 1275–1287. https://doi.org/10.1007/s10803-013-1991-8
Harris, B., & McClain, M. (2024). Best practices in school-based autism assessment and identification. In P. Harrison, A. Thomas, & S. Proctor (Eds.), *Best practices in school psychology*. National Association of School Psychologists.
Harris, B., McClain, M. B., Schwartz, S., & Haverkamp, C. R. (2020). Knowledge of autism spectrum disorder among school psychology graduate students. *Contemporary School Psychology, 24*(2), 239–247. https://doi.org/10.1007/s40688-019-00266-9
Harris, B., Vega, D., Peterson, L. S., & Newell, K. W. (2021). Critical issues in the training of bilingual school psychologists. *Contemporary School Psychology, 25*(3), 273–287.
Hauwadhanasuk, T. (2020). *Advocacy of Chinese-speaking families for the education of their children with autism Spectrum disorder*. Doctoral dissertation, Saint Louis University.
Herrera, S. G., & Murry, K. G. (2011). *Mastering ESL and bilingual methods* (2nd ed.). Pearson Education.
Howard, K. B., Katsos, N., & Gibson, J. L. (2019). The school experiences of bilingual children on the autism spectrum: An interpretative phenomenological analysis. *Research in Developmental Disabilities, 87*, 9–20.
Howard, K. B., Katsos, N., & Gibson, J. L. (2021). Practitioners' perspectives and experiences of supporting bilingual pupils on the autism spectrum in two linguistically different educational settings. *British Educational Research Journal, 47*(2), 427–449.
Hyman, S. L., Levy, S. E., Myers, S. M., & Council on Children with Disabilities, Section on Developmental and Behavioral Pediatrics. (2020). Identification, evaluation, and management of children with autism spectrum disorder. *Pediatrics, 145*(1), e20193447. https://doi.org/10.1542/peds.2019-3447
Kim, H., Kim, S. A., Lee, H., & Dodds, R. (2024). Korean immigrant mothers and the journey to autism diagnosis and services for their child in the United States. *Journal of Autism and Developmental Disorders, 54*(12), 4624–4636.
Kim, I., Wang, Y., Dababnah, S., & Betz, G. (2021). East Asian American parents of children with autism: A scoping review. *Review Journal of Autism and Developmental Disorders, 8*(3), 312–320. https://doi.org/10.1007/s40489-020-00221-y
Lee, B. K., Eyles, D. W., Magnusson, C., Newschaffer, C. J., McGrath, J. J., Kvaskoff, D., Ko, P., Dalman, C., Karlsson, H., & Gardner, R. M. (2021). Developmental vitamin D and autism

spectrum disorders: findings from the Stockholm Youth Cohort. *Molecular Psychiatry, 26*(5), 1578–1588.

Lee, R., & Zhu, Y. (2021). Diagnosis as a sociocultural practice: Critical personal narratives of Asian immigrant mothers with Autism-Spectrum Disorder children in Canada. *Disability & Society, 36*(10), 1643–1662.

Lim, N., & Charlop, M. H. (2018). Effects of English versus heritage language on play in bilingually exposed children with autism spectrum disorder. *Behavioral Interventions, 33*(4), 339–351.

Lipkin, P. H., Macias, M. M., Baer Chen, B., Coury, D., Gottschlich, E. A., Hyman, S. L., Sisk, B., Wolfe, A., & Levy, S. E. (2020). Trends in pediatricians' developmental screening: 2002-2016. *Pediatrics, 145*(4), e20190851. https://doi.org/10.1542/peds.2019-0851

Maenner, M. J., Warren, Z., Williams, A. R., Amoakohene, E., Bakian, A. V., Bilder, D. A., Durkin, M. S., Fitzgerald, R. T., Furnier, S. M., Hughes, M. M., Ladd-Acosta, C. M., McArthur, D., Pas, E. T., Salinas, A., Vehorn, A., Williams, S., Esler, A., Grzybowski, A., Hall-Lande, J., … Shaw, K. A. (2023). Prevalence and characteristics of autism spectrum disorder among children aged 8 years—Autism and developmental disabilities monitoring network, 11 sites, United States, 2020. *Morbidity and Mortality Weekly Report. Surveillance Summaries (Washington, D.C.: 2002), 72*(2), 1–14. https://doi.org/10.15585/mmwr.ss7202a1.

Magnusson, C., Rai, D., Goodman, A., Lundberg, M., Idring, S., Svensson, A., Koupil, I., Serlachius, E., & Dalman, C. (2012). Migration and autism spectrum disorder: population-based study. *The British Journal of Psychiatry, 201*(2), 109–115.

Makrygianni, M. K., & Reed, P. (2010). A meta-analytic review of the effectiveness of behavioural early intervention programs for children with autistic spectrum disorders. *Research in Autism Spectrum Disorders, 4*(4), 577–593.

Mapp, K. L., & Kuttner, P. J. (2013). *Partners in education: A dual capacity-building framework for family-school partnerships*. SEDL.

Matson, J. L., Matheis, M., Burns, C. O., Esposito, G., Venuti, P., Pisula, E., Misiak, A., Kalyva, E., Tsakiris, V., Kamio, Y., Ishitobi, M., & Goldin, R. (2017). Examining cross-cultural differences in autism spectrum disorder: A multinational comparison from Greece, Italy, Japan, Poland, and the United States. *European Psychiatry, 42*, 70–76.

Matsumoto, D., Yoo, S. H., & Fontaine, J. (2008). Mapping expressive differences around the world: The relationship between emotional display rules and individualism versus collectivism. *Journal of Cross-Cultural Psychology, 39*(1), 55–74.

McClain, M. B., Harris, B., Schwartz, S. E., & Golson, M. E. (2021). Differential item and test functioning of the autism spectrum rating scales: A follow-up evaluation in a diverse, nonclinical sample. *Journal of Psychoeducational Assessment, 39*(2). https://doi.org/10.1177/0734282920945529

Monsrud, M., Rydland, V., Geva, E., Thurmann-Moe, A. C., & Lyster, S. H. (2019). The advantages of jointly considering first and second language vocabulary skills among emergent bilingual children. *International Journal of Bilingual Education and Bilingualism, 25*(1), 42–58. https://doi.org/10.1080/13670050.2019.1624685

Morgan, C. H., Abdul-Chani, M., Sherrod, G. M., King, K. P., & Guest, K. C. (2023). The influence of Spanish language on autism spectrum disorder screening: A systematic review. *International Journal of Developmental Disabilities, 70*(8), 1343–1366. https://doi.org/10.1080/20473869.2023.2193490

National Center for Education Statistics (NCES). (2024, May). English learners in public schools. Retrieved from https://nces.ed.gov/programs/coe/indicator/cgf/english-learners

Nolte, K., Fletcher-Watson, S., Sorace, A., Stanfield, A., & Digard, B. G. (2021). Perspectives and experiences of autistic multilingual adults: A qualitative analysis. *Autism in Adulthood, 3*(4), 310–319.

Office of English Language Acquisition (OELA). (2024). The economic benefits of multilingualism. Retrieved from https://ncela.ed.gov/sites/default/files/2024-07/econbenefitsmultilingualism-508.pdf

Peña, E. D., Bedore, L. M., & Kester, E. S. (2016). Assessment of language impairment in bilingual children using semantic tasks: Two languages classify better than one. *International Journal of Language & Communication Disorders, 51*(2), 192–202.

Pham, H. H., Sandberg, N., Trinkl, J., & Thayer, J. (2022). Racial and ethnic differences in rates and age of diagnosis of autism spectrum disorder. *JAMA Network Open, 5*(10), e2239604. https://doi.org/10.1001/jamanetworkopen.2022.39604

Primo, P., Weber, C., Posada De la Paz, M., Fellinger, J., Dirmhirn, A., & Holzinger, D. (2020). Explaining age at autism spectrum diagnosis in children with migrant and non-migrant background in Austria. *Brain Sciences, 10*(7), 448.

Rathje, S. (2009). The definition of culture: An application-oriented overhaul. *Online-Zeitschrift für interkulturelle Studien, 8*(8), 35–58.

Ratto, A. B., Reznick, J. S., & Turner-Brown, L. (2016). Cultural effects on the diagnosis of autism spectrum disorder among Latinos. *Focus on Autism and Other Developmental Disabilities, 31*(4), 275–283.

Rhodes, R. L., Ochoa, S. H., & Ortiz, S. O. (2005). *Assessing culturally and linguistically diverse students: A practical guide*. Guilford Press.

Rivard, M., Millau, M., Magnan, C., Mello, C., & Boulé, M. (2019). Snakes and ladders: Barriers and facilitators experienced by immigrant families when accessing an autism spectrum disorder diagnosis. *Journal of Developmental and Physical Disabilities, 31*, 519–539.

Robins, D. L., Barton, M., & Fein, D. (2014). *Modified checklist for autism in toddlers, revised with follow-up (M-CHAT-R/F)* [Database record]. APA PsycTests. https://doi.org/10.1037/t67574-000.

Romero, P. A., & Branscome, J. (2014). Acculturation and sociocognitive factors. In A. B. Clinton (Ed.), *Assessing bilingual children in context: An integrated approach* (pp. 191–214). American Psychological Association. https://doi.org/10.1037/14320-009

Romo, H. D., Thomas, K. J. A., & García, E. E. (2018). Changing demographics of dual language learners and English Learners: Implications for school success. *Social Policy Report, 31*(2), 1–35. https://doi.org/10.1002/j.2379-3988.2018.tb00028.x

Schwartz, I. S., & Davis, C. A. (2014). Best practices in early identification and services for children with Autism Spectrum Disorders. In P. Harrison & A. Thomas (Eds.), *Best practices: Data-based and collaborative decision making* (pp. 417–432). National Association of School Psychologists.

Shahidullah, J. D., Roberts, H., Parkhurst, J., Ballard, R., Mautone, J. A., & Carlson, J. S. (2023). State of the evidence for use of psychotropic medications in school-age youth. *Children, 10*(9), 1454. https://doi.org/10.3390/children10091454

Squires, J., & Bricker, D. (2009). *Ages & Stages Questionnaires®, Third edition (ASQ®-3): A parent-completed child monitoring system*. Paul H. Brookes.

Sullivan, A. L., Kulkarni, T., & Chhuon, V. (2020). Making visible the invisible: Multistudy investigation of disproportionate special education identification of US Asian American and Pacific Islander students. *Exceptional Children, 86*(4), 449–467.

Taras, V. (2007). Instruments for measuring acculturation. Unpublished manuscript, University of Calgary. Retrieved October 1, 2008, from http://ucalgary.ca/~taras/_private/Acculturation_Survey_Catalogue.pdf.

Trelles, M. P., & Castro, K. (2019). Bilingualism in autism spectrum disorder: Finding meaning in translation. *Journal of the American Academy of Child and Adolescent Psychiatry, 58*(11), 1035–1037. https://doi.org/10.1016/j.jaac.2019.05.027

U.S. Department of Education. (2016, November 29). Non-regulatory guidance: English learners and Title III of the Elementary and Secondary Education Act (ESEA), as amended by the Every Child Succeeds Act (ESSA). Retrieved from https://www.ed.gov/sites/ed/files/policy/elsec/leg/essa/essatitleiiiguidenglishlearners92016.pdf

U.S. Department of Education Dear Colleague Letter. (2025, January 8). Dear colleague letter: Resources for ensuring equal access to education for immigrant students. Retrieved from https://

www.ed.gov/laws-and-policy/key-policy-letters/dear-colleague-letter-resources-ensuring-equal-access-education-immigrant-students

Uono, S., & Hietanen, J. K. (2015). Eye contact perception in the west and east: A cross-cultural study. *PLoS One, 10*(2), e0118094.

Vanegas, S. B. (2021). Examining factors related to the age of diagnosis of children with autism spectrum disorder from immigrant and non-immigrant backgrounds in a diverse clinical sample. *Autism Research, 14*(6), 1260–1270.

Voelkel, H., LeCroy, C. W., Williams, L. R., & Holschuh, J. (2013). The full spectrum: Hispanic understanding of autism. *Best Practices in Mental Health: An International Journal, 9*(1), 31–46.

Wang, H.-T., & Casillas, N. (2013). Asian American parents' experiences of raising children with autism: multicultural family perspective. *Journal of Asian & African Studies, 48*(5), 594–606. https://doi.org/10.1177/0021909612467421. Sage.

WIDA ACCESS. (2025). ACCESS for ELLs. Retrieved from https://wida.wisc.edu/assess/accessBal

Wiggins, L. D., Durkin, M., Esler, A., Lee, L. C., Zahorodny, W., Rice, C., Yeargin-Allsopp, M., Dowling, N. F., Hall-Lande, J., Morrier, M. J., Christensen, D., Shenouda, J., & Baio, J. (2020). Disparities in documented diagnoses of autism spectrum disorder based on demographic, individual, and service factors. *Autism Research, 13*(3), 464–473.

Woods, T., & Hanson, D. (2016). *Over half of children of immigrants are bilingual.* The Urban Institute. Retrieved from https://www.urban.org/urban-wire/over-half-children-immigrants-are-bilingual#:~:text=The%20recently%20updated%20Children%20of,other%20than%20English%20at%20home.

Wu, Y. (2019). Review of Chinese English learners' prosodic acquisition. *English Language Teaching, 12*(8), 89–94. https://doi.org/10.5539/elt.v12n8p89

Xu, G., Strathearn, L., Liu, B., & Bao, W. (2018). Prevalence of autism spectrum disorder among US children and adolescents, 2014-2016. *The Journal of the American Medical Association, 319*(1), 81–82.

You, H.-K., & Rosenkoetter, S. E. (2014). Listening to Korean immigrant mothers: meanings of raising a child with a disability. *Multiple Voices for Ethnically Diverse Exceptional Learners, 14*(1), 30–41.

Zuckerman, K., Lindly, O. J., & Chavez, A. E. (2017). Timeliness of autism spectrum disorder diagnosis and use of services among US elementary school-aged children. *Psychiatric Services, 68*(1), 33–40.

Zuckerman, K. E., Sinche, B., Mejia, A., Cobian, M., Becker, T., & Nicolaidis, C. (2014). Latino parents' perspectives on barriers to autism diagnosis. *Academic Pediatrics, 14*(3), 301–308.

Chapter 15
Assessing Emergent Bilingual Students for Dyslexia

Marlene Sotelo-Dynega and Izabela Konopko

The number of emergent bilingual (EB) students enrolled in schools across the United States has increased over the years, with the most recent data indicating approximately 5 million EBs (roughly 10% of the school population; National Center for Education Statistics [NCES], 2024a). Seventy-six percent of EBs speak Spanish, making it the most common home language (NCES, 2024a). Arabic (2.5%), Chinese (1.8), Vietnamese (1.4%), Portuguese (1%), Russian (0.7%), Haitian (0.6%), Hmong (0.6%), and Urdu (0.5%) are among the top ten home languages of EBs as well (NCES, 2024a). Despite the increasing diversity of our nation's public schools, educators and academics continue to debate how to educate and assess the effectiveness of instruction and interventions among our linguistically minoritized students. Often, educators struggle to differentiate whether learning difficulties result from language differences or underlying disorders among this population, which sometimes leads to a referral to the local educational agency's (LEA) Committee on Special Education (CSE; Sullivan & Ball, 2013).

According to the NCES (2024b), the number of students classified as students with a disability under the Individuals with Disabilities Education Act (IDEA, 2004) was 7.5 million, or 15% of students enrolled in our nation's public schools. More specifically, within that 15% of students, 32% were classified as a student with a specific learning disability (SLD), and 19% with a speech or language impairment (SLI; NCES, 2024b). Further, it has been estimated that the number of students who are classified under IDEA with SLD and SLI does not accurately represent the number of children nationally with learning disabilities. According to the most recent edition of the Diagnostic and Statistical Manual of Mental Disorders (DSM), between 5 and 15% of school-aged children have a learning disability, and of that

M. Sotelo-Dynega (✉) · I. Konopko
Department of Psychology, St. John's University, Queens, NY, USA
e-mail: sotelodm@stjohns.edu

D. Vega, J. N. Wolf (eds.), *Culturally and Linguistically Responsive Intervention and Assessment Practices with Emergent Bilingual Students*,
https://doi.org/10.1007/978-3-032-02084-0_15

15%, it has been estimated that 80% have an impairment in reading, also referred to as dyslexia (American Psychiatric Association [APA], 2022). Additionally, it has been estimated that approximately 10–30% of school-age children may have some form of learning disability in writing (dysgraphia; Chung et al., 2020), and 3–6% of students may have a learning disability in mathematics (dyscalculia; Shalev et al., 2000).

Considering that SLDs and SLIs are language-based disabilities, it is more likely that EBs who do not have a disability would be at higher risk of meeting the classification criteria for these disabilities, especially if the members of the multidisciplinary team are not adequately trained in differentially assessing whether the learning differences are the result of acquiring another language or an underlying disability. According to the U.S. Department of Education's EDFacts Data Warehouse (2020–21), EBs were more likely than non-EBs to be classified with an SLD, SLI, and intellectual disability (ID) and less likely than non-EBs to be classified under other health impaired (OHI), autism, or emotional disturbance (ED). Of the 35% of school-age children between the ages of 5–21 classified with an SLD, 45% were EB; of the 18% classified with SLI, 19% were EBs, and of the 6% with ID, 7% were EBs. Notably, data regarding the number of EBs classified who are referred to the CSE and not found eligible for services are not reported. Unfortunately, when evaluated, EB students are more likely to be incorrectly identified or not identified as having a disability because of the limited preparation among practitioners regarding the nature of bilingualism and the impact of their bilingualism and multiculturalism on standardized test performance (Artiles & Ortiz, 2002; Klingner & Artiles, 2006; Ortiz & Yates, 2001; Sullivan, 2011).

This chapter aims to provide practitioners with a clear understanding of how dyslexia can manifest among the EB population; recommendations will be made to facilitate the diagnostic decision making associated with the determination of whether academic difficulties are the result of language differences that are associated with the typical acquisition of a second language, or dyslexia so that more targeted programming and intervention can be made if warranted. Before transitioning to this discussion, defining key terms relevant to this topic is essential.

Heterogeneity of Bilingualism and Dyslexia

Bilingualism

Emergent bilinguals are commonly treated as a "monolithic group, particularly with respect to English" (Ortiz & Wong, 2020, p. 3). Regardless of their actual linguistic development (i.e., limited proficiency vs. fluent speaker), they tend to instead be categorized in terms of race, ethnicity, age, or "simply as a function of non-native English-speaking status" (Ortiz & Wong, 2020, p. 3). Instead, bilinguals should be conceptualized as a heterogeneous group. Everyone within this group will present with a unique constellation of language development in their first (L1) and second languages (L2) based on their personal experiences. Pearson (2007) demonstrated that input, language status, access to literacy, family language usage, and community support influence whether an individual exposed to two languages will learn them both. Although knowledge of these social factors is essential when conceptualizing *how* an individual became bilingual and should be part of a thorough intake, proficiencies in their L1 and L2 must be assessed to more accurately comprehend *why* a bilingual is struggling with reading.

Dyslexia

According to the International Dyslexia Association (IDA, 2002):

> dyslexia is a specific learning disability that is neurobiological in origin. It is characterized by difficulties with accurate and/or fluent word recognition and by poor spelling and decoding abilities. These difficulties typically result from a deficit in the phonological component of language that is often unexpected in relation to other cognitive abilities and the provision of effective classroom instruction. Secondary consequences may include problems in reading comprehension and reduced reading experience that can impede growth of vocabulary and background knowledge.

There is much confusion regarding who can "diagnose" dyslexia, often leading families to seek services from private practitioners, which can be exceptionally time-consuming and financially daunting. Notably, as stated in the IDA (2002) definition, dyslexia is a "specific learning disability." This term is synonymous with the IDEA (2004) definition of a SLD, which also lists dyslexia as a synonymous term. According to IDEA (2004), SLD is:

> a disorder in one or more of the basic psychological processes involved in understanding or in using language, spoken, or written, which disorder may manifest itself in the imperfect ability to listen, think, speak, read, spell, or do mathematical calculations. Such a term includes such conditions as perceptual disabilities, brain injury, minimal brain dysfunction, ***dyslexia***, and developmental aphasia. Such a term does not include a learning problem that is primarily the result of visual, hearing, or motor disabilities; of mental retardation; of emotional disturbance; or of environmental, cultural, or economic disadvantage (IDEA, 2004, §602.30. Definitions).

Like with bilingualism, dyslexics are also often categorized as a group of individuals with reading difficulties without consideration given to the heterogeneity among this population (Erbeli et al., 2021; Zoubrinetzky et al., 2014), which then precludes an understanding of *why* an individual may be struggling with reading. Therefore, the identification of dyslexia among linguistically minoritized individuals warrants a multi-dimensional approach that not only considers the individual's unique cultural and linguistic history but also includes an understanding of how the brain acquires reading, how the extant literature has specified that reading should be taught and whether or not, the individual has had access to scientifically supported reading curricula and interventions.

Most reading disorders stem from neuropsychological differences affecting at least one aspect of the reading process (Hulme & Snowling, 2016). While IDEA (2004) and its Part B (2006) regulations classify reading issues into categories such as SLD in basic reading skills, reading comprehension, and reading fluency, these classifications only describe some of the academic manifestations of the disorder and do not address the underlying causes. Understanding the root cause of a child's reading difficulties is crucial for implementing targeted interventions, program modifications, and testing accommodations.

Dual-Route Model (DRM)

The DRM is a widely supported and frequently used model of basic reading skill acquisition (Castles & Coltheart, 1993; Castles et al., 2006; Coltheart et al., 2001). Specifically, the model specifies how an individual acquires, stores, and retrieves a language's orthography or spelling system. Initially, when presented with an unfamiliar word, the individual utilizes the sub-lexical route of word recognition by sounding out the word using their acquired grapheme-phoneme correspondence knowledge. Repeated exposure to unfamiliar words makes them familiar and allows for long-term storage in the mental lexicon. Once in long-term storage, these familiar words can be accessed automatically via the lexical route. Over time, repetition of this process leads to automatic word recognition and reading fluency. Reading fluency allows the reader to think about what they are reading and connect the content to their prior knowledge, which allows for comprehension (National Institute for Literacy, 2006). Notably, fluent readers use sub-lexical and lexical strategies to decode unfamiliar words throughout the lifespan.

Dyslexia Subtypes

Dyslexia can result from disruptions in the DRM's lexical and/or sublexical routes due to brain injury or illness, known as acquired dyslexia, which can occur at any time in life (Coslett, 2000) or due to an unexpected difficulty in reading among individuals with the necessary intelligence, motivation, and schooling, referred to as developmental dyslexia (Shaywitz, 1998). Subtypes of reading disorders, based on the DRM, suggest that weaknesses in cognitive and neuropsychological processes related to word recognition routes can inhibit reading fluency and comprehension (Bosse et al., 2007; Castles & Coltheart, 1993; Coltheart et al., 2001; Ramus & Ahissar, 2012; Zoubrinetzky et al., 2014).

Dyslexia can be categorized into two main types: phonological and orthographic. Phonological dyslexia involves difficulties with the sublexical route of word recognition, which leads to problems with learning the sounds/phonemes associated with letters/graphemes. According to Mather and Goldstein (2008), these individuals can present weaknesses in phonemic awareness, phonics, and decoding words and nonwords (pseudowords), often relying on context clues and their sight word vocabulary via the lexical route. They may also exhibit a history of articulation difficulties and struggle with reading fluency.

Orthographic dyslexia, or surface dyslexia, involves a potential dysfunction in the lexical route of word recognition. These individuals struggle with visually memorizing and retrieving words, leading to difficulties with spelling, recognizing irregular words, and automatizing word recognition, forcing them to decode words by guessing at them, over-relying on contextual cues and sublexical route strategies by sounding words out, even when the words are familiar. They may also experience writing problems that include spelling errors of omission and commissions, letter and number reversals and transpositions, a disregard for punctuation, mathematical calculation errors, and difficulties with automatizing math facts (Mather & Goldstein, 2008). When individuals have weaknesses in both routes, it is referred to as mixed dyslexia, which indicates that their reading and writing impairments may be more pronounced due to limited compensatory strategies from the more robust route.

Language Difference or Disorder

Examining reading and writing strengths and weaknesses according to the DRM can help teachers and practitioners determine where a student is having difficulty. Still, considering an EB student's unique linguistic history must be central to understanding why they struggle to acquire basic reading skills. Specifically, while phonological processing deficits are a core characteristic of dyslexia in monolingual students, EBs may perform below expectations on measures of these functions because of developmental and experiential factors unrelated to dyslexia, such as incomplete English language acquisition (i.e., awareness of the phonemes of a language), primary language loss, or limited bilingual instruction (Ijalba et al., 2020).

Dyslexia as a Cross-Linguistic Perspective

According to the IDA (2020a), the prevalence of dyslexia affects 15–20% of the population worldwide, and the incidence of the disorder is not significantly different across various writing systems (Goswami, 2010; Yang et al., 2022), although differences do exist and can impact the severity and manifestation of the disorder (Caravolas, 2005; Goswami, 2010). The research on this topic is complex due to the systematic differences in language systems that result in convoluted comparative analyses. According to Frost (2005), an opaque or deep orthography is a writing system with irregular and inconsistent letter-sound relationships, making pronunciations less predictable from spelling (e.g., English). Additionally, a transparent or shallow orthography is a writing system where letters consistently correspond to specific sounds, making pronunciation predictable from spelling (e.g., Spanish).

Languages and their respective orthographies can be categorized into three main types: (1) alphabetic orthographies, which use letters and letter clusters to represent phonemes (e.g., English, Czech, and Dutch); (2) syllabic orthographies, which use symbols to represent syllables (e.g., Japanese, Kanji, and Hindi); and (3) logographic orthographies, which use characters to represent spoken words at the monosyllabic morpheme level (e.g., Chinese; Caravolas, 2005). Current cross-cultural research suggests "universality in the neurobiological and neurocognitive underpinnings of dyslexia. However, cross-cultural specificity exists in the manifestation of those underpinnings, with the same biological liability being more likely to cause significant impairment in some languages than in others" (Peterson & Pennington, 2012, p. 3).

The characteristics of dyslexia must be present in both the primary and secondary languages to be consistent with the disorder's characteristics. In their review of dyslexia across various languages, Smythe and Salter (2004) posit that dyslexia is a universal neurobiological condition that affects language processing abilities, regardless of the language; therefore, it is unlikely that reading issues will present only after learning the L2, especially if the individual had already received academic instruction, without issue in their L1. The Linguistic Coding Deficit Hypothesis (LCDH; Ganschow & Sparks, 1995) posits that an individual who presents with a history of learning difficulties in their L1 will likely manifest those difficulties while acquiring the L2. However, the problems may manifest differently in the second language, depending on its orthography.

Further, classification and diagnostic criteria for dyslexia specify exclusionary criteria that invalidate a diagnosis if the learning issues are primarily the result of language proficiency and access to adequate instruction. According to 34 CFR § 300.309(a)(3), when considering a classification of SLD (synonymous with dyslexia): "The group must ensure that its findings are not primarily the result of—(i) a visual, hearing, or motor disability; (ii) intellectual disability; (iii) emotional disturbance; (iv) cultural factors; (v) environmental or economic disadvantage; or (vi) Limited English proficiency" (U.S. Department of Education, 2006, para. a3). The same is true when following the criteria provided by the DSM (APA, 2022) for a SLD: "The learning difficulties are not better accounted for by intellectual disabilities, uncorrected visual or auditory acuity, other mental or neurological disorders, psychosocial adversity, lack of proficiency in the language of academic instruction, or inadequate educational instruction" (p. 77).

Nonetheless, research has shown that children learning opaque languages are more likely to experience ingrained challenges with decoding and encoding than children learning transparent languages. Children learning transparent languages are likely to achieve higher reading accuracy but may work slower than their peers (Brunswick et al., 2010). This is critical information, especially if an EB's L1 is Spanish, and they proceeded through their early grades in their L1 without complication; if they have a weakness with the phonetic aspects of decoding, then transitioning to L2 instruction of an opaque language like English may yield academic difficulties that may not have been encountered in a transparent language like Spanish.

Individuals with dyslexia typically share common cognitive difficulties across languages (Goswami, 2010). Specifically, difficulty with phonological processing (i.e., detecting and manipulating speech sounds in language), verbal short-term memory/phonological memory, and rapid automatized naming (RAN) are hallmark characteristics of dyslexia that interfere with decoding, regardless of the language system (Caravolas, 2005; Goswami, 2010; Goswami et al., 2011). More recently, research has shown the impact of visual processes on the acquisition of reading, specific to the visual attention span (VAS; the number of visual elements that are simultaneously processed in a multielement array) that is also associated with the acquisition of decoding skills; dyslexic individuals have been shown to present with significantly weak VAS compared to typical readers (Tang et al., 2023). Additionally, orthographic challenges involving difficulties with visual language representations have been shown to significantly impact both computational mathematical and writing tasks in addition to reading (Berninger et al., 2002; Geary, 2004; Mammarella et al., 2018; Richards et al., 2009).

The extent to which specific cognitive processes are involved/impaired is in part determined by the structure of the language system and the mode of instruction (Caravolas, 2005; Tang et al., 2023). For example, individuals who learn new characters via rote memorization (such as in the Chinese language) may depend more on visual strategies and memory processes than children who read using a phonemic-based strategy (Caravolas, 2005). Notably, the type of writing system (e.g., alphabetic vs. characters) significantly moderates VAS deficit in dyslexia, with greater severity in alphabetic languages (Tang et al., 2023). Additionally, some studies in languages with transparent orthographies (e.g., German, Dutch, Czech) show that difficulty with phonemic awareness is time-limited, as it tends to resolve by a specific age/grade (i.e., second grade)—but other studies contradict this, indicating that although general cognitive features are similar, nuances exist on a deeper level and require further investigation (Caravolas, 2005).

Similarities are further seen in correlates in brain activation among dyslexics during reading tasks (Li & Bi, 2022; Pollack et al., 2015; Siok et al., 2004). Researchers have consistently demonstrated that left temporoparietal areas, the left middle-superior temporal cortex, and the left inferior temporo-occipital gyrus function atypically and maintain an anomalous structure in individuals with dyslexia (Hadzibeganovic et al., 2010; Siok et al., 2004). However, other studies indicate differences in brain region utilization based on language, leading to mixed findings in the field (Richlan, 2014). The visual-word form area (i.e., posterior region of the brain), specifically the extrastriate cortex of the occipital lobes around the fusiform gyrus in the left hemisphere, is under-activated in individuals struggling with decoding and RAN across many languages (Feifer & Della Toffalo, 2007).

Furthermore, in a study involving tasks of rhyming or reading (letters or words) in various alphabetic languages (i.e., English, Dutch, Italian, German, French, or Norwegian), Pollack et al. (2015) found that typically developing readers demonstrated activation in only left lateralized regions (i.e., the inferior frontal area, precentral area, and middle temporal gyrus). In contrast, atypical readers showed activation not only in the left inferior frontal area and precentral region but also in the right hemisphere, including the superior, medial, and inferior frontal regions, lingual gyrus, and the inferior occipital area. These results support the "universality of a signature pattern of brain activation in dyslexia across alphabetic languages" (Pollack et al., 2015, pp. 6–7). In addition, although complex and inconsistent, some evidence supports that individuals with dyslexia across languages have reduced gray matter volume in the left thalamus (Jednoróg et al., 2015).

Additional research included the Chinese language in comparative analyses, and results highlight that dyslexic individuals across writing systems have a "universal attention-related dysfunction" with hypoactivation in the left inferior frontal cortex (IFC) and the anterior cingulate cortex (ACC; Li & Bi, 2022). However, dyslexic children who read alphabetic languages showed hypoactivation in the left occipital-temporo-parietal regions. In contrast, Chinese dyslexic children showed hyperactivation in the right postcentral gyrus, the left rectus, and the right middle temporal gyrus (Li & Bi, 2022). Furthermore, another study demonstrated commonalities in the cognitive manifestation of dyslexia with neuroimaging studies that indicated less than usual activation in the left angular gyrus and in left middle frontal, posterior temporal, and occipitotemporal regions for both English and Chinese dyslexics (Hu et al., 2010). Recent research demonstrates that although there are many similarities in cognitive and neuropsychological processes in dyslexics across world languages, minor nuances seem dependent on the respective language system.

In summary, weaknesses in specific neuropsychological and cognitive processes have been identified across various languages for individuals with dyslexia. However, the severity and manifestation of difficulties in reading based on weaknesses in these processes differ based on the specific language system and its inherent neuropsychological demands.

Proposed Model for the Identification of Dyslexia Among Emergent Bilinguals

The following section highlights a suggested framework for assessing emergent bilinguals who present with decoding, encoding, language comprehension, and mathematical difficulties that are associated with dyslexia.

Comprehensive Developmental History

A thorough developmental history is a critical component of any evaluation. The goal of this phase in the assessment process is to understand better how the individual arrived at this point in their life where their learning differences are being evaluated to rule out or confirm eligibility for special education. Typically, the practitioner will meet with parents and can follow either an unstructured or structured interview format. It has been well-documented that a significant obstacle for school practitioners has been the lack of caregiver participation in school-based psychological services (Bohanon & Wu, 2011; Crooks et al., 2013; Langley et al., 2010; Santiago et al., 2013; Weist et al., 2003, 2014). The practitioner is encouraged to identify potential barriers to caregiver involvement throughout this process, as the caregiver perspective is critical for case conceptualization.

Baker et al. (2016) identified several factors and solutions for increasing caregiver involvement and engagement with the school, two of which are directly relevant to the assessment process with emergent bilinguals and their families: improving communication and making time. If the family communicates in a language other than English, and the practitioner is not fluent, then interpretation and translation services should be secured. Interpreters should be fluent in the family's language and English and knowledgeable about the topics of discussion (see Arroyos et al., 2018, for a summary of best practices in collaborating with interpreters). Additionally, caregivers' employment schedules may not align with school personnel availability; it is recommended that school personnel reach out to families to identify times that work for them and potentially arrange for flexible scheduling time with the school district that allows for scheduled sessions (e.g., via web or phone) that are outside of the typical school day.

Developmental History

The Behavior Assessment System for Children—Third Edition (BASC-3; Reynolds & Kamphaus, 2015) offers a Structured Developmental History (SDH) form that can be administered as a questionnaire in paper-pencil or digital formats or used as an interview guide for practitioners. This process allows the practitioner to utilize the individual's and their family's perspective on the presenting problem to form more educated hypotheses to be tested, ensuring a more targeted and tailored evaluation and potential treatment course (Youngstrom & Prinstein, 2020).

Language History

Although the BASC-3 SDH includes some language history questions, a more comprehensive approach is required when investigating the impact of an individual's linguistic and educational history in multiple languages. The Language History Questionnaire (LHQ3; Li et al., 2020), now in its third edition, is a free online instrument available in 43 languages that provides estimates of language proficiency, language dominance, and language immersion levels. The LHQ3 also includes questions regarding the rater's education in L1 and L2 and their self-ratings of proficiency with language and listening, speaking, reading, and writing.

Educational History

In addition to determining if the emergent bilingual has ever received formal education in a language other than English, the quality of educational programming the individual received is paramount. History should also include a review of records, including report cards, and collateral interviews with others who can speak to the child's academics in all languages. As discussed previously, although the literature has consistently urged schools to engage in evidence-based instructional and intervention practices, what manifests in the classroom sometimes is not aligned with the science of reading. Notably, according to the federal regulations that detail the procedures for determining if a student has an SLD, it states that the school district:

> must demonstrate that the learning difficulties are not due to a lack of appropriate instruction in reading (appropriate instruction in reading must include the essential components of reading instruction defined in the No Child Left Behind Act Elementary and Secondary Education Act of 1965 § 1208[3]) or math, that the child was provided appropriate instruction in regular education settings, delivered by qualified personnel and data-based documentation of repeated assessments of achievement at reasonable intervals, reflecting formal assessment of student progress during instruction, which was provided to the student's parents. [34 CFR 300.309, para. b] [20 U.S.C. 1221e-3; 1401(30); 1414(b)(6)]

Assessment of Emergent Bilinguals

The information gathered from the comprehensive developmental history is essential for determining how a practitioner should proceed with selecting measures that will comprise the thorough assessment of the emergent bilingual. The language(s) of assessment should be determined based on the individual's language history results, L1 or L2 data that may already be available to the practitioner from state or local standardized testing, and the linguistic characteristics of the practitioner and/or interpreter. Ideally, the assessment of an emergent bilingual would involve assessment in both languages (if warranted) by a practitioner who is also bilingual, using measures that were adequately standardized in each language and that adequately represent the individual that is being assessed. Unfortunately, this combination of characteristics is impossible due to the minimal number of bilingual practitioners (Sotelo-Dynega, 2015) and the limitations associated with the standardization procedures and use of tests among bilinguals (Ortiz, 2002). Instead, utilizing a comprehensive, systematic framework with a broad range of information collection and evaluation methods is the best practice for nondiscriminatory assessment (Ortiz, 2002). Table 15.1 presents suggestions for assessing the previously discussed areas of cognitive and academic functions associated with dyslexia (Table 15.2).

Once standardized testing is complete, Ortiz and Oganes (2022) propose a step-by-step process for multilingual testing of bilingual learners that begins with testing in English (L2). The practitioner is then advised to examine the results to identify any performances below expectation and indicative of a weakness. If a weakness is

Table 15.1 Suggested cognitive measures for the assessment of dyslexia

Domain	Suggested assessment instrument
Sound discrimination	ASA; Auditory Skills Assessment: Speech Discrimination in Noise, Tonal Patterning (Geffner & Goldman, 2010)
Auditory/phonological processing	ASA; Auditory Skills Assessment: Blending (Geffner & Goldman, 2010)
Performance fluency/rapid automatized naming	WISC-V; Wechsler Intelligence Scale for Children, 5th Edition: Naming Speed Color-Object, Naming Speed Letter Number, Naming Speed Literacy, Naming Speed Quantity, Naming Speed Size-Color-Object (Wechsler, 2014)
Immediate verbal memory	WISC-V; Wechsler Intelligence Scale for Children, 5th Edition Digit Span Forward (Wechsler, 2014)
Selective/focused and sustained attention	CATA; Conners Continuous Auditory Test of Attention-Third Edition (Conners, 2014)
Verbal working memory	WISC-V; Wechsler Intelligence Scale for Children, 5th Edition: Arithmetic, Digit Span Backward, Letter-Number Sequencing (Wechsler, 2014)
Sensory functions	Developmental Eye Movement Test (Richman & Garzia, 2016)
Fine-motor functions	NEPSY-II: Fingertip Tapping, Imitating Hand Positions, Hand Motor Sequences (Korkman et al., 2007)
Visual-motor integration	Beery VMI; Beery Buktenica Developmental Test of Visual Motor Integration, Sixth Ed.: Visual Perception, Motor Coordination (Beery et al., 2010)
Gross-motor functions	Movement Assessment Battery, 2nd Edition (Henderson et al., 2007)
Visual spatial perception	DTVP-3; Developmental Test of Visual Perception, Third Edition (Hammill et al., 2013)
Immediate visual memory	NEPSY-II: Memory for Designs Total (Korkman et al., 2007)
Verbal-visual associative Learning and recall/orthographic processing	WISC-V; Wechsler Intelligence Scale for Children, 5th Edition Immediate Symbol Translation (Wechsler, 2014)
Visual working memory	WISC-V; Wechsler Intelligence Scale for Children, 5th Edition Picture Span (Wechsler, 2014)

determined, the practitioner is encouraged to evaluate the potential effect of cultural and linguistic factors on test performance. An instrument like the Culture-Language Interpretative Matrix and the respective Culture-Language Test Classifications (Flanagan et al., 2013, 2017) are practical resources that can facilitate this process. If the performance is deemed to result from the influence of culture and language, then the interpretations follow suit. If the results are not deemed to have been attenuated by the influence of culture and language on test performance, the practitioner is encouraged to proceed to the third step, which involves reevaluating the areas of weakness using the L1. If the scores in L2 are consistently low when administered in L1, then these results can be interpreted as areas of weakness. Finally, Ortiz and Oganes (2022) recommend establishing ecological validity by connecting the low scores with the reason for the referral.

Table 15.2 Suggested academic measures for the assessment of dyslexia

Domain	Examples of suggested assessment instruments
Basic reading skills	TOD-C; Test of Dyslexia-Comprehensive: Irregular Word Reading, Pseudoword Reading (Mather et al., 2024) WJ V ACH: Woodcock Johnson Tests of Achievement, 5th Edition: Letter-Word Identification, Word Attack (McGrew et al., 2025)
Reading fluency	TOD-C; Test of Dyslexia-Comprehensive: Word Reading Fluency, Oral Reading Efficiency (Mather et al., 2024) WJ V ACH: Woodcock Johnson Tests of Achievement, 5th Edition: Sentence Reading Fluency, Word Reading Fluency (McGrew et al., 2025)
Sight word acquisition	TOD-C; Test of Dyslexia-Comprehensive: Letter and Word Choice, Irregular Word Reading, Rapid Irregular Word Reading (Mather et al., 2024)
Phonics knowledge	TOD-C; Test of Dyslexia-Comprehensive: Pseudoword Reading, Rapid Pseudoword Reading (Mather et al., 2024)
Phonemic awareness	WJ V ACH: Woodcock Johnson Tests of Achievement, 5th Edition: Sound Deletion, Sound Blending, Sound Substitution (McGrew et al., 2025)
Decoding efficiency	TOD-C; Test of Dyslexia-Comprehensive: Rapid Irregular Word Reading, Rapid Pseudoword Reading (Mather et al., 2024)
Vocabulary	TOD-C; Test of Dyslexia-Comprehensive: Picture Vocabulary, Listening Vocabulary (Mather et al., 2024)
Reading comprehension	TOD-C; Test of Dyslexia-Comprehensive: Silent Reading Efficiency (Mather et al., 2024) WJ V ACH: Woodcock Johnson Tests of Achievement, 5th Edition: Passage Comprehension, Paragraph Reading Comprehension (McGrew et al., 2025)
Spelling	TOD-C; Test of Dyslexia-Comprehensive: Irregular Word Spelling, Regular Word Spelling (Mather et al., 2024)

Connecting Assessment Findings to Evidence-Based Interventions

The final step in the assessment process is to connect the findings with evidence-based suggestions for recommendations aligned with the referral's initial reason. Considering that EB students present with unique challenges because of their experiences with two (or more) languages, according to the IDA (2020b), effective reading instruction for students with dyslexia must address the development of phonology, sound-symbol associations, syllable instruction, morphology, syntax, and semantics, instruction must be systematic and cumulative, involve explicit instruction, and diagnostic teaching that incorporates continuous assessment.

Effective interventions often include adaptations that consider the specific linguistic features of both the L1 and the L2, addressing orthographic depth differences (Kahn-Horwitz, 2015). Research also suggests that skills learned in one language can transfer to the other, particularly when the languages share similar phonological structures (Sparks et al., 2008). Moreover, culturally and contextually relevant interventions are more effective, using materials and examples meaningful to the student's experiences (Jiménez et al., 2007). Combining direct instruction in both languages with strategies that promote metacognitive skills, such as self-monitoring and strategy use, can lead to better outcomes, highlighting the promise of integrated approaches that address both cognitive and linguistic aspects of dyslexia (Swanson et al., 2006).

Recommendations can also include suggestions for instruction, intervention, additional assessment, and relevant program modifications and testing accommodations. Flanagan et al. (2024) developed and released a digital *intervention library* that includes "instructional, environmental, curricular, remedial, skill-building, and compensatory strategies and supports" (Flanagan et al., n.d.). Practitioners are encouraged to select recommendations aligned with the science of reading and appropriate for emerging bilinguals.

Conclusion

In conclusion, with approximately 10% of the school population consisting of EBs, school personnel must be competent in the differential identification of language differences versus underlying disorders. Consideration of the EB's unique cultural, linguistic, educational, and experiential background, combined with knowledge of the DRM and the identification of dyslexia subtypes, allows for non-discriminatory and culturally responsive decision-making and intervention determinations. Regardless of the outcome of an assessment of an EB, effective interventions should always be tailored based on the EB's unique, linguistic, and experiential trajectory. Incorporating systematic, explicit instruction in phonology, sound-symbol associations, morphology, syntax, and semantics is always vital. Therefore, by engaging in comprehensive assessment practices and promoting evidence-based interventions, school personnel can better support the academic success of this growing and diverse student population.

References

American Psychiatric Association. (2022). *Diagnostic and statistical manual of mental disorders, fifth edition-text revision (DSM-5-TR)*. American Psychiatric Association.

Arroyos, E., Diaz, D., & Torres, I. (2018). Best practices in collaborating with interpreters: Lessons learned. *Communique, 46*, 29–30.

Artiles, A. J., & Ortiz, A. A. (2002). *English language learners with special education needs: Identification, assessment, and instruction*. Center for Applied Linguistics and Delta Systems.

Baker, T. L., Wise, J., Kelley, G., & Skiba, R. J. (2016). Identifying barriers: Creating solutions to improve family engagement. *School Community Journal, 26*, 161–184.

Beery, K. E., Buktenica, N., & Beery, N. A. (2010). *Beery-Buktenica developmental test of visual-motor integration* (6th ed.). Pearson.

Berninger, V. W., Abbott, R. D., Abbott, S. P., Graham, S., & Richards, T. (2002). Writing and reading: Connections between language by hand and language by eye. *Journal of Learning Disabilities, 35*(1), 39–56.

Bohanon, H., & Wu, M. J. (2011). Can prevention programs work together? An example of school-based mental health with prevention initiatives. *Advances in School Mental Health Promotion, 4*, 35–46.

Bosse, M. L., Tainturier, M. J., & Valdois, S. (2007). Developmental dyslexia: The visual attention span deficit hypothesis. *Cognition, 100*, 198–230.

Brunswick, N., McDougall, S., & Davies, P. M. (Eds.). (2010). *Reading and dyslexia in different orthographies*. Psychology Press.

Caravolas, M. (2005). The nature and causes of dyslexia in different languages. In M. J. Snowling & C. Hulme (Eds.), *Science of reading: A handbook* (pp. 336–356). Blackwell.

Castles, A., Bates, T., & Coltheart, M. (2006). John Marshall and the developmental dyslexias. *Aphasiology, 20*, 871–892.

Castles, A., & Coltheart, M. (1993). Varieties of developmental dyslexia. *Cognition, 47*, 149–180.

Chung, P. J., Patel, D. R., & Nizami, I. (2020). Disorder of written expression and dysgraphia: definition, diagnosis, and management. *Translational Pediatrics, 9*(Suppl 1), S46–S54. https://doi.org/10.21037/tp.2019.11.01

Coltheart, M., Rastle, K., Perry, C., Langdon, R., & Ziegler, J. (2001). DRC: A dual route cascaded model of visual word recognition and reading aloud. *Psychological Review, 108*, 204–256.

Conners, C. K. (2014). *Conners' continuous performance test* (3rd ed.). MHS.

Coslett, H. B. (2000). Acquired dyslexia. *Seminars in Neurology, 20*(4), 419–426.

Crooks, C. V., Chiddo, D., Zwarych, S., Hughes, R., & Wolfe, D. A. (2013). Predicting implementation of success of an evidence-based program to promote healthy relationships among students two to eight years after teacher training. *Canadian Journal of Community Mental Health, 32*, 125–138.

Erbeli, F., Rice, M., & Paracchini, S. (2021). Insights into dyslexia genetics research from the last two decades. *Brain Sciences, 12*(1), 27. https://doi.org/10.3390/brainsci12010027

Feifer, S. G., & Della Toffalo, D. A. (2007). The orthographic processor: Establishing the neural code for automaticity and fluency. In S. G. Feiferm & D. A. Della Toffalo (Eds.), *Integrating RTI with cognitive neuropsychology: A scientific approach to reading* (1st ed., pp. 63–79). School Neuropsych Press.

Flanagan, D. P., Mascolo, J. T., Ortiz, S. O., & Alfonso, V. C. (2024). *Intervention library: Resources for instruction and intervention*. CAI/Cross-Battery Assessment.

Flanagan, D. P., Mascolo, J. T., Ortiz, S. O., & Alfonso, V. C. (n.d.). *IL: FIRST bridging the assessment-intervention gap*. Intervention Library. https://www.wiley.com/learn/interventionlibrary/

Flanagan, D. P., Ortiz, S. O., & Alfonso, V. C. (2013). *Essentials of cross-battery assessment* (3rd ed.). Wiley.

Flanagan, D. P., Ortiz, S. O., & Alfonso, V. C. (2017). *Cross-battery assessment software system 2.0*. Wiley.

Frost, R. (2005). Orthographic systems and skilled word recognition processes in reading. In M. J. Snowling, & C. Hulme (Eds.), *The science of reading: A handbook* (pp. 272–295). Blackwell.

Ganschow, L., & Sparks, R. L. (1995). Effects of direct instruction in Spanish phonology on the native-language skills and foreign-language aptitude of at-risk foreign-language learners. *Journal of Learning Disabilities, 28*(2), 107–120.

Geary, D. C. (2004). Mathematics and learning disabilities. *Journal of Learning Disabilities, 37*(1), 4–15.

Geffner, D., & Goldman, R. (2010). *Auditory skills assessment*. Pearson.

Goswami, U. (2010). Typical reading development and developmental dyslexia across languages. In D. Coch, G. Dawson, & K. W. Fischer (Eds.), *Human behavior, learning, and the developing brain: Atypical development* (pp. 145–167). Guilford Press.

Goswami, U., Wang, H.-L. S., Cruz, A., Fosker, T., Mead, N., & Huss, M. (2011). Language-universal sensory deficits in developmental dyslexia: English, Spanish, and Chinese. *Journal of Cognitive Neuroscience, 23*(2), 325–337. https://doi.org/10.1162/jocn.2010.21453

Hadzibeganovic, T., Van Den Noort, M., Bosch, P., Perc, M., Van Kralingen, R., Mondt, K., & Coltheart, M. (2010). Cross-linguistic neuroimaging and dyslexia: A critical view. *Cortex, 46*(10), 1312–1316. https://doi.org/10.1016/j.cortex.2010.06.011

Hammill, D. D., Pearson, N. A., & Voress, J. K. (2013). *Developmental test of visual perception* (3rd ed.). Pearson.

Henderson, S. E., Sugden, D. A., & Barnett, A. (2007). *Movement assessment battery for children* (2nd ed.). Pearson.

Hu, W., Lee, H. L., Zhang, Q., Liu, T., Geng, L. B., Seghier, M. L., Shakeshaft, C., Twomey, T., Green, D. W., Yang, Y. M., & Price, C. J. (2010). Developmental dyslexia in Chinese and English populations: Dissociating the effect of dyslexia from language differences. *Brain, 133*(6), 1694–1706. https://doi.org/10.1093/brain/awq106

Hulme, C., & Snowling, M. J. (2016). Reading disorders and dyslexia. *Current Opinion in Pediatrics, 28*, 731–735.

Ijalba, E., Bustos, A., & Romero, S. (2020). Phonological-orthographic deficits in developmental dyslexia in three Spanish-English bilingual students. *American Journal of Speech-Language Pathology, 29*(3), 1133–1151. https://doi-org.jerome.stjohns.edu/10.1044/2020_AJSLP-19-00175

Individuals with Disabilities Education Act. (2004). *20 U.S.C. § 1400.*

International Dyslexia Association. (2002). *Definition of dyslexia.* Retrieved from https://dyslexiaida.org/definition-of-dyslexia/

International Dyslexia Association. (2020a). *Dyslexia basics.* https://dyslexiaida.org/dyslexia-basics/

International Dyslexia Association. (2020b). *Effective reading instruction for students with dyslexia.* https://dyslexiaida.org/effective-reading-instruction-for-students-with-dyslexia/

Jednoróg, K., Marchewka, A., Altarelli, I., Monzalvo Lopez, A. K., van Ermingen-Marbach, M., Grande, M., Grabowska, A., Heim, S., & Ramus, F. (2015). How reliable are gray matter disruptions in specific reading disability across multiple countries and languages? Insights from a large-scale voxel-based morphometry study. *Human Brain Mapping, 36*(5), 1741–1754. https://doi.org/10.1002/hbm.22734

Jiménez, J. E., Siegel, L. S., & López, P. (2007). The relationship between IQ and reading disabilities in English-speaking Canadian and Spanish-speaking children. *Journal of Learning Disabilities, 36*(1), 15–23.

Kahn-Horwitz, J. (2015). English as a foreign language spelling: Comparisons between good and poor spellers. *Journal of Research in Reading, 38*(1), 1–18.

Klingner, J. K., & Artiles, A. J. (2006). English language learners struggling to learn to read: Emergent scholarship on linguistic differences and learning disabilities. *Journal of Learning Disabilities, 39*(5), 386–389. https://doi.org/10.1177/00222194060390050201

Korkman, M., Kirk, U., & Kemp, S. (2007). *NEPSY | Second edition*. Pearson.

Langley, A. K., Nadeem, E., Kataoka, S. H., Stein, B. D., & Jaycox, L. H. (2010). Evidence-based mental health programs in schools: Barriers and facilitators of successful implementation. *School Mental Health, 2*, 105–113.

Li, P., Zhang, F., Yu, A., & Zhao, X. (2020). Language History Questionnaire (LHQ3): An enhanced tool for assessing multilingual experience. *Bilingualism: Language and Cognition, 23*(5), 938–944. https://doi.org/10.1017/S1366728918001153

Li, Y., & Bi, H.-Y. (2022). Comparative research on neural dysfunction in children with dyslexia under different writing systems: A meta-analysis study. *Neuroscience & Biobehavioral Reviews, 137*, 104650. https://doi.org/10.1016/j.neubiorev.2022.104650

Mammarella, I. C., Caviola, S., Giofrè, D., & Borella, E. (2018). Separating math from anxiety: The role of inhibitory mechanisms. *Applied Neuropsychology: Child, 7*(4), 342–353.

Mather, N., & Goldstein, S. (2008). *Learning disabilities and challenging behaviors: A guide to intervention and classroom management* (2nd ed.). Brookes.

Mather N., McCallum R. S., Bell S. M., & Wendling B. J. (2024). *Tests of dyslexia.* Western Psychological Services.

McGrew, K. S., Mather, N., LaForte, E. M., & Wendling, B. J. (2025). Woodcock-Johnson V. Riverside Assessments, LLC.

National Center for Education Statistics. (2024a). English learners in public schools. *Condition of education*. U.S. Department of Education, Institute of Education Sciences. Retrieved February 23, 2025, from https://nces.ed.gov/programs/coe/indicator/cgf.

National Center for Education Statistics. (2024b). Students with disabilities. *Condition of education*. U.S. Department of Education, Institute of Education Sciences. Retrieved February 13, 2025, from https://nces.ed.gov/programs/coe/indicator/cgg.

National Institute for Literacy. (2006). *Put reading first, kindergarten through grade 3* (3rd ed.). Author.

Ortiz, A. A., & Yates, J. R. (2001). A framework for serving English language learners with disabilities. *Journal of Special Education Leadership, 14*(2), 72–80.

Ortiz, S. O. (2002). Best practices in nondiscriminatory assessment. In A. Thomas & J. Grimes (Eds.), *Best practices in school psychology IV* (pp. 1321–1336). National Association of School Psychologists.

Ortiz, S. O., & Oganes, M. (2022). Nondiscriminatory, cross-cultural school neuropsychological assessment. In D. Miller, D. Maricle, C. Bedford, & J. Gettman (Eds.), *Best practices in school neuropsychology* (2nd ed.). Wiley.

Ortiz, S. O., & Wong, J. Y. T. (2020, October 1). Fairness in tests and test score interpretation with English learners. *The Score*. https://www.apadivisions.org/division-5/publications/score/2020/10/assessing-english-learners.

Pearson, B. Z. (2007). Social factors in childhood bilingualism in the United States. *Applied Psycholinguistics, 28*, 399–410.

Peterson, R. L., & Pennington, B. F. (2012). Developmental dyslexia. *Lancet, 379*(9830), 1997–2007. https://doi.org/10.1016/S0140-6736(12)60198-6

Pollack, C., Luk, G., & Christodoulou, J. A. (2015). A meta-analysis of functional reading systems in typically developing and struggling readers across different alphabetic languages. *Frontiers in Psychology, 6*. https://doi.org/10.3389/fpsyg.2015.00191

Ramus, F., & Ahissar, M. (2012). Developmental dyslexia: The difficulties of interpreting poor performance, and the importance of normal performance. *Cognitive Neuropsychology, 29*(1–2), 104–122.

Reynolds, C. R., & Kamphaus, R. W. (2015). *Behavior assessment for children: Third edition (BASC-3)* [Assessment instrument]. Pearson.

Richards, T. L., Berninger, V. W., & Fayol, M. (2009). fMRI activation differences between 11-year-old good and poor spellers' access in working memory to temporary and long-term orthographic representations. *Journal of Neurolinguistics, 22*(4), 327–353.

Richlan, F. (2014). Functional neuroanatomy of developmental dyslexia: The role of orthographic depth. *Frontiers in Human Neuroscience, 8*. https://doi.org/10.3389/fnhum.2014.00347siok

Richman, J. E., & Garzia, R. P. (2016). *Developmental eye movement test*. Bernell.

Santiago, C. D., Kaltman, S., & Miranda, J. (2013). Poverty and mental health: How do low-income adults and children fare in psychotherapy? *Journal of Clinical Psychology, 69*, 115–126.

Shalev, R. S., Auerbach, J., Manor, O., & Gross-Tsur, V. (2000). Developmental dyscalculia: Prevalence and prognosis. *European Child & Adolescent Psychiatry, 9*(Suppl 2), II58–II64. https://doi.org/10.1007/s007870070009

Shaywitz, S. E. (1998). Dyslexia. *New England Journal of Medicine, 338*, 307–312.

Siok, W. T., Perfetti, C. A., Jin, Z., & Tan, L. H. (2004). Biological abnormality of impaired reading is constrained by culture. *Nature, 431*, 71–76.

Smythe, I., & Salter, R. (2004). Introduction, dyslexia—Different contexts, same problems. In I. Smythe, J. Everatt, & R. Salter (Eds.), *International book of dyslexia* (pp. 1–4). Wiley.

Sotelo-Dynega, M. (2015). What is a bilingual school psychologist? A national survey of the credentialing bodies of school psychologists: Implications for the assessment of bilinguals. *Journal of Psychoeducational Assessment, 33*(3), 247–258. https://doi.org/10.1177/0734282914550811

Sparks, R. L., Patton, J., Ganschow, L., & Humbach, N. (2008). Long-term cross-linguistic transfer of skills from L1 to L2. *Language Learning, 58*(3), 411–449.
Sullivan, A. L. (2011). Disproportionality in special education identification and placement of English language learners. *Exceptional Children, 77*(3), 317–334. https://doi.org/10.1177/001440291107700304
Sullivan, A. L., & Ball, A. (2013). Disproportionality in special education: Effects of individual and school variables on disability risk. *Exceptional Children, 79*(4), 475–494.
Swanson, H. L., Sáez, L., & Gerber, M. (2006). Growth in literacy and cognition in bilingual children at risk or not at risk for reading disabilities. *Journal of Educational Psychology, 98*(2), 247–264.
Tang, J., Ma, X., Peng, P., Cha, K., Yao, Y., & Zhao, J. (2023). Visual attention span deficit in developmental dyslexia: A meta-analysis. *Research in Developmental Disabilities, 141*, 104590. https://doi.org/10.1016/j.ridd.2023.104590
U.S. Department of Education. (2006). Assistance to states for the education of children with disabilities, 34 C.F.R. § 300.309(a)(3). Retrieved from https://www.ecfr.gov/current/title-34/subtitle-B/chapter-III/part-300/subpart-D/subject-group-ECFR0f22fac7ad954f5/section-300.309.
U.S. Department of Education, EDFacts Data Warehouse (EDW). IDEA part B child count and educational environments collection, 2020–21. Retrieved February 17, 2024, from https://sites.ed.gov/idea/osep-fast-facts-educational-environments-school-aged-children-disabilities/
Wechsler, D. (2014). *Wechsler Intelligence Scale for Children | Fifth edition*. Pearson.
Weist, M. D., Evans, S. W., & Lever, N. A. (2003). *Handbook of school mental health: Advancing practice and research*. Springer.
Weist, M. D., Youngstrom, E. A., Stephan, S., Lever, N., Fowler, J., Taylor, L., & Hoagwood, K. (2014). Challenges and ideas from a research program on high-quality, evidence-based practice in school mental health. *Journal of Clinical Child and Adolescent Psychology, 43*, 244–255.
Yang, L., Li, C., Li, X., Zhai, M., An, Q., Zhang, Y., Zhao, J., & Weng, X. (2022). Prevalence of developmental dyslexia in primary school children: A systematic review and meta-analysis. *Brain Sciences, 12*(2). https://doi.org/10.3390/brainsci12020240
Youngstrom, E. A., & Prinstein, M. J. (2020). Introduction to evidence-based assessment: A recipe for success. In E. A. Youngstrom, M. J. Prinstein, E. J. Mash, & R. A. Barkley (Eds.), *Assessment of childhood and adolescence* (5th ed.). Guilford Press.
Zoubrinetzky, R., Bielle, F., & Valdois, S. (2014). New insights on developmental dyslexia subtypes: Heterogeneity of mixed reading profiles. *PLoS One, 9*(6), e99337. https://doi.org/10.1371/journal.pone.0099337

Index

D. Vega, J. N. Wolf (eds.), *Culturally and Linguistically Responsive Intervention and Assessment Practices with Emergent Bilingual Students*,
https://doi.org/10.1007/978-3-032-02084-0

L

M

N

O

MIX
Papier aus verantwortungsvollen Quellen
Paper from responsible sources
FSC® C105338

If you have any concerns about our products,
you can contact us on
ProductSafety@springernature.com

In case Publisher is established outside the EU,
the EU authorized representative is:
Springer Nature Customer Service Center GmbH
Europaplatz 3, 69115 Heidelberg, Germany

Printed by Libri Plureos GmbH
in Hamburg, Germany